Complications of Percutaneous Coronary Interventions

Samuel M. Butman, MD, FACC, FSCAI

Associate Professor of Medicine, Section of Cardiology, University of Arizona Sarver Heart Center, Tucson, Arizona

Editor

Complications of Percutaneous Coronary Interventions

Forewords by Joseph S. Alpert, MD,
and Antonio Colombo, MD

With 92 Illustrations in 233 Parts, 13 in Full Color

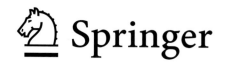 Springer

Samuel M. Butman, MD, FACC, FSCAI
Associate Professor of Medicine
Section of Cardiology
University of Arizona Sarver Heart Center
Tucson, AZ 85724
USA

Library of Congress Control Number: 2005924412

ISBN 10: 0-387-24468-9   Printed on acid-free paper.
ISBN 13: 978-0387-24468-6

Printed in the United States of America.   (BS/MVY)

9 8 7 6 5 4 3 2 1   SPIN 10938560

springeronline.com

How and when my parents instilled my concern for my many patients
and for those whom others care for, I may never know.
This work is dedicated to you, Mom and Dad.
Wherever you are, be proud of what you continue to do for many, many patients.

Foreword I

Every physician hates to have a patient develop a complication. Nevertheless, we also know that when a problem does develop, one needs a clear corrective strategy to minimize the effect of the complication and thereby prevent a major morbid event. The most frightening of all cardiologic complications occur in the catheterization laboratory. Indeed, Lewis Dexter, one of my mentors, told me about his first, accidental catheterization of the pulmonary artery. When he saw, under the fluoroscope, that the catheter was dancing back and forth in the lung, Dr. Dexter was convinced that he had perforated the patient's heart while trying to thread the catheter through the right atrium to the renal veins. However, after some thought and observation, he realized that he had not encountered a complication; instead he had tripped upon the opportunity to diagnose and understand various forms of heart diseases. Clinical cardiac catheterization had been born!

The 14 chapters in this book have various real-life complications that have occurred during coronary intervention. They also describe various strategies for avoiding or managing them. The chapters take the reader sequentially through a variety of situations, any one of which would make for a potentially "bad day" in the catheterization laboratory. Starting with medication problems, the authors work their way from the groin to the coronary arteries, detailing unpleasant situations and how to deal with them. All types of intervention and every device employed are considered, including balloon angioplasty, guidewires, stents, brachytherapy, and closure devices for sealing off peripheral arterial access. Other forms of complication are also considered, such as the no-reflow phenomenon and early versus late complications. Finally, the legal and liability concerns of these complications are examined, as are resuscitation and the reporting of adverse events.

This highly complete, readable, and useful text will be of inestimable value to catheterization personnel.

Joseph S. Alpert, MD
Robert S. and Irene P. Flinn Professor of Medicine
Head, Department of Medicine
University of Arizona Health Science Center
Tucson, Arizona

Foreword II

No procedures: no complications.

In most conferences of interventional cardiology, the sessions dealing with "Complications" are usually the ones where few or no empty seats are available. The most effective way to dramatically reduce and truly eliminate the risk for complications is not to perform a procedure. In real life this approach translates into what we call "patient selection." The experience accumulated in almost 30 years of percutaneous coronary interventions has given us some useful information to enable us to estimate the risk of complications according to the characteristics of the patient and of the lesion. A very common evaluation we all perform before any intervention is to estimate the risk versus the benefit of the procedure we plan to perform. A procedure is considered appropriate when the risk of complications is far below the potential clinical advantage. In some circumstances, such as in percutaneously treating a patient with cardiogenic shock, we are ready to accept a very high risk of complications in the face of a much higher risk associated with the natural history of the untreated condition.

Besides these foreseeable complications there are a group of complications that are very rare and almost never occur (less than 1%). Nevertheless, on an "unlucky day" we may experience one of these. These complications are the worst because they are totally unexpected, and they may occur with the operator unprepared and not trained to deal with them (the very reason why this patient, a low-risk case, was selected). The operator not infrequently has an initial sense of bewilderment, which may further delay an effective management.

The truth of the matter is that no matter what strategy an interventional cardiologist is going to use, in no way is he liberated from the occurrence of complications. Perhaps one of the highest risk periods in the practice of interventional cardiology occurs following long intervals in which many procedures were successfully performed and no complications occurred.

The point of this discussion is that familiarity with most complications (never all, as there is always the complication not yet described), their associated factors, their pathophysiology, their treatment, and ways to minimize their occurrence are essential in the education of every interventional cardiologist. These are the reasons that I consider the work of Samuel Butman a laudable contribution to the field. Even though a lot has been written about complications and journals frequently describe case reports and reviews, it is very useful to have a single book that systematically approaches the issue of complications that may occur in performing coronary interventions. It is important to keep in mind that as devices evolve the potential for even newer complications arises as well. We now treat more complex patients because we feel more experienced and have better devices and because we are not afraid to deal with undilatable lesions or to attempt to reopen total occlusions considered untreatable in the past. The result of this more aggressive approach, which gives more options to patients, is the emergence of new complications or familiar complications presenting in a different way. It is quite different to deal with a coronary perforation in a patient on heparin compared to one receiving IIb/IIIa inhibitors or bivalirudin.

For these reasons there is need for an updated approach to complications. I think this work fulfills these requirements. Each chapter is introduced by a detailed case presentation describing the occurrence of and, at times unsuccessful, solution to a specific complication. A review of the literature with cases, the pathophysiology of the complication, and the various proposed treatments are then presented. There are some important and novel chapters—"Legal Complications of Percutaneous Coronary Procedures" and "Adverse Event Reporting: Physicians, Manufacturers, and the Food and Drug Administration"—interesting for both practitioners and the many ancillary people involved in these procedures. All the contributors are very experienced and provide a reliable and very credible evaluation of each topic.

I cannot conclude this introduction without mentioning that besides my profound interest in reading and learning about complications, I am absolutely delighted to write these words because my association with Sam dates to the time when I was a cardiology fellow at the Veterans Administration Hospital in California and I performed my first angioplasties under his direction. More than anything else, I am happy to see a tool that many interventionalists will find very useful. Careful and critical reading of this book may ultimately help to effectively prevent some complications, and even if the complications occur, the reader may feel more confident and capable of instituting the most appropriate treatment.

Antonio Colombo, MD
Director, Interventional Cardiology
Columbus Hospital and San Raffaele University Hospital
Milan, Italy

Preface

In the first 125 interventional procedures I performed in the early 1980s, using primitive equipment, no patient had a myocardial infarction, none required urgent surgery, and none died. That run did not last, of course, and now having performed over 2,200 percutaneous coronary interventions, I know better. Perhaps it is simply a wish to pass along the idea of "knowing better" that has led me to this task.

The **idea** for writing this book came not from a particular untimely event during an interventional procedure. Rather, it arose from a combination of factors: occasional reviews of legal files, where complications occur in laboratories far away and by cardiologists I do not know; events discussed at our weekly conferences; and complications I have witnessed or been a party to.

It appears that at times we are unaware of some of the risks to which we subject ourselves, and more importantly our patients. While most of us would prefer that complications simply not occur, this is not the case. Complications are an unfortunate but real part of percutaneous coronary interventions.

The **purpose** of this book is to put as many of the complications reported and experienced by many in this field under one cover, to serve as a tool and resource for trainees, for technical staff, for laboratories, and for cardiologists alike. As is true with most things in life, better education and dissemination of the information can only improve on what we do. The authors contributing to this book are dedicated to bettering interventional cardiovascular care by minimizing the number of complications, always a source of angst for all.

This book is organized in a familiar proximal (skin) to distal (coronary intervention) approach, with several additional chapters rounding out its scope. Information into both legal ramifications and government responsibilities provides further insight into the risks and benefits of the devices and the procedure more and more of our patients continue to embrace.

My background as an interventional cardiologist is straightforward. After having learned the basics in the early 1980s, I was proctored, and then I developed a coronary interventional program at the Veteran's Administration Medical Center in Long Beach, California. Later, I moved to Arizona where, as director of the Cardiac Catheterization Laboratories, I developed a state-of-the-art active multivessel interventional program at the University of Arizona in Tucson. We have had an outstanding success rate, combined with a very low complication rate during my tenure as director, nearly 20 years.

I could not have written this book without the open and honest assistance of my coauthors—who all agreed to lead their chapters with an unfortunate case of their own—and the daily support of the excellent CCL staff who are not only well trained but a pleasure to come to in the morning and reluctantly meet, as we do at times, during the odd hours of the night. My editor at Springer, Robert Albano, and his developmental editor, Stephanie Sakson, were supportive and generous with their time and patience. Finally, a special note of gratitude to Eva, my partner, and a co-author, as well. Next time I will not take my work with me on vacations.

Samuel M. Butman, MD, FACC, FSCAI

Contents

Contributors

Peter Akmajian, Esq
Chandler, Udall PC, Tucson, AZ 85701, USA

William L. Ballard, MD, FACC
Director, Cardiac Catheterization Laboratory and Interventional Cardiology, Cardiology of Georgia, Fuqua Heart Center of Atlanta, Piedmont Hospital, Atlanta, GA 30309, USA

Gurpreet Baweja, MD
Cardiology Fellow, University of Arizona Sarver Heart Center, Tucson, AZ 85724, USA

Samuel M. Butman, MD, FACC, FSCAI
Associate Professor of Medicine, Section of Cardiology, University of Arizona Sarver Heart Center, Tucson, AZ 85724, USA

Antonio J. Chamoun, MD
Director, Interventional Cardiology Fellowship, Brandywine Valley Cardio-vascular Associates, Thorndale, PA 19372, USA

Albert W. Chan, MD, MSc, FRCP(C), FACC, FSCAI
Associate Director, Catheterization Laboratory, Department of Cardiology, Ochsner Clinic Foundation, New Orleans, LA 70121, USA

H.M. Omar Farouque, MBBS (Hons), PhD, FRACP
Interventional Cardiologist, Department of Cardiology, Austin Health, Victoria, Australia

Richard R. Heuser, MD, FACC, FSCAI
Director of Cardiovascular Research, St. Joseph's Hospital and Medical Center, Clinical Professor of Medicine, University of Arizona, College of Medicine, Phoenix Heart Center, Phoenix, AZ 85013, USA

Raghunandan Kamineni, MD
Salem Cardiology Associates, Salem, OR 97302, USA

Karl B. Kern, MD
Professor of Medicine, University of Arizona Sarver Heart Center, Tucson, Arizona 85724, USA

David P. Lee, MD
Assistant Professor of Medicine (Cardiovascular), Associate Director, Cardiac Catheterization and Coronary Intervention Laboratories, Stanford Interventional Cardiology, Stanford, CA 94305, USA

Eva B. Manus, RT
Product Surveillance Manager, Intralase Corporation, Irvine, CA 92618, USA

Paul E. Nolan, Jr., PharmD, FCCP, FASHP
Professor, Department of Pharmacy Practice and Science, College of Pharmacy and Senior Clinical Scientist, University of Arizona Sarver Heart Center, Tucson, AZ 85721, USA

Ashish Pershad, MD, FACC, FSCAI
Interventional Cardiologist, Heart and Vascular Center of Arizona, Phoenix, AZ 85006, USA

Hoang M. Thai, MD, FACC
Assistant Professor of Medicine, Department of Cardiology, University of Arizona College of Medicine, SAVAHCS Medical Center, Tucson, AZ 85723, USA

Toby C. Trujillo, PharmD, BCPS
Clinical Coordinator—Cardiovascular Specialist, Director, Pharmacy Residency Programs, Department of Pharmacy, Boston Medical Center, Boston, MA 02118, USA

Barry F. Uretsky, MD, FACC, FSCAI
John Sealy Centennial Chair, Professor of Medicine, Director, Interventional Cardiology, Division of Cardiology, University of Texas Medical Branch, Galveston, TX 77555, USA

Christopher J. White, MD, FACC, FESC, FSCAI
Chairman, Department of Cardiology, Ochsner Clinic Foundation, New Orleans, LA 70121, USA

1
Introduction

Samuel M. Butman

"Complications: It's just as important to share the cases that don't go according to plan"

From the cover of Endovascular Today, Volume 3, July/August 2004

There is gratification in performing a high-risk intervention in a patient wary of general anesthesia, surgery, and a prolonged recovery (Figure 1-1). Unfortunately, this can be easily offset when an unexpected complication occurs during a seemingly straightforward intervention, necessitating additional and unplanned interventions to avert disaster (Figure 1-2). This is the reality of day-to-day percutaneous coronary interventions performed, on average, in 25% of patients undergoing diagnostic coronary angiography.

Why write a seemingly negatively charged book? Which, if any, interventionalists would agree to contribute cases, let alone a chapter? The answer to the first question is simple: With the reality that the majority of procedures are uncomplicated, it is easy to go through training, work in a busy cardiac catheterization laboratory, and practice for some time doing a moderate number of interventions, and not be aware of the myriad of complications that can occur or, more importantly, that may be averted. More information and a greater dissemination of the information can only further improve outcomes—the goal of this book of bad things that can happen to good people.

Indeed, it was somewhat difficult to find experienced cardiologists willing to contribute, not so much due to the subject matter, but because so many of us are simply too busy. However, all agreed with the aim in publishing this book of complications, accepting that they occur, albeit infrequently, that they may be avoidable, and that they are more readily managed when we know more about them. As I write this introduction with all the contributing chapters finalized, novel complications are being reported.

Approximately one million percutaneous interventional procedures were performed in 2003 in the United States, with twice that number performed worldwide.[1] An estimated 7500 interventional cardiologists in the United States and another 11,000 worldwide performed these complex and high-risk procedures in 1500 U.S. and foreign hospitals.[2] The numbers continue to increase with expanding indications, improved tools, and better long-term outcomes with drug-coated stents, which reduce the incidence of restenosis.[3,4] The incidence of significant adverse events is very low, with recent reports describing overall complication rates between 1% and 5%.[5,6] There are an increasing number of physicians performing percutaneous coronary intervention, and while many perform a low volume of procedures, success rates of over 97% are still expected.

With hundreds of procedures being performed worldwide daily, even a 2%–3% complication risk is an important consideration to both the physician and the patient involved in a procedure, more so if an actual adverse event occurs during the procedure. Complications range from the minor bruise postprocedure to the rare but life-threatening pulmonary hemorrhage due to glycoprotein IIb/IIIa inhibitor therapy,[7] aortic dissection from an ostial vessel dilatation,[8] or death after failure of resuscitative efforts. This book is a compilation of many published reports, data freely available from U.S. Food and Drug Administration websites, personal experiences of my colleague–authors, and my own database of events, with the hope that knowledge of potential and real missteps and a better identification of the early signs of compromise will lead to even better outcomes for all.

Models of risk prediction and stratification of higher risk patients were reported early in the percutaneous coronary balloon angioplasty experience. These continue to be reported regularly from many sources, reflecting both the growing library of experience and the newer and more novel technologies.[9–11] While of moderate use in prediction and patient selection, the ever-improving and

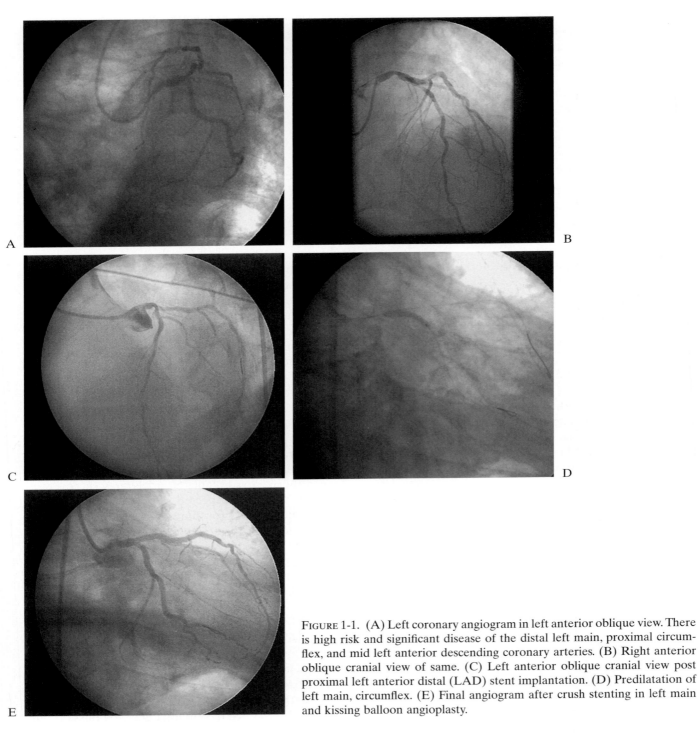

FIGURE 1-1. (A) Left coronary angiogram in left anterior oblique view. There is high risk and significant disease of the distal left main, proximal circumflex, and mid left anterior descending coronary arteries. (B) Right anterior oblique cranial view of same. (C) Left anterior oblique cranial view post proximal left anterior distal (LAD) stent implantation. (D) Predilatation of left main, circumflex. (E) Final angiogram after crush stenting in left main and kissing balloon angioplasty.

changing tools and drugs available have minimized the real effect of these reports on patient selection on a day-to-day basis. Since the advent of coronary stenting, type B and C coronary lesions do not portend the same risk as they did during the era of "plain old balloon angioplasty." Conversely, most clinicians who have experienced severe no-reflow during the treatment of a degenerated vein graft or during the course of an acute infarct vessel angioplasty have learned to both be aware of the potential and, from the literature, know how to treat it. We now have a better understanding of who is at risk and what works to avoid and treat the no-reflow event. The continuing reports in our specialty journals, the wisdom of those with large experiences in textbooks on interventional cardiology, and our own clinical experience are all invaluable in affecting the care we provide our patients.

The risks have remained low, but even an occasional bad event should cause us to stop and reconsider what we do. The availability of an alternate therapy, be it medical or surgical, should always be an option considered. Coronary perforations are uncommon today, but there is still a risk as we develop better or more aggressive interventions to open chronic total occlusions.[12,13] As

we begin to more frequently consider interventions in patients with left main coronary artery stenoses, untoward events will continue to occur in the coronary artery, in the groin, or postprocedure and range from nuisance to life threatening.[14] This is an ever-changing landscape with continual improvements and new potential problems as we leave the older technology for newer and improved tools.

Success in the cardiac catheterization laboratory is dependent not only on proper selection of patients, but also on skilled and focused technical staff and better-than-adequate imaging equipment. Better imaging

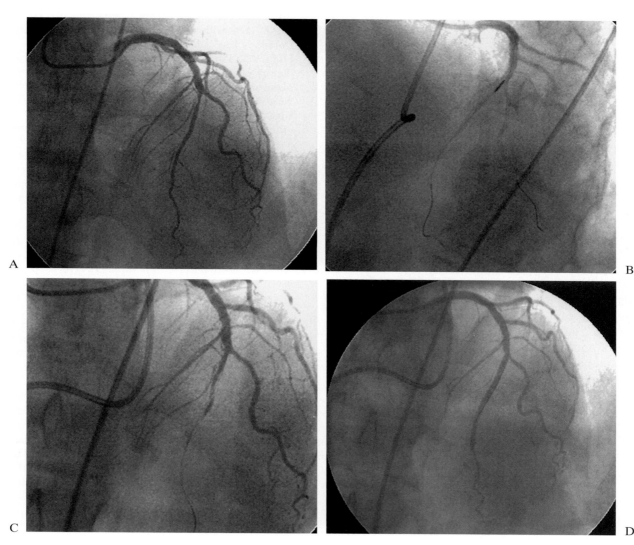

A

B

C

D

FIGURE 1-2. (A) Left coronary angiogram in the apical cranial view. High-grade disease is seen in the mid left anterior descending artery just distal to the origin of a diagonal branch. (B) Left anterior oblique cranial view with the intravascular ultrasonographic catheter at the lesion. A second wire is in the diagonal branch. (C) After balloon dilatation with a second, larger, cutting balloon, inadvertently oversized to the proximal vessel from intravascular ultrasound data, there is dissection of the LAD with reduced blood flow. (D) Additional unplanned stents were successfully placed with a good final angiographic result.

equipment is critical, and the manufacturers continue to move forward with us in this regard. The increasing body mass of our aging population, the growing number of procedures being performed, and the need for better visualization as we attack more complex anatomy all demand the best imaging equipment as well as improved wires, balloons, and guide catheters. The catheterization laboratory technical staff may not always make or break a case, but they can assist or distract a physician from the task at hand. How easily an exchange wire is kept in place, rather than inadvertently moved, or how quickly an expanding hematoma or coronary dissection is recognized makes a difference. Having a dedicated, stable, and focused team is key to facile, safe, and more frequently successful outcomes.

A final note to ponder, both ethical and legal, is how we approach our patients before they reach the laboratory, specifically the manner in which they are asked to sign their consent forms. Are our patients being properly informed about the risks and benefits of coronary revascularization, be it percutaneous or surgical? The answer comes from a recent poll of patients.[15] In this report, 42% of the patients could not identify the risk of percutaneous coronary intervention, and a similar number could not identify the possible benefits of the procedure! While the numbers were slightly worse for surgical revascularization, two-thirds could not quantify the risks inherent during percutaneous coronary intervention. One can only wonder what number of interventional cardiologists might fare similarly. This figure should not be surprising given the ad hoc, frequently routine approach of percutaneous coronary intervention today. Do we tell our patients that the risk of coronary perforation and death is higher when we are dealing with a more complex lesion or a total occlusion, or when we are using a bigger balloon or a more complex device?[16] Are we describing the myriad of noncoronary complications that may occur?[17] What about alternative approaches and their risks? Are they honestly and openly discussed with the patient? Would our surgical colleagues agree? Should we postpone a potential same-day intervention when other options exist, or when particularly high-risk anatomy is present? How often do we ask a surgeon to discuss options with the patient before possible percutaneous intervention?

The book is organized in the manner that we perform the interventions, from "skin to skin," with a few additional chapters. Of note, the chapter on the legal aspects of percutaneous coronary intervention is not meant to be a distraction or cause for alarm, but rather it is aimed at a better understanding of what can and cannot be done to prevent further suffering if an untoward event does occur. Specific approaches to treating complications are dealt with in each chapter to some degree, but are not the focus of this book. They have been described in several general textbooks on coronary intervention. It is the hope of all contributors that anticipating or recognizing a problem or minor mishap earlier as a result of reading this book will lead to less serious adverse events and better outcomes for both our readers and our patients.

References

1. Millennium Research Group. US, European, and Japan markets for interventional cardiology. 2002–2003.
2. Personal communication, Guidant Corporation, 2004.
3. Schofer J, Schuter M, Gershlick AH, et al. Sirolimus-eluting stents for treatment of patients with long atherosclerotic lesions in small coronary arteries: double-blind, randomized controlled trial (E-SIRIUS). Lancet. 2003;362:1093–1099.
4. Morice M-C. A randomized comparison of a sirolimus-eluting stent with a standard stent for coronary revascularization. N Engl J Med. 2002;346:1773–1780.
5. Hong MK, Popma JJ, Baim DS, et al. Frequency and predictors of major in-hospital ischemic complications after planned and unplanned new-device angioplasty from the New Approaches to Coronary Intervention (NACI) registry. Am J Cardiol. 1997;80:40K–49K.
6. Altmann DB, Racz M, Battleman DS, et al. Reduction in angioplasty complications after the introduction of coronary stents: results from a consecutive series of 2242 patients. Am Heart J. 1996;132:503–507.
7. Ali A, Hashem M, Rosman HS, et al. Use of glycoprotein IIb/IIIa inhibitors and spontaneous pulmonary hemorrhage. J Invasive Cardiol. 2003;15:186–188.
8. Goldstein JA, Casserly IP, Katsiyiannis WT, et al. Aorto-coronary dissection complicating a percutaneous coronary intervention. J Invasive Cardiol. 2003;15:89–92.
9. Ross, MJ, Herrmann HC, Moliterno DJ, et al. Angiographic variables predict increased risk for adverse ischemic events after coronary stenting with glycoprotein IIb/IIIa inhibition. J Am Coll Cardiol. 2003;42:981–988.
10. Singh M, Rihal CS, Selzer F, et al. Validation of a Mayo Clinic risk adjustment model for in-house complications after percutaneous coronary interventions, using the National Heart, Lung, and Blood Institute dynamic registry. J Am Coll Cardiol. 2003;42:1722–1728.
11. De Feyter PJ, McFadden E. Risk score for percutaneous coronary intervention: is forewarned forearmed? J Am Coll Cardiol. 2003;42:1729–1730.
12. Witzke CF, Matin-Herrero F, Clarke SC, Pomerantzev E, Palacios IF. The changing pattern of coronary perforation in the new device era. J Invasive Cardiol. 2004;16:297–301.
13. Kandzari DE. The challenge of chronic total occlusions: an old problem in a new perspective. J Interv Cardiol. 2004;17:259.
14. Kar B, Butkevich A, Civitello AB, et al. Hemodynamic support with a percutaneous left ventricular assist device during stenting of an unprotected left main coronary artery. Tex Heart Inst J. 2004;31:84–86.
15. Alexander KP, Harding T, Coombs L, Peterson E. Are patients properly informed prior to revascularization decisions [abstract]? J Am Coll Cardiol. 2003;41(suppl A):535A.

16. Stankovic G, Orlic D, Corvaja N, et al. Incidence, predictors, in-hospital, and late outcomes of coronary artery perforations. Am J Cardiol. 2004;93:213–216.

17. Wiley JM, White CJ, Uretsky BF. Noncoronary complications of coronary intervention. Cathet Cardiovasc Diag. 2002;57:257–265.

2
Complications of the Medications

Paul E. Nolan, Jr. and Toby C. Trujillo

In the United States nearly 600,000 percutaneous coronary interventions (PCI) are performed annually.[1] Adjunctive pharmacologic therapies are used to facilitate and assure favorable patient outcomes in the setting of PCI.[2-4] However, complications, some severe, occur with the use of these adjunctive therapies. This chapter will discuss selected complications, including their prevention and treatment.

1. Case 1. An Unusual Bleeding Complication

A 28-year-old male presented to the emergency department complaining of chest discomfort and shortness of breath that began 1 hour prior to arrival. The past medical history was significant for three orthotopic heart transplantations. He also had a history of mild chronic renal insufficiency. His medications included cyclosporine, azathioprine, prednisone, diltiazem, and pantoprazole. The initial electrocardiographic readings revealed sinus tachycardia at a rate of 105 beats per minute (bpm) and marked ST-segment depression in leads V4–V6. During the ensuing cardiac catheterization, a high-grade coronary stenosis of the left circumflex artery was found and mild pulmonary hypertension was documented. He was given 4000 U heparin intravenously (IV) and a 180 μg/kg IV bolus of eptifibatide, followed by a continuous IV infusion at 2.0 μg/kg/min. Following angioplasty and implantation of a drug-eluting stent, there was no residual stenosis. The patient was prescribed 325 mg aspirin and 75 mg clopidogrel, after a loading dose of 300 mg was given in the cardiac catheterization laboratory. Baseline laboratory values included hemoglobin of 10.7 g/dL, hematocrit of 31%, platelet count of 249,000/mm³, and a serum creatinine of 1.9 mg/dL. Six hours postintervention, the patient began complaining of shortness of breath, was noted to be hypoxic, and devel-

oped hemoptysis of about 100 mL. The eptifibatide infusion was stopped and the patient was transferred to the cardiovascular intensive care unit for observation. The initial chest X-ray revealed haziness throughout both lungs, bilateral pleural effusions, and cardiomegaly. A second X-ray performed 9 hours later revealed alveolar and interstitial edema and an increase in the right pleural effusion. In the ensuing 72 hours, hemoglobin levels fell to 8.7 g/dL and the platelet count fell to 177,000/mm³. The remainder of the hospital course was one of recovery and he was subsequently discharged home with a diagnosis of pulmonary hemorrhage related to eptifibatide.

2. Bleeding Complications

Hemorrhagic complications represent a worrisome, relatively common, acute adverse event associated with PCI and its attendant pharmacotherapy. In clinical trials hemorrhagic complications generally have been classified as major, moderate, or minor according to definitions originally used either in the Thrombolysis in Myocardial Infarction (TIMI) or Global Utilization of Streptokinase or tPA Outcomes (GUSTO) trials.[5] However, these arbitrary definitions, which were originally conceived for thrombolytic trials, may underestimate the true incidence of clinically important hemorrhagic complications following PCI in the modern era of combined anticoagulant and triple antiplatelet therapy.[5,6] Registries reflecting routine clinical practice commonly report greater hemorrhagic rates as compared to clinical trials.[5] Major hemorrhagic complications generally occur at vascular access sites, but also include gastrointestinal, intraocular, intracranial, and retroperitoneal bleeding.[5,6] Myocardial ischemic complications may also occur as the result of bleeding.[6] Risk factors for periprocedural hemorrhage include advanced age, female gender, renal impairment, hepatic dysfunction, diabetes, and post-PCI heparin use (Table 2-1).[5,6] Additional predictors of bleeding include

TABLE 2-1. Risk factors for bleeding post-PCI.

Advanced age
Female gender
Renal impairment
Hepatic dysfunction
Diabetes
Postprocedure heparin use

when PCI is used as a rescue coronary intervention for ongoing infarction after thrombolytic therapy, in the presence of cardiogenic shock, or in the setting of a platelet count nadir of less than 150,000/mm³.[7]

Renal insufficiency is a particularly important clinical risk factor for bleeding given that platelet dysfunction frequently develops as a consequence of reduced renal function.[8] Furthermore, the kidney serves as an important organ of elimination for several pharmacological agents used during PCI including enoxaparin; the glycoprotein (GP) IIb/IIIa antagonists, eptifibatide and tirofiban; the direct thrombin antagonists, hirudin and to a lesser degree, bivalirudin and agatroban; as well as unfractionated heparin to a limited extent.[8-11] Hepatic and intestinal drug-metabolizing activity also may be diminished in the setting of chronic renal impairment.[12] The patient in Case 1 presented with a history of mild, chronic renal insufficiency and an admission serum creatinine of 1.9 mg/dL. Employing the commonly used Cockcroft and Gault formula: {[140 − age (in years)] [total body weight (kg)]/(72 × Scr)}, his estimated creatinine clearance was about 57 mL/min.[13] Thus, his renal dysfunction was seemingly safe enough to administer full-dose eptifibatide. However, this formula appears to overestimate actual glomerular filtration rate in transplant recipients receiving long-term cyclosporine therapy.[14]

The patient experienced pulmonary hemorrhage (Figure 2-1), an uncommon but potentially lethal adverse effect that has been described following the administration of each of the three currently available GP IIb/IIIa receptor antagonists,[15-19] clopidogrel,[20] and thrombolytic agents.[21] In addition to the chronic renal dysfunction and the administration of full-dose eptifibatide, the patient's elevated pulmonary pressures may have contributed to the occurrence of pulmonary hemorrhage. Elevated pulmonary pressures as well as underlying pulmonary disease have been frequently associated with GP IIb/IIIa inhibitor-related pulmonary hemorrhage.[15-19] Other possible contributors to the patient's hemorrhagic complication even include aspirin, which is more likely to prolong the bleeding time in patients with renal impairment,[22] and diltiazem, which the patient was taking chronically prior to PCI, and which can also inhibit platelet activation.[23]

To minimize the risk of severe hemorrhagic complications in patients undergoing PCI, especially those with renal dysfunction, appropriate initial reductions in the dosages of agents that are renally eliminated should be undertaken, followed by careful monitoring of anticoagulant therapy, and perhaps even periprocedural platelet function monitoring to guide GP IIb/IIIa dosing.[8,9,24] The direct thrombin antagonist bivalirudin may represent an alternative therapy to GP IIb/IIIa antagonists even in patients with renal dysfunction.[25,26] The use of heparin-coated stents also may have a role in higher risk patients.[27] Efforts to minimize the risk of transfusion-requiring bleeding should be emphasized in that there may be an increased risk of mortality in patients with acute coronary syndromes who receive transfusions.[27a]

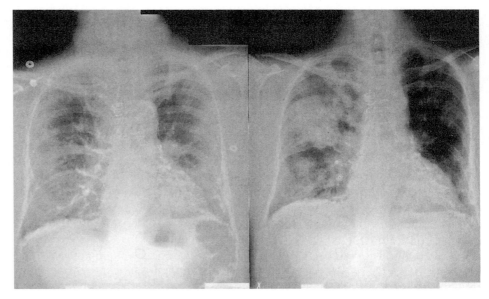

FIGURE 2-1. Radiographs of a patient who developed alveolar hemorrhage following the administration of abciximab. The radiograph on the left was obtained on admission. The radiograph on the right shows a dense right upper lobe consolidation and faint left upper lobe infiltrates that were noted 2 hours after receiving abciximab. (From Kalra et al.[15])

3. Treatment of Major Hemorrhage

The approach to bleeding at the access site and retroperitoneal bleeding, as well as specific risk factors for this major area of concern, is more extensively discussed in Chapter 11.

However, any treatment of major hemorrhagic complications should immediately include cessation of any anticoagulant and GP IIb/IIIa antagonist therapy.[28,29] Anticoagulant therapy with unfractionated heparin may be quickly reversed by appropriate doses of protamine sulfate.[28] However, protamine only partially reverses low-molecular-weight heparins.[28,29] Reversal of direct thrombin antagonists represents a unique challenge given the lack of specific antidotes for these agents.[28] Replacement of clotting factors with fresh frozen plasma or cryoprecipitate or the administration of desmopressin, recombinant factor VIIa, or prothrombin complex concentrates represents several different, but inadequately studied strategies for reversing direct thrombin antagonists.[28] With respect to emergent reversal of GP IIb/IIIa receptor antagonists, platelet transfusions are generally recommended for abciximab.[29] However, platelet transfusions alone may be insufficient for reversing eptifibatide and tirofiban.[29] Fibrinogen supplementation in the form of fresh frozen plasma or cryoprecipitate in combination with platelet transfusion may be more suitable for reversing the antiplatelet effects of the small-molecule, competitive GP IIb/IIIa antagonists.[30] Platelet or red blood cell transfusions may be useful in reversing the antiplatelet effects of aspirin or clopidogrel.[29,31]

4. Case 2. Acute Stent Thrombosis: Possible Role of Suboptimal Pharmacological Therapy

A 60-year-old, 90-kg man with a history of hypertension, type II diabetes mellitus, hyperlipidemia, and chronic lumbar pain was admitted to the hospital with unstable angina and evidence of inferolateral ST-segment depression. Medications on admission included 81 mg/day aspirin, 10 mg/day lisinopril, 25 mg/day hydrochlorothiazide, 40 mg/day atorvastatin, 10 mg/bid glyburide, and 600 mg/tid ibuprofen. All laboratory values including troponin I and creatine kinase were within normal limits except a serum glucose of 150 mg/dL. Coronary angiography revealed significant high-grade stenoses of the right and left circumflex arteries. Prior to PCI he was given 325 mg aspirin, 300 mg clopidogrel, 5000 IU bolus of heparin, and a bolus and infusion of tirofiban. Bare-metal stents were placed in the right coronary and circumflex arteries with a good angiographic result.

Approximately 10 hours post-PCI, the patient again experienced anginal pain and an ECG revealed sinus tachycardia at 130 bpm with ST-segment elevation in leads II, III, and aVF. Emergency coronary angiography revealed a clot totally occluding the stent in the right coronary artery (RCA). Thrombectomy and intracoronary infusion of tissue plasminogen activator were utilized successfully. The peak creatine kinase was 750 IU/L, with an MB fraction of 7.5% and a troponin I level of 7.17 ng/mL.

Acute or subacute coronary stent thrombosis following PCI and stent placement with bare-metal stents (Figure 2-2) is a relatively uncommon clinical phenomenon in the current era of double or triple antiplatelet therapy, generally occurring at a rate less than or equal to 1%, but up to 3%.[27,32–34] While generally considered a problem of inadequate stent deployment or proper anticoagulant, antiplatelet therapy, or adherence, clinical risk factors predisposing to coronary stent thrombosis include persistent dissection, total stent length, final lumen diameter, number of stents, history of congestive heart failure, older age, female gender, and a history of diabetes mellitus.[32–34] Catastrophic clinical outcomes including death and nonfatal myocardial infarction can result from coronary stent thrombosis.

In this case study, could suboptimal pharmacological therapy have contributed to the occurrence of coronary stent thrombosis? This patient could have aspirin resistance as a result of poorly controlled diabetes. Platelets in patients with type 2 diabetes may manifest a reduced sensitivity to aspirin.[35] Alternatively, a pharmacodynamic drug–drug interaction between aspirin and the nonselective, nonaspirin, nonsteroidal anti-inflammatory agent ibuprofen may also elicit aspirin resistance.[36–39] Ibuprofen, particularly when administered prior to aspirin therapy, may prevent aspirin from gaining access to its target site on platelet cyclooxygenase-1, thereby diminishing aspirin's antiplatelet and cardioprotective effects.[36,37] The risk of the antagonistic effects of ibuprofen may be greater with increased frequency of dosing.[38,39] Diclofenac and acetaminophen appear to have a reduced propensity to antagonize the antiplatelet effects of aspirin as compared to ibuprofen, and, therefore, may serve as alternative therapies for patients requiring anti-inflammatory medications for noncardiac conditions.[36] Naproxen may also be a suitable alternative to ibuprofen provided that simultaneous administration with aspirin is avoided.[39,39a] The use of COX-2 inhibitors should be discouraged because of the potential risk for cardiovascular complications.[39b] The use of a single, high, loading dose of aspirin (1000 mg) added to a pre-PCI regimen of daily, low-dose aspirin, although not formally tested in the setting of concomitant use of ibuprofen, appears to significantly reduce platelet activation pre- and post-PCI.[40]

In addition, this patient may have had clopidogrel resistance as a consequence of combined therapy with

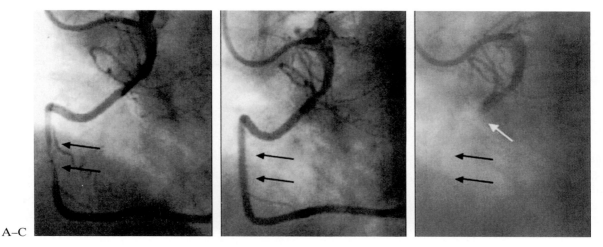

FIGURE 2-2. Angiography demonstrating a case of subacute stent thrombosis in a bare-metal stent. (A) Angiography before stent implantation. (B) Angiography after stent implantation. (C) Subacute stent thrombosis of implanted stent 1 day after stent implantation. (From Gupta et al.[27])

atorvastatin.[41–43] Clopidogrel is a prodrug that requires metabolic conversion to the active metabolite that inhibits adenosine diphosphate (ADP)-induced platelet aggregation.[41,44] The metabolic conversion to the active metabolite occurs via the action of the hepatic isozyme, cytochrome P-450 3A4 (CYP3A), which may be inhibited by atorvastatin and other inhibitors of CYP3A4.[41–43] The clinical significance of this interaction is uncertain given the post hoc report from the Clopidogrel for the Reduction of Events During Observation (CREDO) trial.[45] This trial showed a benefit in the 1-year composite endpoint of death, acute myocardial infarction (AMI), or stroke in the patients randomized to pre-PCI treatment with 300 mg clopidogrel, coupled with 1-year post-PCI treatment with 75 mg/day clopidogrel. However, careful examination of the 1-year composite endpoint showed a lower absolute event rate, 5.4%, in the patients taking statins not metabolized by CYP3A4 versus 7.6% in the patients taking statins metabolized by CYP3A4.[45] The clinical importance of this potential drug–drug interaction is still unknown at this time, however,[46] and whether a higher loading of 600 mg clopidogrel would circumvent this possible interaction remains unknown.[47]

Another aspect of this case related to suboptimal clopidogrel pharmacotherapy centers around the importance of timing following a loading dose of clopidogrel. The longer delay to PCI may permit greater conversion of clopidogrel to its active metabolite. Resistance to the antiaggregatory effects of clopidogrel may be greatest within the first 2 hours following a 300-mg loading dose.[48,49] Other investigators also have reported highly variable as well as frequent, suboptimal platelet inhibition within 2.5 hours following a 300-mg loading dose of clopidogrel.[50] The patient in Case 2 received a loading dose of clopidogrel just 1 hour prior to the start of PCI. A higher loading dose of clopidogrel (600 mg) may shorten the time to platelet inhibition as noted previously[47] and may be necessary to achieve adequate antiplatelet effects in overweight patients, such as in the patient in this case study, who undergo PCI and stenting.[51]

A meta-analysis of randomized-controlled clinical trials demonstrates that intravenously administered GP IIb/IIIa receptor antagonists confer a significant reduction in mortality in patients undergoing PCI.[52] This meta-analysis further extends their proven benefit in reducing periprocedural infarction. Furthermore, these agents may be particularly effective in reducing mortality in patients with preexisting diabetes and non–ST-elevation myocardial infarction (NSTEMI) acute coronary syndromes.[53–56] However, a conflicting report from the New York State PCI Database Registry showed a significant 57% relative increase in in-hospital major adverse coronary events that consisted of a composite of death, urgent coronary artery bypass surgery, postprocedural AMI, abrupt closure, and stent thrombosis in a cohort of patients receiving intravenous GP IIb/IIIa antagonists as compared to a matched cohort not receiving these agents.[57] Alarmingly, the increase in the primary endpoint was largely the result of significant increases in the three thrombosis-associated endpoints, postprocedural AMI, abrupt closure, and stent thrombosis. These findings may possibly reflect the pro-thrombotic potential of GP IIb/IIIa receptor antagonists.[58,59] Optimal dosing of GP IIb/IIIa receptor antagonists, guided by appropriate technology to monitor the degree of inhibition of platelet function, as noted in the GOLD study, may be indicated to reduce the risk for post-PCI major adverse coronary event (MACE).[60] This patient did not undergo monitoring of his platelet function following administration of tirofiban, where current bolus dosing recommendations for tirofiban may result in suboptimal inhibition of platelet aggregation.[61]

5. Case 3. Thrombocytopenia

A 60-year-old woman with a history of coronary artery disease presented to the hospital emergency room with chest pain. The electrocardiogram revealed ST-segment depression and T-wave inversion in leads V1–V6. Medications at the time of admission included 81 mg aspirin, 25 mg atenolol, 40 mg hydrochlorothiazide, and 40 mg pravastatin. At coronary angiography, a 90% occlusion of the mid-left anterior descending coronary artery and high-grade occlusion of the circumflex artery were found. Other baseline, pre-PCI laboratory values were within normal limits including a platelet count of 250,000/mm³. Prior to successful PCI the patient was administered a 3000 IU bolus of IV heparin, 0.25 µg/kg abciximab IV bolus followed by a continuous infusion of 0.125 µg/kg/min, 325 mg aspirin, and 300 mg clopidogrel. Initial troponin I and creatine kinase values were suggestive of acute NSTEMI.

Twelve hours post-PCI, the hematocrit was minimally reduced, but the platelet count was 60,000/mm³. A repeat blood sample was immediately obtained and the platelet count repeated using both citrate-containing (i.e., blue-top tube) and EDTA-containing (i.e., purple-top tube) sample tubes. The platelet counts from the citrate-containing and EDTA-containing tubes were 210,000/mm³ and 75,000/mm³, respectively. A diagnosis of abciximab-induced pseudothrombocytopenia (PTCP) was made. The patient had an uneventful post-PCI course and was discharged.

5.1. Pseudothrombocytopenia

Pseudothrombocytopenia (PTCP) is an in vitro phenomenon that generally results as a consequence of blood collection in EDTA-containing sample tubes.[62–64] Ethylenediaminetetraacetic acid is a calcium chelator that via calcium binding may alter the conformation of the GP IIb receptor on the surface of the platelet, and may expose a neoepitope that is recognized by IgG or IgM autoantibodies, resulting in artifactual clumping of platelets. Pseudothrombocytopenia also can result when blood is collected in either citrate-containing or heparin-containing sample tubes.[62,63] Therefore, in addition to an evaluation of the automated platelet count in both citrate- and EDTA-containing tubes, microscopic examination of a peripheral blood smear should be performed

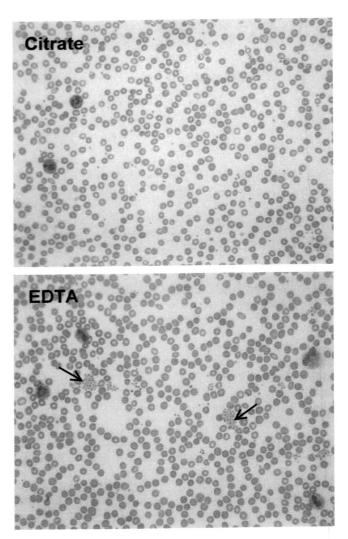

FIGURE 2-3. Example of a peripheral blood smear that was collected in an EDTA-containing tube (bottom), and taken from a patient who was administered abciximab. The smear reveals prominent platelet clumping consistent with pseudothrombocytopenia. The second smear (top) is from the same patient, but collected in a citrate-containing blood tube, and it is normal. (Reprinted with permission from Holmes et al.[64])

to distinguish between PTCP, with its typical large platelet aggregates, genuine thrombocytopenia, or heparin-induced thrombocytopenia (HIT), if unfractionated heparin, as in this case, or low-molecular-weight heparin, has been used (Figure 2-3).[62–64] An analysis of four randomized, placebo-controlled trials of abciximab revealed an overall incidence of abciximab-associated PTCP of 2.1%.[62] This rate was significantly greater than that of the placebo-treated group (0.6%). Pseudothrombocytopenia was responsible for over one-third of the low platelet counts noted in patients undergoing coronary interventions in these studies, but was not associated with adverse outcomes.

5.2. True Thrombocytopenia

In large, placebo-controlled clinical trials, the rate of occurrence of thrombocytopenia as compared to placebo was significantly more frequent in abciximab- and tirofiban-, but not in eptifibatide-, treated patients.[63] Nonetheless, thrombocytopenia has been reported to occur following administration of eptifibatide with or without prior exposure.[65,66] In comparative trials of GP IIb/IIIa receptor antagonists, thrombocytopenia is significantly observed more frequently following the administration of abciximab when compared to either tirofiban[67] or eptifibatide.[68] Unlike pseudothrombocytopenia, true thrombocytopenia developing in the setting of acute coronary syndromes is associated with a higher incidence of major adverse clinical events including hemorrhage, death, and myocardial infarction.[69]

Heparin-Induced Thrombocytopenia

Heparin-induced thrombocytopenia (HIT) must also be suspected when a patient's post-PCI platelet count is less than normal, and the patient has been administered either unfractionated heparin (UFH) or a low-molecular-weight heparin (LMWH) periprocedurily.[70,71] Although HIT typically occurs 4 or more days after the start of UFH[70] or 7 days after beginning treatment with LMWH,[71] prior administration of UFH, particularly within 100 days of the index administration, can result in a rapid onset (i.e., within 2–18 h) of HIT.[70] This patient had received UFH during cardiac catheterization 2 months prior to undergoing PCI.

Heparin-induced thrombocytopenia type 2 is a condition caused by heparin-dependent IgG antibodies formed against platelet factor 4.[72] The resultant IgG/platelet factor 4/heparin immune complexes then bind to platelets initiating platelet activation and aggregation and generating platelet microparticles, which can trigger the formation of arterial or venous thrombi including acute stent thrombosis.[73] Also, in patients presenting with NSTEMI and the history of a high likelihood of prior heparin exposure, and who were then given UFH during the index event, the subsequent presence of antiplatelet factor 4/heparin antibodies, even in the absence of thrombocytopenia, served as an independent predictor of myocardial infarction or death occurring at 1 month following the presentation of NSTEMI.[69]

To avoid the possibility of HIT or the development of platelet factor 4/heparin antibodies in the setting of PCI, especially in patients with prior heparin exposure, direct thrombin antagonists, particularly the bivalent thrombin inhibitors, hirudin and bivalirudin, may serve as alternatives to UFH or LWMH.[25,74] Direct thrombin inhibitors also serve as useful alternative anticoagulants for patients with a history of HIT undergoing PCI.[72,75]

6. Contrast-Induced Nephropathy

Contrast-induced nephropathy (CIN) has been reported to occur in 1%–6% of hospitalized patients and may be as high as 50% in patients who are considered high risk.[76] Risk factors for CIN include underlying renal insufficiency, diabetes, heart failure, dehydration, and the concomitant use of nonsterodial anti-inflammatory agents, diuretics, aminoglycosides, and possibly angiotensin-converting enzyme (ACE) inhibitors (Table 2-2). The volume of contrast administered also has a direct impact in the incidence of CIN. The most widely accepted hypothesis for the mechanism of CIN is believed to be a combination of direct renal tubular epithelial cell toxicity and renal medullary ischemia. Renal medullary ischemia is likely a result of decreased renal blood flow secondary to vasoconstriction from contrast media. In addition, hyperosmolar stress from contrast media can lead to the generation of oxygen free radicals that may cause direct toxicity.[76–78]

Although the definition of CIN has varied over time, it is now generally accepted that a 25% increase in serum creatinine or a rise of 0.5 mg/dL over baseline constitutes CIN. This increase typically occurs 24–48 hours after contrast administration. Most cases of CIN are nonoliguric and reversible within 7–10 days. The use of either low-osmolar or iso-osmolar contrast has been demonstrated to reduce the risk of CIN when compared to high-osmolar compounds.[76–78]

Several pharmacologic strategies have been investigated for prophylaxis, but most have not been shown to decrease the incidence of CIN. Theophylline, calcium channel blockers, diuretics, dopamine, atrial natriuretic peptide, and endothelin antagonists all have been demonstrated to be ineffective in reducing the incidence of CIN.[76] Recently fenoldopam, a dopamine-1 receptor agonist that produces renal arterial vasodilatation, in a placebo-controlled, randomized, double-blind trial

TABLE 2-2. Risk factors for contrast-induced nephropathy.

Renal insufficiency
Proteinuria
Diabetes mellitus
Heart failure
Dehydration
Nonsterodial anti-inflammatory agents
Aminoglycosides
Angiotensin-converting enzyme inhibitors
High volume of contrast agent
High-osmolar contrast agents

involving 315 patients undergoing invasive cardiac procedures with preexisting renal dysfunction, was shown to be no better than placebo in preventing CIN.[79]

One pharmacologic agent that has been demonstrated to decrease the incidence of CIN is N-acetylcysteine (NAC). It is thought that NAC's effect in reducing CIN is secondary to the drug's abilities to produce vasodilatation in the kidney and also to scavenge oxygen free radicals. Multiple medium-sized randomized trials have demonstrated that NAC, when given at a dose of 600 mg/bid on the day before and the day of the procedure, significantly reduces the incidence of CIN.[76] However, conflicting reports are emerging regarding its efficacy, although its safety seems high.

The most effective intervention to date for preventing CIN is pre- and postprocedural hydration with saline. At-risk patients should be hydrated with 1 mL/kg/h of 0.45% saline to 12 hours prior to the procedure and 12 hours postprocedurally when possible.[77] The administration of adequate hydration should be the cornerstone of any strategy to prevent CIN, and it is important that any other strategy (such as NAC) employed to prevent CIN is done in conjunction with, not in place of, adequate hydration. Recently it has been suggested that sodium chloride is not the optimal solution to provide adequate hydration in patients receiving contrast media.[80] With sodium chloride (154 mEq/L in 5% dextrose) or sodium bicarbonate (154 mEq/L in 5% dextrose), both given as a 3 mL/kg/h bolus 1 hour prior to contrast injection and then continued as a 1 mL/kg/h infusion for 6 hours afterwards, the incidence of CIN was significantly decreased (1.7% vs. 13.6%, $P = 0.02$). Further data is needed before sodium bicarbonate becomes the standard of practice for hydration in association with contrast media administration.

7. Treatment of the No-Reflow Phenomenon

Multiple mechanisms appear to be at play in the no-reflow phenomenon. In addition to mechanical issues, these include endothelial swelling and myocyte edema in the ischemic zone followed by heightened adrenergic tone and mechanical plugging by leukocytes, platelets, and fibrin following reperfusion, all of which contribute to increased downstream resistance.[81,82] Patients who experience no-reflow have a higher risk of MI and death.[82]

The intracoronary administration of several different pharmacologic agents to either treat or prevent the no-reflow phenomenon has become a common practice in the catheterization laboratory. Potential choices to treat no-reflow include the calcium channel blockers verapamil, diltiazem, and nicardipine; the direct and indirect

TABLE 2-3. Potential adverse effects of no-reflow drug therapy.

Adverse effect	Hypotension	Bradycardia/ heart block	Dyspnea
Drug			
Nitric oxide donors			
Nitroglycerin	•		
Nitroprusside	••		
Calcium channel blocker			
Verapamil	•	••	
Diltiazem	••	•	
ATP channel openers			
Adenosine	•	•	•
Nicorandil	•		

Abbreviation: ATP, adenosine triphosphate.
• mild potential
•• frequent

nitric-oxide donors nitroprusside and nitroglycerin; adenosine; the respective alpha-1 and alpha-2 adrenergic blockers urapidil and yohimbine; and the adenosine triphosphate (ATP)-sensitive potassium channel opener, nicorandil.[81–89] Although some clinical information is available for each of these agents regarding their ability to ameliorate the no-reflow phenomenon, overall there is a lack of comparative, randomized trial data regarding their ability to improve myocardial perfusion and clinical outcomes. The reader is referred to a recent review for typical doses used for several of the more commonly used agents.[82] Furthermore, combination therapy may lead to resolution in resistant instances.[86]

In addition to concerns regarding the beneficial effects of these agents on clinical outcomes, the clinician must be concerned regarding the potential for causing systemic adverse effects following the intracoronary administration of each of these agents. Once again, the available literature addressing these safety concerns is sparse and a general rule should be to monitor for typical side effects seen with intravenous administration of each agent (Table 2-3).

7.1. Nitroprusside

Based on available information, the administration of intracoronary nitroprusside appears to be the most effective agent. Administration of a median dose of 200 µg (range, 50–1000 µg) effectively improved angiographic flow without producing any significant hypotension or other adverse effects.[83]

7.2. Adenosine

Adenosine is known to prevent many of the underlying biochemical and physiologic changes mediating ischemia-reperfusion injury, and subsequently would be expected to prevent no-reflow in the setting of PCI. Of particular concern with the intracoronary administration of adenosine is the potential to produce significant brady-cardia and heart block, especially in the setting of active ischemia. Adenosine may also produce difficulty in breathing. When administered via the intracoronary route in patients receiving PCI for AMI, adenosine significantly reduced the incidence of no-reflow as compared to a saline placebo.[84] No episodes of arteriovenous (AV) block were seen, nor was there an increase in chest pain in patients receiving adenosine. It is important to note that this study occurred in the setting of AMI and the high level of sympathetic drive may have prevented any significant heart block from adenosine.

7.3. Calcium Channel Blockers

While several different calcium channel blockers have been studied in the treatment of no-reflow during PCI, there is little information to suggest which of these agents would be the best agent in terms of efficacy and safety.[85–87] In a study comparing the effects of intracoronary administration of nicardipine, diltiazem, and verapamil on coronary blood flow in minimally diseased left anterior descending or left circumflex arteries (<30% stenosis), all three agents significantly increased flow.[85] However, nicardipine appeared to increase flow to a greater degree than either diltiazem or verapamil in the doses studied. No patients experienced changes in heart rate or mean arterial blood pressure with any drug, but two patients experienced type 1 second-degree AV block after receiving diltiazem as opposed to none with either nicardipine or verapamil. It important to note that these patients were undergoing diagnostic catheterization and administration into the right coronary artery was excluded.

8. Agents Used to Produce Conscious Sedation

Conscious sedation can be described as a state that allows the patient to tolerate unpleasant procedures while maintaining adequate cardiopulmonary function and the ability to respond purposely to verbal commands or physical stimuli.[90,91] This level of sedation is often appropriate for patients undergoing angiography and/or PCI.

8.1. Benzodiazepines

The most common sedatives used for conscious sedation are the benzodiazepines, such as midazolam, diazepam, or lorazepam.[91] All of these agents cause anxiolysis, antegrade amnesia, and hypnosis. Of these agents, midazolam is often favored due to its rapid onset, short duration of action (45–60 min) leading to rapid recovery, low risk of respiratory depression, and antegrade amnestic effects.

Midazolam should be given in 1–3 mg bolus and then titrated by 1-mg increments every 5–10 minutes until the desired response is achieved. In patients who are elderly or debilitated, or who are also receiving other CNS-active medications such as opiates, the bolus dose and titration dose should be lowered by 50%. Midazolam should not be used on patients with known benzodiazepine hypersensitivity or acute narrow-angle glaucoma. Adverse reactions from IV administration include hiccups, nausea, vomiting, oversedation, headache, coughing, and pain at the injection site.

8.2. Opioid Analgesics

Opioid analgesics can be used in conjunction with sedatives in the provision of conscious sedation, especially during procedures where pain is a factor.[91] Fentanyl is often favored due to its quick onset, short duration of action, and lack of active metabolites as compared to other opioid analgesics such as meperidine or morphine. Fentanyl should be given as a 50–100 μg bolus and titrated in increments of 25 μg to the desired effect. In elderly patients or patients receiving concomitant sedatives, the dose should be decreased by 25%. Rapid IV administration can lead to a rigid chest wall and difficulty breathing.

Of greatest concern with the agents used for conscious sedation is the occurrence of respiratory depression. Policies should be in place that specify the frequency and duration of monitoring, the appropriate use of reversal agents (naloxone and flumazenil), and the threshold for intubation to protect the patient's airway.[90,91] Patients with chronic obstructive pulmonary disease, obese patients, and elderly patients are at particularly high risk for developing respiratory adverse events.[91] Other important adverse effects for which clinicians must monitor include orthostatic circulatory depression, nausea/vomiting/constipation and urinary retention, and pruritis/urticaria.[91] Hypotension is another complication of conscious sedation. Hypotension may be easily corrected by placing the patient in the head-down position while simultaneously giving IV fluids. If this intervention does not improve the blood pressure, more aggressive drug therapy is immediately needed.

Finally, it is vital that for at least 24 hours postprocedure the patient not be permitted to drive a car, operate machinery or power tools, drink any alcoholic beverages, make any important decisions, or sign legal papers.

9. Conclusions

Adjunctive pharmacological therapy plays an important role in the provision of favorable PCI and post-PCI clinical outcomes. However, to optimize the use of these agents, the clinician must recognize how patients' concurrent medical conditions and associated medical therapy can contribute to the occurrence of either suboptimal outcomes or adverse effects.

References

1. American Heart Association. Heart disease and stroke statistics—2004 update. Dallas, TX: American Heart Association; 2003.
2. Braunwald E, Antman EM, Beasley JW, et al. Management of patients with unstable angina and non-ST-segment elevation myocardial infarction update. J Am Coll Cardiol. 2002;40:1366–1374.
3. Philipp R, Grech ED. ABC of interventional cardiology. Interventional pharmacotherapy. Br Med J. 2003;327:43–46.
4. Kereiakes DJ. Adjunctive pharmacotherapy before percutaneous coronary intervention in non-ST-elevation acute coronary syndromes: the role of modulating inflammation. Circulation. 2003;108(suppl III);III-22–III-27.
5. Moscucci M. Frequency and costs of ischemic and bleeding complications after percutaneous coronary interventions: rationale for new antithrombotic agents. J Invasive Cardiol. 2002;14(suppl B):55B–64B.
6. Lopez LM. Clinical challenges of bleeding in percutaneous coronary intervention. Am J Health Syst Pharm. 2003; 60(suppl 3):S8–S14.
7. Dauerman HL, Andreou C, Perras MA, et al. Predictors of bleeding complications after rescue coronary interventions. J Thromb Thrombolysis. 2000;10:83–88.
8. Rammohan C, Fintel D. Dosing considerations and monitoring of low molecular weight heparin and glycoprotein IIb/IIIa antagonists in patients with renal insufficiency. Curr Cardiol Rep. 2003;5:303–309.
9. Reddan D, Szczech LA, O'Shea S, et al. Anticoagulation in acute cardiac care in patients with chronic kidney disease. Am Heart J. 2003;145:586–594.
10. Arpino PA, Hallisey RK. Effect of renal function on the pharmacodynamics of argatroban. Ann Pharmacother. 2004;38:25–29.
11. Kandrotas RJ. Heparin pharmacokinetics and pharmacodynamics. Clin Pharmacokinet. 1992;22:359–374.
12. Pichette V, Leblond FA. Drug metabolism in chronic renal failure. Curr Drug Metab. 2003;4:91–103.
13. Cockcroft DW, Gault MH. Prediction of creatinine clearance from serum creatinine. Nephron. 1976;6:31–41.
14. Goral S, Ynares C, Shyr Y, et al. Long-term renal function in heart transplant recipients receiving cyclosporine therapy. J Heart Lung Transplant. 1997;16:1106–1112.
15. Kalra S, Bell MR, Rihal CS. Alveolar hemorrhage as a complication of treatment with abciximab. Chest. 2001;120:126–131.
16. Khanlou H, Tsiodras S, Eiger G, et al. Fatal alveolar hemorrhage and abciximab (ReoPro) therapy for acute myocardial infarction. Catheter Cardiovasc Intervent. 1998;44:313–316.
17. Ali A, Patil S, Grady KJ, et al. Diffuse alveolar hemorrhage following administration of tirofiban or abciximab: a nemesis of platelet glycoprotein IIb/IIIa inhibitors. Catheter Cardiovasc Intervent. 2000;49:181–184.
18. Ali A, Hashem M, Rosman HS, et al. Use of platelet glycoprotein IIb/IIIa inhibitors and spontaneous pulmonary hemorrhage. J Invasive Cardiol. 2003;15:186–188.
19. Orford JL, Fasseas P, Holmes DR, et al. Alveolar hemorrhage associated with periprocedural eptifibatide. J Invasive Cardiol. 2004;16:341–342.
20. Kilaru PK, Schweiger MJ, Kozman HA, et al. Diffuse alveolar hemorrhage after clopidogrel use. J Invasive Cardiol. 2001;13:535–537.
21. Awadh N, Ronco JJ, Bernstein V, et al. Spontaneous pulmonary hemorrhage after thrombolytic therapy for acute myocardial infarction. Chest. 1994;106:1622–1624.
22. Gaspari F, Vigano G, Orisio S, et al. Aspirin prolongs bleeding time in uremia by a mechanism distinct from platelet cyclooxygenase inhibition. J Clin Invest. 1987; 79:1788–1797.
23. Dai H, Chen J, Tao Q, et al. Effects of diltiazem on platelet activation and cytosolic calcium during percutaneous transluminal coronary angioplasty. Postgrad Med J. 2003;79: 522–526.
24. Mukherjee D, Chew DP, Robbins M, et al. Clinical application of procedural platelet monitoring during percutaneous coronary intervention among patients at increased bleeding risk. J Thromb Thrombolysis. 2001;11:151–154.
25. Lincoff AM, Bittl JA, Harrington RA, et al. Bivalirudin and provisional glycoprotein IIb/IIIa blockade compared with heparin and planned glycoprotein IIb/IIIa blockade during percutaneous coronary intervention. REPLACE-2 randomized trial. JAMA. 2003;289:853–863.
26. Chew DP, Bhatt DL, Kimball W, et al. Bivalirudin provides increasing benefit with decreasing renal function: a meta-analysis of randomized trials. Am J Cardiol. 2003;92: 919–923.
27. Gupta V, Aravamuthan BR, Baskerville S, et al. Reduction of subacute stent thrombosis (SAT) using heparin-coated stents in a large-scale, "real world" registry. J Invasive Cardiol. 2004;16:304–310.
27a. Rao SV, Jollis JG, Harrington RA, et al. Relationship of blood transfusion and clinical outcomes in patients with acute coronary syndromes. JAMA. 2004;292:1555–1562.
28. Warkentin TE, Crowther MA. Reversing anticoagulants both old and new. Can J Anaesth. 2002;49(suppl):S11–S25.
29. Schroeder WS, Gandhi PJ. Emergency management of hemorrhagic complications in the era of glycoprotein IIb/IIIa receptor antagonists, clopidogrel, low molecular weight heparin, and third-generation fibrinolytic agents. Curr Cardiol Rep. 2003;5:310–317.
30. Li YF, Spencer FA, Becker RC. Comparative efficacy of fibrinogen and platelet supplementation on the in vitro reversibility of competitive glycoprotein IIb/IIIa receptor-directed platelet inhibition. Am Heart J. 2002;143:725–732.
31. Rocca B, Fitzgerald GA. Simple read: erythrocytes modulate platelet function. Should we rethink the way we give aspirin? Circulation. 1997;95:11–13.
32. Cutlip DE, Baim DS, Ho KKL, et al. Stent thrombosis in the modern era. A pooled analysis of multicenter coronary stent clinical trials. Circulation. 2001;103:1967–1971.

33. Orford JL, Lennon R, Melby S, et al. Frequency and correlates of coronary stent thrombosis in the modern era. J Am Coll Cardiol. 2002;40:1567–1572.

34. Reynolds MR, Rinaldi MJ, Pinto DS, et al. Current clinical characteristics and economic impact of subacute stent thrombosis. J Invasive Cardiol. 2002;14:364–368.

35. Watala C, Golanski J, Pluta J, et al. Reduced sensitivity of platelets from type 2 diabetic patients to acetylsalicylic acid (aspirin)—its relation to metabolic control. Thromb Res. 2004;113:101–113.

36. Catella-Lawson F, Reilly MP, Kapoor SC, et al. Cyclooxygenase inhibitors and the antiplatelet effects of aspirin. N Engl J Med. 2001;345:1809–1817.

37. MacDonald TM, Wei L. Effect of ibuprofen on cardioprotective effect of aspirin. Lancet. 2003;361:573–574.

38. Kurth T, Glynn RJ, Walker AM, et al. Inhibition of clinical benefits of aspirin on first myocardial infarction by nonsteroidal antiinflammatory drugs. Circulation. 2003;108: 1191–1195.

39. Kimmel SE, Berlin JA, Reilly M, et al. The effects of nonselective non-aspirin non-steroidal anti-inflammatory medications on the risk of nonfatal myocardial infarction and their interaction with aspirin. J Am Coll Cardiol. 2004;43:985–990.

39a. Capone ML, Sciulli MG, Tacconelli S, et al. Pharmacodynamic interaction of naproxen with low-dose aspirin in health subjects. J Am Coll Cardiol. 2005;45:1295–1301.

39b. Drazen JM. COX-2 inhibitors – a lesson in unexpected problems. N Engl J Med. 2005;352:1131–1132.

40. Ten Berg JM, Gerritsen WBM, Haas FJLM, et al. High-dose aspirin in addition to daily low-dose aspirin decreases platelet activation in patients before and after percutaneous coronary intervention. Thromb Res. 2002;105:385–390.

41. Clarke TA, Waskell LA. Clopidogrel is metabolized by human cytochrome P450 3A and inhibited by atorvastatin. Drug Metab Dispos. 2003;31:53–59.

42. Lau WC, Waskell LA, Watkins PB, et al. Atorvastatin reduces the ability of clopidogrel to inhibit platelet aggregation. A new drug–drug interaction. Circulation. 2003;107:32–37.

43. Neubauer H, Günesdogan B, Hanefeld C, et al. Lipophilic statins interfere with the inhibitory effects of clopidogrel on platelet function—a flow cytometry study. Eur Heart J. 2003;24:1744–1749.

44. Lau WC, Gurbel PA, Watkins PB, et al. Contribution of hepatic cytochrome P450 3A4 metabolic activity to the phenomenon of clopidogrel resistance. Circulation. 2004;109: 166–171.

45. Saw J, Steinhubl SR, Berger PB, et al., for the Clopidogrel for the Reduction of Events During Observation Investigators. Lack of adverse clopidogrel-atorvastatin clinical interaction from secondary analysis of a randomized, placebo-controlled clopidogrel trial. Circulation. 2003;108: 921–924.

46. Cannon CP, Brauwald E, McCabe CH, et al. Intensive versus moderate lipid lowering with statins after acute coronary syndromes. N Engl J Med. 2004;350:1495–1504.

47. Müller I, Besta F, Schulz C, et al. Effects of statins on platelet inhibition by a high loading dose of clopidogrel. Circulation. 2003;108:2195–2197.

48. Steinbuhl SR, Berger PB, Mann JT, et al. Early and sustained dual oral antiplatelet therapy following percutaneous coronary intervention. A randomized controlled trial. JAMA. 2002;288:2411–2420.

49. Gurbel PA, Bliden KP, Hiatt BL, et al. Clopidogrel for coronary stenting. Response variability, drug resistance, and the effect of pretreatment platelet reactivity. Circulation. 2003;107:2908–2913.

50. Lepäntalo A, Virtanen KS, Heikkilä J, et al. Limited early antiplatelet effect of 300 mg clopidogrel in patients with aspirin therapy undergoing percutaneous coronary interventions. Eur Heart J. 2004;25:476–483.

51. Angiolillo DJ, Fernández-Ortiz A, Bernardo E, et al. Platelet aggregation according to body mass index in patients undergoing coronary stenting: should clopidogrel loading-dose be weight adjusted? J Invasive Cardiol. 2004;16:169–174.

52. Karvouni E, Datritsis DG, Ioannidis JPA. Intravenous glycoprotein IIb/IIIa receptor antagonists reduce mortality after percutaneous coronary interventions. J Am Coll Cardiol. 2003;41:26–32.

53. Lincoff MA. Important triad in cardiovascular medicine. Diabetes, coronary intervention, and platelet glycoprotein IIb/IIIa receptor blockade. Circulation. 2003;107:1556–1559.

54. Corpus RA, George PB, House JA, et al. Optimal glycemic control is associated with a lower rate of target vessel revascularization in treated type II diabetic patients undergoing elective percutaneous coronary intervention. J Am Coll Cardiol. 2004;43:8–14.

55. Bhatt DL, Marso SP, Lincoff AM, et al. Abciximab reduces mortality in diabetics following percutaneous coronary intervention. J Am Coll Cardiol. 2000;35:922–928.

56. Roffi M, Chew DP, Mukherjee D, et al. Platelet glycoprotein IIb/IIIa inhibitors reduce mortality in diabetic patients with non-ST-segment-elevation acute coronary syndromes. Circulation. 2001;104:2767–2771.

57. Vakili BA, Kaplan RC, Slater JN, et al. A propensity analysis of the impact of platelet glycoprotein IIb/IIIa inhibitor therapy on in-hospital outcomes after percutaneous coronary intervention. Am J Cardiol. 2003;91:946–950.

58. Quinn MJ, Plow EF, Topol EJ. Platelet glycoprotein IIb/IIIa inhibitors. Recognition of a two-edged sword? Circulation. 2002;106:379–385.

59. Nannizzi-Alaimo L, Alves VL, Phillips DR. Inhibitory effects of glycoprotein IIb/IIIa antagonists and aspirin on the release of soluble CD40 ligand during platelet stimulation. Circulation. 2003;107:1123–1128.

60. Steinhubl SR, Talley JD, Braden GA, et al. Point-of-care measured platelet inhibition correlates with a reduced isk of an adverse cardiac event after percutaneous coronary intervention. Results of the GOLD (Au-Assessing Ultegra) multicenter study. Circulation. 2001;103:2572–2578.

61. Soffer D, Moussa I, Karatepe M, et al. Suboptimal inhibition of platelet aggregation following tirofiban bolus in patients undergoing percutaneous coronary intervention for unstable angina pectoris. Am J Cardiol. 2003;91: 872–875.

62. Sane DC, Damaraju LV, Topol EJ, et al. Occurrence and

clinical significance of pseudothrombocytopenia during abciximab therapy. J Am Coll Cardiol. 2000;36:75–83.

63. Greinacher A, Eichler P, Lubenow N, et al. Drug-induced and drug-dependent immune thrombocytopenias. Rev Clin Exp Hematol. 2001;5:166–200.

64. Holmes MB, Kabbani S, Watkins MW, et al. Abciximab-associated pseudothrombocytopenia. Circulation. 2000;101:938–939.

65. Paradiso-Hardy FL, Madan M, Radhakrishnan S, et al. Severe thrombocytopenia possibly related to readministration of eptifibatide. Catheter Cardiovasc Intervent. 2001;54:63–67.

66. Bougie DW, Wilker PR, Wuitschick ED, et al. Acute thrombocytopenia after treatment with tirofiban or eptifibatide is associated with antibodies specific for ligand-occupied GPIIb/IIIa. Blood. 2002;100:2071–2076.

67. Topol EJ, Moliterno DJ, Herrmann HC, et al., for the TARGET Investigators. Comparison of two platelet glycoprotein IIb/IIIa inhibitors, tirofiban and abciximab, for the prevention of ischemic events with percutaneous coronary revascularization. N Engl J Med. 2001;344:1888–1894.

68. Fahdi IE, Saucedo JF, Hennebry T, et al. Incidence and time course of thrombocytopenia with abciximab and eptifibatide in patients undergoing percutaneous coronary intervention. Am J Cardiol. 2004;93:453–455.

69. Williams RT, Damaraju LV, Mascelli MA, et al. Anti-platelet factor 4/heparin antibodies. An independent predictor of 30-day myocardial infarction after acute coronary ischemic syndromes. Circulation. 2003;107:2307–2312.

70. Warkentin TE, Kelton JG. Temporal aspects of heparin-induced thrombocytopenia. N Engl J Med. 2001;344:1286–1292.

71. Gruel Y, Pouplard C, Nguyen P, et al. Biological and clinical features of low-molecular-weight heparin-induced thrombocytopenia. Br J Haematol. 2003;121:786–792.

72. Hirsch J, Heddle N, Kelton JG. Treatment of heparin-induced thrombocytopenia. Arch Intern Med. 2004;164:361–369.

73. Sakai K, Oda H, Honsako A, et al. Obstinate thrombosis during percutaneous coronary intervention in a case with heparin-induced thrombocytopenia with thrombosis syndrome successfully treated by argatroban anticoagulant therapy. Catheter Cardiovasc Intervent. 2003;59:351–354.

74. The Direct Thrombin Inhibitor Trialists' Collaborative Group. Direct thrombin inhibitors in acute coronary syndromes: principal results of a meta-analysis based on individual patients' data. Lancet. 2002;359:294–302.

75. Mahaffey KW, Lewis BE, Wildermann MN, et al. The anticoagulant therapy with bivalirudin to assist in the performance of percutaneous coronary intervention in patients with heparin-induced thrombocytopenia (ATBAT) study: main results. J Invasive Cardiol. 2003;15:611–616.

76. Cox CD, Tsikouris JP. Preventing contrast nephropathy: what is the best strategy? A review of the literature. J Clin Pharmacol. 2004;44:327–337.

77. Levine GN, Kern MJ, Berger PB, et al. Management of patients undergoing percutaneous coronary revascularizations. Ann Intern Med. 2003;139:123–136.

78. Gerlach AT, Pickworth KK. Contrast medium-induced nephrotoxicity: pathophysiology and prevention. Pharmacotherapy. 2000;20:540–548.

79. Stone GW, McCullough PA, Tumlin JA, et al. Fenoldapam mesylate for prevention of contrast-induced nephropathy. JAMA. 2003;290:2284–2291.

80. Merten GJ, Burgess WP, Gray LV, et al. Prevention of contrast-induced nephropathy with sodium bicarbonate. JAMA. 2004;291:2328–2334.

81. Rezkalla SH, Kloner RA. No-reflow phenomenon. Circulation. 2002;105:656–662.

82. Gibson CM. Has my patient achieved adequate myocardial perfusion? Circulation. 2003;108:504–507.

83. Hillegass WB, Dean NA, Liao L, et al. Treatment of no-reflow and impaired flow with the nitric oxide donor nitroprusside following percutaneous coronary interventions: initial human clinical experience. J Am Coll Cardiol. 2001;37:1335–1343.

84. Marzilli M, Orsini E, Marraccini P, Testa R. Beneficial effects of intracoronary adenosine as an adjunct to primary angioplasty in acute myocardial infarction. Circulation. 2000;101:2154–2159.

85. Fugit MD, Rubal BJ, Donovan DJ, et al. Effects of intracoronary nicardipine, diltiazem and verapamil on coronary blood flow. J Invasive Cardiol. 2000;12:80–85.

86. Dillon WC, Hadian D, Ritchie ME. Refractory no-reflow successfully treated with local infusion of high-dose adenosine and verapamil—a case report. Angiology. 2001;52:137–141.

87. Kaplan BM, Benzuly KH, Kinn JW, et al. Treatment of no-reflow in degenerated saphenous vein graft interventions: comparison of intracoronary verapamil and nitroglycerin. Catheter Cardiovasc Diagn. 1996;39:113–118.

88. Gregorini L, Marco J, Farah B, et al. Effects of selective alpha-1 and alpha-2 adrenergic blockade on coronary flow reserve after coronary stenting. Circulation. 2002;106:2901–2907.

89. Tsubokawa A, Ueda K, Sakamoto H, et al. Effect of intracoronary nicorandil administration on preventing no-reflow/slow flow phenomenon during rotational atherectomy. Circulation. 2002;66:119–123.

90. Gross JB, et al. Practice guidelines for sedation and analgesia by non-anesthesiologists. Anesthesiology. 2002;96:1004–1017.

91. Martin ML, Lennox PH. Sedation and analgesia in the interventional radiology department. J Vasc Interv Radiol. 2003;14:1119–1128.

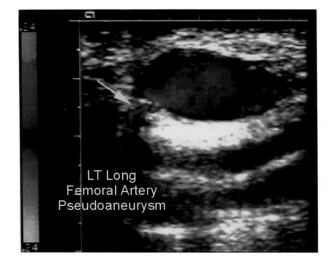

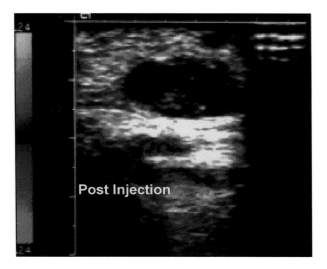

FIGURE 3-1. Color Doppler view of pseudoaneurysm in long axis. The common femoral artery is deep to the pseudoaneurysm. The neck is shown with an arrow.

FIGURE 3-3. Thrombosed pseudoaneurysm. Echogenic thrombus is visible within the pseudoaneurysm, with no detectable flow signal.

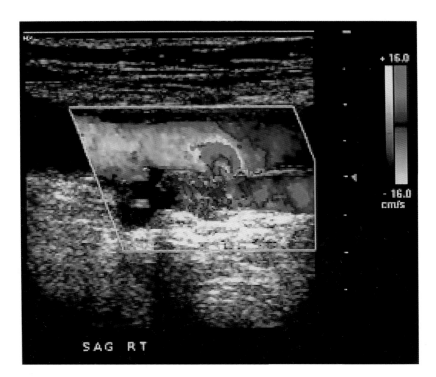

FIGURE 3-4. Arteriovenous fistula between right superficial femoral artery (bottom) and femoral vein (top). Color Doppler demonstrates the abnormal connection between the artery and vein.

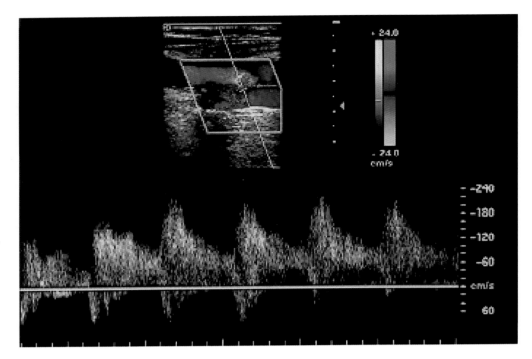

FIGURE 3-5. Doppler waveform showing arterialization of the venous Doppler tracing.

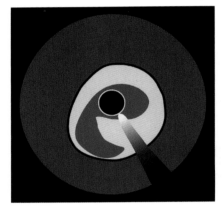

FIGURE 4-3. Schematic represention of IVUS of LAD dissection postangioplasty.

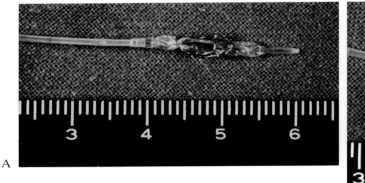

A

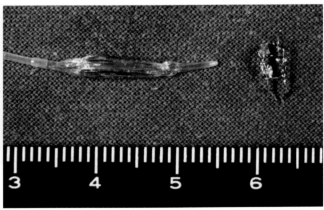

B

FIGURE 6-6. (A) Close-up image of the avulsed Be Bravo stent struts wrapping around the cutting balloon. (B) After manual removal from the cutting balloon, the avulsed and distorted stent struts are seen on the right. (From Wang et al.[14] Copyright ©2002, reprinted with permission of Wiley-Liss, Inc., a subsidiary of John Wiley & Sons, Inc.)

FIGURE 8-3. The pores can be clearly seen in the polyurethane filter. Postprocedural cardiac enzymes were within normal limits, and the patient was discharged home after an uneventful in-hospital course.

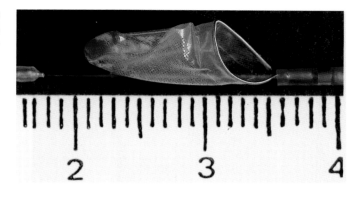

FIGURE 10-4. This 48-year-old woman underwent two stent placements within a month. Photograph of left mid back 2 months after last procedure shows well-marginated focal erythema and desquamation. (Reprinted with permission from Stone et al. J Am Acad Derm. 1998;38:333–336.)

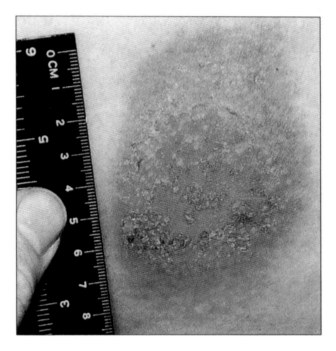

FIGURE 10-5. This 69-year-old man with history of angina underwent two angioplasties of left coronary artery within 30 hours. Photograph taken 1 to 2 months after last procedure shows secondary ulceration over left scapula. (Reprinted with permission from Granel et al. Ann Dermat Venereol. 1998;125:405–407.)

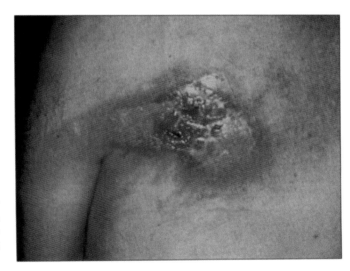

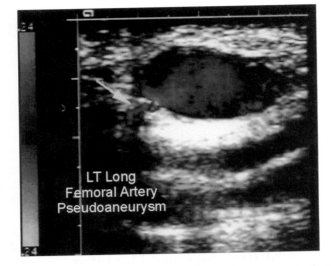

FIGURE 3-1. Color Doppler view of pseudoaneurysm in long axis. The common femoral artery is deep to the pseudo-aneurysm. The neck is shown with an arrow. (See color plate.)

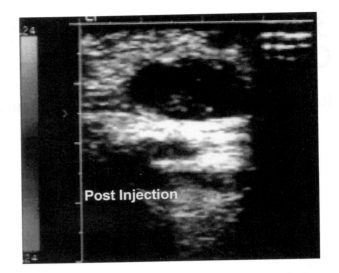

FIGURE 3-3. Thrombosed pseudoaneurysm. Echogenic thrombus is visible within the pseudoaneurysm, with no detectable flow signal. (See color plate.)

in the femoral artery above the inguinal ligament, the hematoma may extend posteriorly, into the retroperitoneal space, and result in more severe blood loss. This bleeding may not be evident from surface inspection but should be suspected if a patient develops unexplained hypotension, tachycardia, fall in hematocrit, or ipsilateral flank pain following a femoral arterial catheterization.

The mainstay in the treatment of groin bleeding is direct manual compression. Mechanical clamp or pneumatic compression, when used to control bleeding, should be applied very cautiously without prolonged (>3 min)

occlusion of distal flow, and with continuous monitoring until control is obtained. These devices should be avoided in patients at higher risk of femoral thrombosis due to peripheral vascular disease, or prior aorto–femoral or

TABLE 3-1. Factors predisposing to vascular access-site bleeding complications.

Anatomic factors
Elderly patient (>70 years)[11]
Obese patient[37]
Female patient[11]
Lower extremity vascular disease[5,11]
Small body surface area (<1.6 m^2)[11]
Procedural factors
Through-and-through puncture
High puncture (above inguinal ligament)
Low puncture (profunda or superficial femoral artery)[12]
Multiple punctures
Large sheath size[5,12]
Prolonged procedure time[12]
Prolonged indwelling sheath time[12]
Venous sheath[13]
Hemodynamic factors
Severe hypertension[37]
Hematologic factors
Multiple platelet antagonists (aspirin, clopidogrel, GP IIb/IIIa antagonists)[11]
Postprocedural antithrombotic agents (heparin, warfarin)[4,5,12]
Thrombolytic agents (tPA, TNKase)[4]
Underlying coagulopathy or thrombocytopenia
Human factors
Operator inexperience[14]
Inability to gain "control" of site upon sheath removal
Short duration of pressure applied to obtain hemostasis

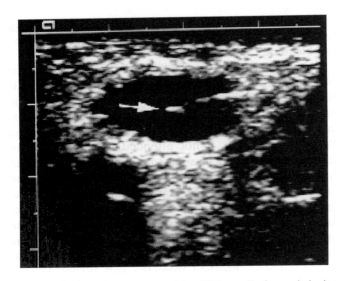

FIGURE 3-2. Pseudoaneurysm with a 25G needle (arrow) during ultrasound-guided thrombin injection.

Abbreviations: TNKase, tenecteplase; tPA, tissue-type plasminogen activator.

fem–popliteal bypass surgery. Large hematomas may require transfusion, but surgical exploration for possible repair is generally not required. Uncontrollable free bleeding around the sheath suggests laceration of the femoral artery. This problem can usually be managed by replacement of the sheath with the next-larger-diameter sheath. Bleeding should be restricted with manual compression around the sheath until the procedure is completed. If heparin is used during the procedure it should be reversed, the sheath removed, and prolonged compression (typically 30–60 min) applied to the access site either manually or with a compression device. In a patient with a large hematoma causing hypotension, stabilization of hemodynamics with rapid volume replacement (crystalloid or blood) is critical. In hypertensive patients, blood pressure should be lowered with appropriate agents. If the bleeding cannot be controlled, urgent surgical exploration with repair of the vascular access site may be required.

The key to avoiding access-site bleeding complications is meticulous attention to the access site, recognition of predisposing factors (Table 3-1), and avoidance of post-procedural heparin. While study design is still debated, the use of bivalirudin, in lieu of the combination of intravenous heparin and GP IIb/IIIa platelet receptor blocker, has been associated with a significant reduction (41%) in bleeding-related complications.[15] These investigators confirmed that lower bleeding complications do result in significant savings, as well. Following interventional procedures, sheaths should be removed when the activated clotting time (ACT) falls to acceptable levels (<170s). Allowing adequate time to compress the access site and achieving complete hemostasis after sheath removal are quintessential in preventing hematomas and subsequent complications.

3. Pseudoaneurysm

A pseudoaneurysm is an encapsulated hematoma that communicates with the artery due to dissolution of the clot plugging the arterial puncture site (Figure 3-1). Blood can flow into the cavity during systole and back into the artery during diastole. Because the hematoma has no arterial wall structures it is referred to as *pseudoaneurysm*. Pseudoaneurysm usually results from inadequate compression and incomplete hemostasis following sheath removal. The factors that are associated with increased risk of pseudoaneurysm formation are shown in Table 3-2.

Distinguishing a pseudoaneurysm from an expanding hematoma is frequently difficult at the bedside. Generally a pseudoaneurysm is a tender, pulsatile mass with an audile bruit over the mass. Large hematomas may look

TABLE 3-2. Factors associated with increased risk of pseudo-aneurysm formation.

Low vascular access in the superficial femoral or profunda artery (i.e., puncture below the bifurcation of the common femoral)[16]
Severe peripheral vascular disease[14]
Large sheaths[16]
Prolonged sheath time[12]
Prolonged anticoagulation[16]
Premature ambulation

exactly the same, and any patient with a large or painful hematoma should be evaluated for pseudoaneurysm. Likewise, pseudoaneurysm should be suspected when a hematoma is associated with femoral nerve palsy. Duplex ultrasound scanning confirms the diagnosis of pseudoaneurysm and angiography is rarely unnecessary.

The natural history of a pseudoaneurysm is uncertain. Spontaneous closure of postcatheterization pseudoaneurysms has been reported;[17] however, the predictors for spontaneous closure are not well defined. Treatment of a pseudoaneurysm depends on the size, the expansion, and the need for anticoagulation. Pseudoaneurysms less than 3 cm can usually be followed clinically and often do not need surgical repair. A follow-up ultrasound in 1–2 weeks after the initial diagnosis is useful to confirm resolution and exclude expansion of the pseudoaneurysm. By this time, spontaneous thrombosis occurs in most cases, requiring no further treatment. However, if progressive hemorrhage, rapid expansion of the pseudoaneurysm, or development of femoral neuralgia or distal ischemia occurs during follow-up, immediate treatment is recommended.[17–19] Techniques used to treat pseudoaneurysms include ultrasound-guided compression,[20] surgical repair, insertion of coils,[21] ultrasound-guided direct thrombin injection (Figures 3-2 and 3-3),[22,23] fluoroscopically guided direct thrombin injection,[1] and covered stents.[24,25] Kang and colleagues[22] reported that 75% of pseudoaneurysms were thrombosed within 15 seconds of using direct thrombin injection.

Of the above-described techniques, ultrasound-guided compression is a common initial therapy in patients with suitable anatomy. Successful compression of pseudoaneurysms with long and thin necks can be expected in 92%–98% of cases when further anticoagulation is not needed.[26] Those needing continued anticoagulation have lower success rates, about 54%–86%.[27–30] Surgical repair is considered for failed ultrasound compression or thrombin injection as well as when the femoral nerve is involved.[31] Also, surgical intervention is usually necessary when severe groin pain limits compression therapies.

The key to avoiding pseudoaneurysm formation is accurate puncture of the common femoral artery and effective initial control of bleeding after sheath removal. Fluoroscopic localization of the skin nick to overlie the inferior border of the femoral head effectively reduces the error of low vascular puncture. Other factors that deserve consideration are use of small sheaths, prompt sheath removal after ACT falls to acceptable level, avoidance of postprocedural anticoagulation, treatment of hypertension at the time of sheath removal, and again, adequate groin compression with complete hemostasis.

4. Retroperitoneal Hemorrhage

The inguinal ligament serves as a barrier between pelvic and infrainguinal spaces. Because effective vessel compression above the bones may not be possible, femoral puncture above the inguinal ligament may result in bleeding that tracks posteriorly into the retroperitoneal space. The reported incidence of retroperitoneal hematoma, while low (<1%), can be catastrophic after an apparently successful angiographic PCI.[7,9]

Such bleeding is not evident from the surface, especially in obese patients. Frequently the diagnosis is suspected when hypotension does not respond to simple measures and a fall in hematocrit is seen. Other clues to the diagnosis are unexplained tachycardia, vague abdominal pain, ipsilateral flank pain,[32,33] and abdominal distention. If the hematoma is adjacent to the psoas muscle, the patient may develop hip pain and inability to flex the hip. Large retroperitoneal hematomas can mimic acute appendicitis with right lower quadrant pain and fever.[34] Severe retroperitoneal hemorrhage can cause hemodynamic collapse, shock, liver and renal failure, and disseminated intravascular coagulation.[35]

Computed tomographic or ultrasound scanning of the abdomen and pelvis can confirm a diagnosis of retroperitoneal hematoma. The treatment is usually expectant but with close attention to vital signs and hemodynamic status. Rapid replacement of volume with crystalloid or blood is important, and heparin should be reversed and any GP IIb/IIIa receptor blocker infusion stopped immediately. Vascular sheaths should be promptly removed followed by prolonged compression of the access site. If the above measures fail, urgent surgical exploration is warranted. If abciximab was used during the PCI, its antiplatelet effect can be reversed with platelet transfusion. Eptifibatide and tirofiban have no antidotes but their antiplatelet effect dissipates within 6 hours.

Careful localization of the femoral artery entry site, accurate single anterior wall puncture, avoidance of excessive anticoagulation, and careful manipulation of the guidewire help prevent retroperitoneal hemorrhage. To reiterate, the inguinal crease is an unreliable marker for deep vascular anatomy, especially in obese patients.[36] A useful guide for femoral artery access site is fluoroscopic localization of the medial third of the femoral head with an understanding that arterial entry is always superior to whatever skin landmarks are used given the angle of puncture.

5. Arteriovenous Fistula

Puncturing the femoral artery and the overlying femoral vein can result in an arteriovenous (AV) fistula after sheath removal. Also, ongoing bleeding from a femoral puncture site may decompress into an adjacent venous puncture site to form an AV fistula. The reported incidence of AV fistula following PCI is 0.1%–1.5%.[5,37] The factors that increase the risk of AV fistula formation are multiple punctures to obtain vascular access, low puncture (superficial femoral or profunda with transection of a small venous branch) or high puncture (common femoral artery and involvement of the lateral femoral circumflex vein), and impaired clotting. Risk factors identified from two studies with over 10,000 consecutive patients who underwent cardiac catheterization and were followed up prospectively over a period of 2–3 years were high heparin dosage, warfarin therapy, puncture of the left groin, systemic arterial hypertension, and female gender for the development of femoral AV fistula. Coronary intervention, size and number of sheaths, age, and body mass index did not significantly affect the incidence of femoral AV fistula.[38,39]

An AV fistula is frequently not clinically evident for days after the femoral catheterization procedure.[40] Clinical signs associated with AV fistulae are to-and-fro continuous bruit over the puncture site, and a swollen, tender extremity due to venous dilatation. The latter is unusual in iatrogenic AV fistulas, however. Ultrasound may demonstrate the abnormal connection between the artery and vein on color Doppler images (Figure 3-4, see color plate) and arterialization of the venous Doppler tracings (Figure 3-5, see color plate). A small AV fistula with low-volume AV flow by Duplex scan can be managed conservatively because many of these close spontaneously.[7] Some authors suggest prompt surgical repair of large AV fistulae due to the fear of developing high-output heart failure if left untreated. However, two reviews of large groups of patients with femoral AV fistulae, followed prospectively for over a period of 2–3 years failed to show an increase of cardiac volume overload or limb damage.[38,39] Surgical repair, if considered, involves excision or division of the fistula, or synthetic grafting of the involved vessels. Nonsurgical techniques such as ultrasound-guided compression[27] and endovascular stent grafting have been reported, but are limited.[24,25]

FIGURE 3-4. Arteriovenous fistula between right superficial femoral artery (bottom) and femoral vein (top). Color Doppler demonstrates the abnormal connection between the artery and vein. (See color plate.)

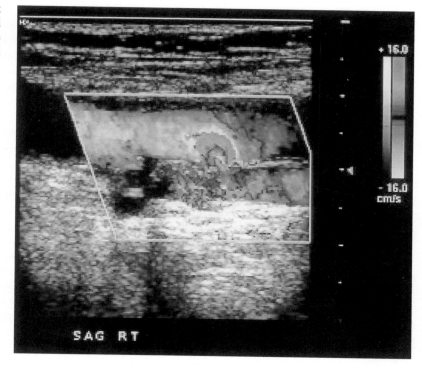

6. Groin Infection

Groin infections after PCI, while rare, are debilitating with the necessary care and associated risk involved. Cleveland and colleagues observed only three infectious complications in 4669 patients who underwent PCI.[41]

Gram-positive organisms, especially *Staphylococcus* species, are the predominant cause of groin abscesses and endarteritis associated with femoral arterial cannulation.[41–44] Risk factors for the development of groin infections after PCI are presence of hematoma or foreign material within the lumen of the artery.[45,46] Groin infec-

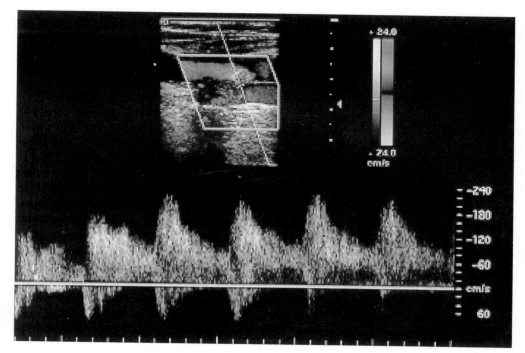

FIGURE 3-5. Doppler waveform showing arterialization of the venous Doppler tracing. (See color plate.)

tions may be more frequent with the use of vascular closure devices compared to manual compression.[47] The braided, polyester suture used in some closure devices may act as a nidus for infection, while the tract following collagen deposition for closure may also serve as a source of bacterial seeding.

Groin infections are usually diagnosed by the presence of access-site erythema, pain, or, more obviously, when exudative drainage appears. Fever and/or rigors indicate systemic involvement and higher risk. A complete blood count and blood cultures should be obtained in all patients to help assess the level of involvement. A local reaction such as phlebitis at the access site responds to hot soaks and elevation of the affected limb, but if cellulitis or exudative drainage is present, systemic antibiotics should be strongly and immediately considered. Abscesses require surgical drainage in addition to the parenteral antibiotic therapy, and surgical exploration to exclude an indolent abscess is also worthy of consideration.

7. Thrombotic Occlusion

Local thrombosis of a normal femoral artery is a rare complication, except in patients with small common femoral artery lumen in whom a large-diameter catheter or sheath has been placed. The reported incidence of femoral artery thrombosis after interventional procedures is less than 1%. However, more commonly patients have preexisting atherosclerotic disease, and femoral artery thrombosis can lead to subsequent complications such as limb ischemia (21%), leg amputation (11%), and death (2%).[48] The risk factors that are associated with thrombotic occlusion of the access site include peripheral vascular disease, advanced age, hypercoaguable state, cardiomyopathy, small-caliber vessels, female gender, and small body habitus. Spasm and local dissection may also contribute to arterial thrombosis.

Femoral artery occlusion results in sudden onset of limb pain, pallor, cyanosis, absence of distal pulse, and a cool extremity. If preexisting peripheral vascular disease is present, the symptoms may not be as sudden, however. Physical examination looking for the above signs and duplex scanning will confirm that femoral artery thrombosis has occurred. Arteriography usually is not needed for confirmation of the diagnosis but is necessary to localize the occlusion and guide therapeutic decisions.

If the vascular sheath itself is causing obstruction to antegrade flow, removal of the sheath may resolve limb ischemia. Persistent limb ischemia with diminished or absent pulses despite removal of vascular sheath suggests femoral artery thrombosis or dissection at the puncture site. This requires urgent surgical consultation while immediate heparinization is begun and urgent thrombectomy is considered to prevent muscle necrosis and possible limb amputation. Thrombectomy by Fogarty catheter or percutaneous rheolysis (Possis® Angioget) have been used to treat femoral artery thrombosis. If thrombectomy fails, surgical thromboendarterectomy or even bypass grafting may be considered to avoid limb dysfunction or loss.

Using small sheaths in high-risk patients with peripheral vascular disease, small vessels, or hypercoaguable states can reduce femoral artery thrombosis. Regular flushing and avoiding delays in vascular sheath removal are essential and if an indwelling sheath is necessary, infusion of pressurized heparinized saline through the sheath may help prevent local thrombosis. Of course, consideration of a brachial or radial approach will avoid this risk in particularly high-risk patients. While not without inherent risk, access-site complications are lower with this approach.[49-53] A recent report of total extraction of the radial artery after coronary angiography illustrates that anything is indeed possible.[54]

8. Arterial Laceration and Perforation

Advancement of guidewires, catheters, or other devices can result in peripheral arterial tear or perforation. Also, deep skin nicks in patients with superficial-lying femoral vessels can also cause arterial laceration. Arterial perforation can occur at the access site or at a site remote from the puncture site. The incidence of arterial perforation remote from the access site is less than 0.1%.[55]

Uncontrollable bleeding around the vascular sheath suggests arterial laceration, while perforation may be suspected if the patient complains of acute pain at the moment of guidewire or catheter manipulation. Continuous bleeding will result in hypotension and potential collapse. Catheter or guidewire withdrawal can cause more discomfort as extravasation increases when the defect gets exposed. Bleeding from guidewire perforation can be less obvious, as the defect is usually small and bleeding is slow. Contrast injection may confirm extravasation of blood, but is typically not diagnostic if the perforation is small. Digital subtraction angiography may be a more sensitive tool, but clinical suspicion and early exploration can be life saving.

Free bleeding around the vascular sheath usually responds to replacement with a next-larger-diameter sheath. However, if the bleeding persists manual compression around the sheath during the procedure is indicated. Most guidewire-induced arterial perforations are benign and resolve spontaneously without significant blood loss. If the bleeding is continuing, any anticoagulation should be stopped and reversed immediately. Lost blood volume should be replaced with crystalloid or blood. Depending on the location and extent of perforation, the perforation can be treated with prolonged balloon inflation,[56] covered stents,[57] therapeutic coil embolization,[56] or surgical repair.[56]

Arterial perforation can be avoided with careful and gentle advancement of guidewires, catheters, or other interventional devices. The tip of the guidewire should always be observed under fluoroscopy during catheter advancement. If resistance is encountered during guidewire advancement it should be withdrawn and redirected.

9. Arterial Dissection

Access-site arterial dissection occurs during the retrograde advancement of guidewires, especially hydrophilic guidewires or catheters. The reported incidence of such dissection with interventional procedures is 0.01%–0.4%.[58–62] However, the true frequency is probably higher, as most minor dissections may go unnoticed or unreported. Patients with peripheral vascular disease are more likely to develop dissection during interventional procedures.

Serious consequences from iatrogenic access-site arterial dissection with interventional procedures are rare. However, unrecognized local dissection at the access site may sometimes lead to development of late thrombosis

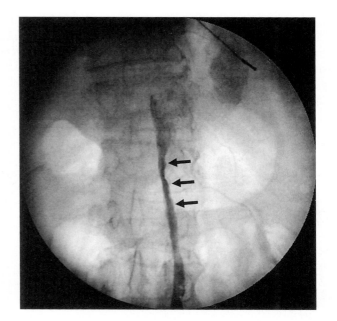

FIGURE 3-7. Retrograde test angiography confirmed apparent total occlusion up to thoracic aorta.

or pseudoaneurysm formation. As most access-site vascular dissections are retrograde from the advancement of guidewires or catheters, antegrade flow will usually "tack down" the flap without need for further therapy. Dissections associated with thrombosis and/or distal flow impairment need immediate surgical or percutaneous treatment with stenting. Forcing the guidewire or catheter to advance when resistance is encountered should never be done as this may result in retrograde dissection or perforation of the vessel. Hydrophilic wires provide poor tactile feedback and should be used very cautiously under fluoroscopic guidance.

In a recent example, a patient underwent a planned diagnostic angiogram to evaluate an abnormal stress study. After an unremarkable femoral arterial catheterization, difficulty was found in advancing various wires past the iliac bifurcation. Due to the patient's age, this was felt to be due to complex peripheral arterial disease (Figure 3-6). Further passage of what was felt to be a total occlusion revealed staining and lack of clearing of the contrast in the abdominal aorta (Figure 3-7). The presumptive diagnosis was severe and diffuse thoracoabdominal atherosclerotic aortic disease. However, after a second attempt at diagnosis, this time from the right radial artery, a widely patent aorta with a significant narrowing only at the right common iliac artery was found (Figures 3-8 and 3-9). This case is a severe example of an arterial dissection and while no clinical adverse event followed, an incorrect diagnosis of disease was initially made.

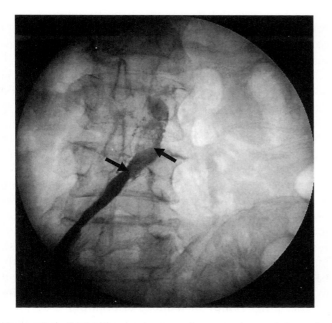

FIGURE 3-6. Right iliac angiogram of apparent complete occlusion in a patient undergoing attempted diagnostic coronary angiography.

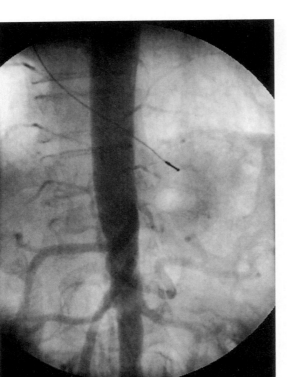

FIGURE 3-8. Antegrade aortogram obtained during radial artery approach revealed a widely patent thoracoabdominal aorta.

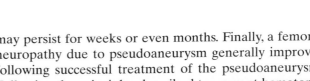

FIGURE 3-9. Antegrade abdominal and iliac aortography revealed disease in the right common iliac artery, confirming the diagnosis of a retrograde dissection.

The principles described to prevent arterial perforation also apply to arterial dissection. In patients with peripheral vascular disease, catheter exchanges should be done with an exchange length (300 cm) guidewire, and dilators and vascular sheaths should always be advanced over a leading guidewire.

10. Femoral Neuropathy

Neuropathy is a rare complication following cardiac catheterization via the femoral route.[63] Femoral neuropathy usually develops from inadvertent direct injury to the femoral nerve with the needle in an attempt to gain vascular access. Femoral neuropathy can also occur due to impingement of the nerve with a large groin hematoma or pseudoaneurysm from femoral artery puncture. A transient femoral neuropathy may also be caused by excess topical or local lidocaine at the access site.

Femoral neuropathy manifests as sensory impairment in the anterolateral aspect of the thigh or as inability to ambulate or bear weight due to quadriceps weakness. Femoral neuropathy due to topical lidocaine resolves in several hours as the effect of lidocaine wears off; however, if due to a large groin hematoma, symptoms

may persist for weeks or even months. Finally, a femoral neuropathy due to pseudoaneurysm generally improves following successful treatment of the pseudoaneurysm. Following the principles described to prevent hematoma or pseudoaneurysm formation can avoid the development of femoral neuropathy as well.

Improved management of the access site is essential in achieving both better patient care and reducing hospital expenses. Attempts to reduce complications related to the access site have included improvements in anticoagulation and antiplatelet regimens following PCI, better identification of patients at risk, lower profile equipment,[64–66] increasing use of transradial interventions,[49–53] and closure devices (discussed in Chapter 11). Regarding the latter, while these devices decrease the discomfort of prolonged compression and allow early ambulation, clinical trials to date have failed to demonstrate significant reduction of major vascular complications compared with manual compression.[67,68] These devices are constantly being improved and hopefully further improvements and experience will eliminate these hemorrhagic access-site complications. Until then operators should be knowledgeable and prepared to handle the various complications associated with vascular access for interventional procedures.

References

1. Samal AK, White CJ, Collins TJ, et al. Treatment of femoral artery pseudoaneurysm with percutaneous thrombin injection. Catheter Cardiovasc Interv. 2001;53:259–263.

2. Popma JJ, Satler LF, Pichard AD, et al. Vascular complications after balloon and new device angioplasty. Circulation. 1993;88:1569–1578.

3. Batchelor WB, Anstrom KJ, Muhlbaier LH, et al. Contemporary outcome trends in the elderly undergoing percutaneous coronary interventions: results in 7,472 octogenarians. National Cardiovascular Network Collaboration. J Am Coll Cardiol. 2000;36:723–730.

4. Oweida SW, Roubin GS, Smith RB 3rd, Salam AA. Postcatheterization vascular complications associated with percutaneous transluminal coronary angioplasty. J Vasc Surg. 1990;12:310–315.

5. Muller DW, Shamir KJ, Ellis SG, Topol EJ. Peripheral vascular complications after conventional and complex percutaneous coronary interventional procedures. Am J Cardiol. 1992;69:63–68.

6. Kalinowski EA, Trerotola SO. Postcatheterization retroperitoneal hematoma due to spontaneous lumbar arterial hemorrhage. Cardiovasc Intervent Radiol. 1998;21: 337–339.

7. Kent KC, Moscucci M, Mansour KA, et al. Retroperitoneal hematoma after cardiac catheterization: prevalence, risk factors, and optimal management. J Vasc Surg. 1994;20: 905–910; discussion 910–913.

8. Omoigui NA, Califf RM, Pieper K, et al. Peripheral vascular complications in the Coronary Angioplasty Versus Excisional Atherectomy Trial (CAVEAT-I). J Am Coll Cardiol. 1995;26:922–930.

9. Grines CL, Glazier S, Bakalyar D, et al. Predictors of bleeding complications following coronary angioplasty. Circulation. 1991;84:II-591.

10. Topol EJ. Toward a new frontier in myocardial reperfusion therapy: emerging platelet preeminence. Circulation. 1998;97:211–218.

11. Piper WD, Malenka DJ, Ryan TJ Jr., et al. Predicting vascular complications in percutaneous coronary interventions. Am Heart J. 2003;145:1022–1029.

12. Davis C, VanRiper S, Longstreet J, Moscucci M. Vascular complications of coronary interventions. Heart Lung. 1997;26:118–127.

13. Saucedo JF, Feldman T, Gershony G, et al. 13th annual symposium on transcatheter cardiovascular therapeutics. September 11–16, 2001. Washington, DC, USA. Abstracts. Am J Cardiol. 2001;88:1G–147G.

14. Hood DB, Mattos MA, Douglas MG, et al. Determinants of success of color-flow duplex-guided compression repair of femoral pseudoaneurysms. Surgery. 1996;120:585–588; discussion 588–590.

15. Lincoff AM, Bittl JA, Harrington RA, et al. Bivalirudin and provisional glycoprotein IIb/IIIa blockade compared with heparin and planned glycoprotein IIb/IIIa blockade during percutaneous coronary intervention: REPLACE-2 randomized trial. JAMA. 2003;289:853–863.

16. Kim D, Orron DE, Skillman JJ, et al. Role of superficial femoral artery puncture in the development of pseudoaneurysm and arteriovenous fistula complicating percutaneous transfemoral cardiac catheterization. Catheter Cardiovasc Diagn. 1992;25:91–97.

17. Kent KC, McArdle CR, Kennedy B, et al. A prospective study of the clinical outcome of femoral pseudoaneurysms and arteriovenous fistulas induced by arterial puncture. J Vasc Surg. 1993;17:125–131; discussion 131–133.

18. Feld R, Patton GM, Carabasi RA, et al. Treatment of iatrogenic femoral artery injuries with ultrasound-guided compression. J Vasc Surg. 1992;16:832–840.

19. Coley BD, Roberts AC, Fellmeth BD, et al. Postangiographic femoral artery pseudoaneurysms: further experience with US-guided compression repair. Radiology. 1995;194:307–311.

20. Agarwal R, Agrawal SK, Roubin GS, et al. Clinically guided closure of femoral arterial pseudoaneurysms complicating cardiac catheterization and coronary angioplasty. Catheter Cardiovasc Diagn. 1993;30:96–100.

21. Pan M, Medina A, Suarez de Lezo J, et al. Obliteration of femoral pseudoaneurysm complicating coronary intervention by direct puncture and permanent or removable coil insertion. Am J Cardiol. 1997;80:786–788.

22. Kang SS, Labropoulos N, Mansour MA, Baker WH. Percutaneous ultrasound guided thrombin injection: a new method for treating postcatheterization femoral pseudoaneurysms. J Vasc Surg. 1998;27:1032–1038.

23. Brophy DP, Sheiman RG, Amatulle P, Akbari CM. Iatrogenic femoral pseudoaneurysms: thrombin injection after failed US-guided compression. Radiology. 2000;214: 278–282.

24. Waigand J, Uhlich F, Gross CM, et al. Percutaneous treatment of pseudoaneurysms and arteriovenous fistulas after invasive vascular procedures. Catheter Cardiovasc Interv. 1999;47:157–164.

25. Thalhammer C, Kirchherr AS, Uhlich F, et al. Postcatheterization pseudoaneurysms and arteriovenous fistulas: repair with percutaneous implantation of endovascular covered stents. Radiology. 2000;214:127–131.

26. Steinkamp HJ, Werk M, Felix R. Treatment of postinterventional pseudoaneurysms by ultrasound-guided compression. Invest Radiol. 2000;35:186–192.

27. Schaub F, Theiss W, Heinz M, et al. New aspects in ultrasound-guided compression repair of postcatheterization femoral artery injuries. Circulation. 1994;90:1861–1865.

28. Moote DJ, Hilborn MD, Harris KA, Elliott JA, MacDonald AC, Foley JB. Postarteriographic femoral pseudoaneurysms: treatment with ultrasound-guided compression. Ann Vasc Surg. 1994;8: 325–331.

29. Cox GS, Young JR, Gray BR, et al. Ultrasound-guided compression repair of postcatheterization pseudoaneurysms: results of treatment in one hundred cases. J Vasc Surg. 1994;19:683–686.

30. Chatterjee T, Do DD, Kaufmann U, Mahler F, Meier B. Ultrasound-guided compression repair for treatment of femoral artery pseudoaneurysm: acute and follow-up results. Catheter Cardiovasc Diagn. 1996;38:335–340.

31. Kazmers A, Meeker C, Nofz K, et al. Nonoperative therapy for postcatheterization femoral artery pseudoaneurysms. Am Surg. 1997;63:199–204.

32. Shires T. Principles of surgery. New York: McGraw Hill; 1984:240–241.

33. Boylis SM LE, Gilas NW. Traumatic retroperitoneal hematoma. Am J Surg. 1962;103:477.

34. Haviv YS, Nahir M, Pikarski A, et al. A late retroperitoneal hematoma mimicking acute appendicitis—an unusual complication of coronary angioplasty. Eur J Med Res. 1996;1:591–592.

35. Sreeram S, Lumsden AB, Miller JS, et al. Retroperitoneal hematoma following femoral arterial catheterization: a serious and often fatal complication. Am Surg. 1993;59: 94–98.

36. Grier D, Hartnell G. Percutaneous femoral artery puncture: practice and anatomy. Br J Radiol. 1990;63:602–604.

37. Waksman R, King SB III, Douglas JS, et al. Predictors of groin complications after balloon and new-device coronary intervention. Am J Cardiol. 1995;75:886–889.

38. Kelm M, Perings SM, Jax T, et al. Incidence and clinical outcome of iatrogenic femoral arteriovenous fistulas: implications for risk stratification and treatment. J Am Coll Cardiol. 2002;40:291–297.

39. Perings SM, Kelm M, Jax T, Strauer BE. A prospective study on incidence and risk factors of arteriovenous fistulae following transfemoral cardiac catheterization. Int J Cardiol. 2003;88:223–228.

40. Smith SM, Galland RB. Late presentation of femoral artery complications following percutaneous cannulation for cardiac angiography or angioplasty. J Cardiovasc Surg (Torino). 1992;33:437–439.

41. Cleveland KO, Gelfand MS. Invasive staphylococcal infections complicating percutaneous transluminal coronary angioplasty: three cases and review. Clin Infect Dis. 1995; 21:93–96.

42. Smith TP, Cruz CP, Moursi MM, Eidt JF. Infectious complications resulting from use of hemostatic puncture closure devices. Am J Surg. 2001;182:658–662.

43. Maki DG, McCormick RD, Uman SJ, Wirtanen GW. Septic endarteritis due to intra-arterial catheters for cancer chemotherapy. I. Evaluation of an outbreak. II. Risk factors, clinical features and management. III. Guidelines for prevention. Cancer. 1979;44:1228–1240.

44. Brummitt CF, Kravitz GR, Granrud GA, Herzog CA. Femoral endarteritis due to Staphylococcus aureus complicating percutaneous transluminal coronary angioplasty. Am J Med. 1989;86:822–824.

45. Frazee BW, Flaherty JP. Septic endarteritis of the femoral artery following angioplasty. Rev Infect Dis. 1991;13: 620–623.

46. Dougherty SH. Pathobiology of infection in prosthetic devices. Rev Infect Dis. 1988;10:1102–1117.

47. Carey D, Martin JR, Moore CA, Valentine MC, Nygaard TW. Complications of femoral artery closure devices. Catheter Cardiovasc Interv. 2001;52:3–7; discussion 8.

48. Humphries AW. Evaluation of the natural history and result of treatment involving the lower extremities. New York: McGraw-Hill; 1973.

49. Lotan C, Hasin Y, Mosseri M, et al. Transradial approach for coronary angiography and angioplasty. Am J Cardiol. 1995;76:164–167.

50. Kiemeneij F, Laarman GJ, Odekerken D, et al. A randomized comparison of percutaneous transluminal coronary angioplasty by the radial, brachial and femoral approaches: the access study. J Am Coll Cardiol. 1997;29: 1269–1275.

51. Kiemeneij F, Laarman GJ, Slagboom T, van der Wieken R. Outpatient coronary stent implantation. J Am Coll Cardiol. 1997;29:323–327.

52. Mann T, Cubeddu G, Bowen J, et al. Stenting in acute coronary syndromes: a comparison of radial versus femoral access sites. J Am Coll Cardiol. 1998;32:572–576.

53. de Belder AJ, Smith RE, Wainwright RJ, Thomas MR. Transradial artery coronary angiography and intervention in patients with severe peripheral vascular disease. Clin Radiol. 1997;52:115–118.

54. Abu-Ful A, Benharroch D, Henkin Y. Extraction of the radial artery during transradial coronary angiography: an unusual complication. J Invasive Cardiol. 2003;15:351–352.

55. Lauk EK. A survey of complications of percutaneous retrograde angiography. Radiology. 1963;81:257–263.

56. Hayes PD, Chokkalingam A, Jones R, et al. Arterial perforation during infrainguinal lower limb angioplasty does not worsen outcome: results from 1409 patients. J Endovasc Ther. 2002;9:422–427.

57. Steinkamp HJ, Werk M, Seibold S, et al. [Treatment of arterial traumas by the Wallgraft endoprosthesis.] Rofo Fortschr Geb Rontgenstr Neuen Bildgeb Verfahr. 2001; 173:97–102.

58. Connors JP, Thanavaro S, Shaw RC, et al. Urgent myocardial revascularization for dissection of the left main coronary artery: a complication of coronary angiography. J Thorac Cardiovasc Surg. 1982;84:349–352.

59. Bourassa MG, Noble J. Complication rate of coronary arteriography. A review of 5250 cases studied by a percutaneous femoral technique. Circulation. 1976;53:106–114.

60. Guss SB, Zir LM, Garrison HB, et al. Coronary occlusion during coronary angiography. Circulation. 1975;52:1063–1068.

61. Feit A, Kahn R, Chowdhry I, et al. Coronary artery dissection secondary to coronary arteriography: case report and review. Catheter Cardiovasc Diagn. 1984;10:177–181.

62. Morise AP, Hardin NJ, Bovill EG, Gundel WD. Coronary artery dissection secondary to coronary arteriography: presentation of three cases and review of the literature. Catheter Cardiovasc Diagn. 1981;7:283–296.

63. Butler R, Webster MW. Meralgia paresthetica: an unusual complication of cardiac catheterization via the femoral artery. Catheter Cardiovasc Interv. 2002;56:69–71.

64. Fitzgerald J, Andrew H, Conway B, et al. Outpatient angiography: a prospective study of 3 French catheters in unselected patients. Br J Radiol. 1998;71:484–486.

65. Steffenino G, Dellavalle A, Ribichini F, et al. Ambulation three hours after elective cardiac catheterisation through the femoral artery. Heart. 1996;75:477–480.

66. Metz D, Chapoutot L, Brasselet C, Jolly D. Randomized evaluation of four versus five French catheters for transfemoral coronary angiography. Clin Cardiol. 1999;22:29–32.

67. Kussmaul WG 3rd, Buchbinder M, Whitlow PL, et al. Rapid arterial hemostasis and decreased access site complications after cardiac catheterization and angioplasty: results of a randomized trial of a novel hemostatic device. J Am Coll Cardiol. 1995;25:1685–1692.

68. Brachmann J, Ansah M, Kosinski EJ, Schuler GC. Improved clinical effectiveness with a collagen vascular hemostasis device for shortened immobilization time following diagnostic angiography and percutaneous transluminal coronary angioplasty. Am J Cardiol. 1998;81:1502–1505.

4
Complications of Plain Old Balloon Angioplasty

David P. Lee

1. Case 1: A Coronary Dissection after Percutaneous Transluminal Coronary Angioplasty

A 68-year-old man with a recent history of new-onset angina and a positive stress thallium showing a reversible anterior defect underwent coronary angiography. The angiogram demonstrated a high-grade stenosis of the left anterior descending artery (Figure 4-1). Percutaneous transluminal coronary angioplasty (PTCA) was attempted using a 2.5 × 15-mm Maverick-2 coronary angioplasty balloon (Boston Scientific, Natick, MA) over a Whisper 0.014″/190-cm coronary guidewire (Cordis, Miami Lakes, FL). One inflation was performed at 8 atm, yielding the results shown in Figure 4-2. An intravascular ultrasound (Figure 4-3, see color plate, part B) was performed to further investigate the angiographic lesion and a coronary artery dissection was confirmed. A 3.0 × 18-mm Express-2 stent (Boston Scientific, Natick, MA) was deployed and yielded an excellent result; no residual dissection was indicated (Figure 4-4) and the patient did well.

2. Case 2: Arterial Rupture after Percutaneous Transluminal Coronary Angioplasty

A 72-year-old woman was admitted with an acute coronary syndrome and underwent coronary angiography that revealed a tight stenosis within the diagonal artery (Figure 4-5). A Balanced MiddleWeight coronary guidewire (Guidant, Santa Clara, CA) was navigated beyond the target lesion and a 2.5 × 15-mm Cross Sail angioplasty balloon (Guidant) was inflated twice, with a highest pressure of 14 atm. The post-PTCA angiogram revealed extensive dye staining into the myocardium (Figure 4-6).

The patient began suffering from chest pain and the procedure was abandoned. An echocardiogram was performed in the catheterization laboratory 4 hours later, showing only a minimal pericardial effusion with no hemodynamic compromise and new lateral wall hypokinesis. The patient's ECG showed evolutionary changes of a lateral wall myocardial infarction over the course of the next 2 days, with eventual resolution of her chest pain and no change in her pericardial effusion by follow-up echocardiography. Her peak creatine kinase was 742.

3. Introduction

The introduction of percutaneous transluminal coronary angioplasty (PTCA) in 1977 by Grüntzig[1] revolutionized the treatment of coronary artery disease. As the technology has evolved, PTCA has remained an important procedure in its own right, now usually as an adjunct to coronary stenting. There have been evolutionary improvements in balloon technology with changes in balloon coatings, design, and catheter delivery techniques, but the basic approach to balloon angioplasty has remained steady.

The mechanism of balloon angioplasty to relieve coronary stenoses has been well studied and reviewed.[2] In summary, balloon dilation induces injury to the coronary endothelium, causing microdissections and plaque splitting at the site of barotraumas that may extend beyond the balloon injury site. The plaque is crushed against the vessel wall, activating local thrombosis and platelets, and the plaque may be physically denuded and embolized distal to the injury site. The stretching and injury of the vessel wall may also initiate a complex pathologic process in which scar tissue eventually forms, clinically evident as a renarrowing of the vessel (restenosis) within 3 to 9 months.

Despite the relative mechanistic inelegance of balloon angioplasty, the procedure has been popular and effec-

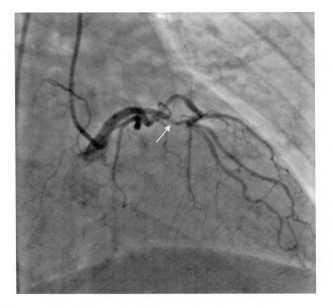

FIGURE 4-1. High-grade left anterior descending coronary artery (LAD) stenosis (arrow) in a 68-year-old man.

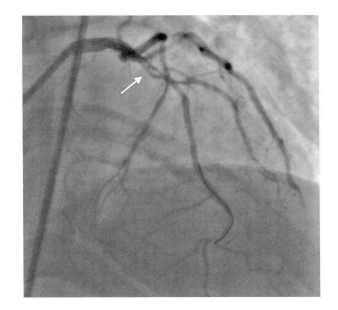

FIGURE 4-2. Left anterior descending coronary artery with type B dissection postangioplasty. Note double lumen (arrow) without flow compromise.

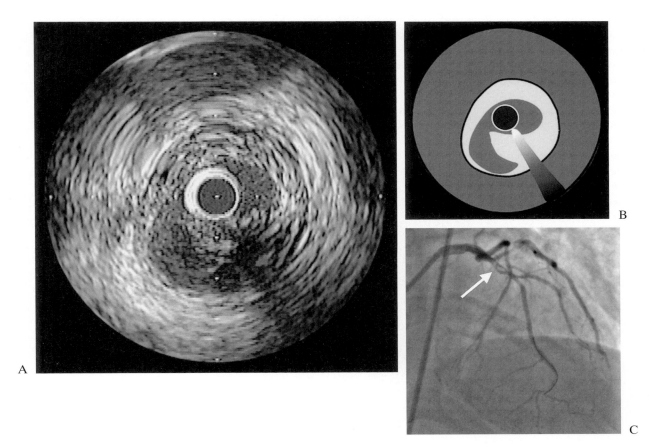

FIGURE 4-3. (A) Intravascular ultrasound of LAD dissection postangioplasty; (B) schematic represention; (C) angiographic comparison. (See color plate, part B only.)

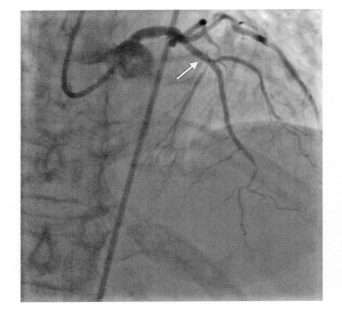

FIGURE 4-4. Left anterior descending coronary artery after stenting (arrow).

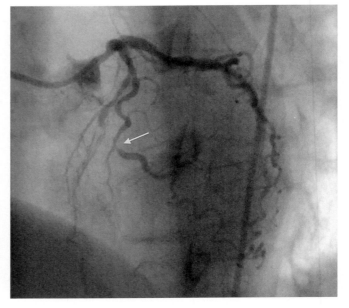

FIGURE 4-5. High-grade diagonal artery stenosis (arrow) in a 72-year-old woman.

tive for the relief of angina. Acute complications, while distressing to all, are generally uncommon with long-term restenosis rates dependent upon the degree of relief of luminal obstruction and the size and length of the treatment area. With the advent of coronary stents, balloon angioplasty has become an adjunct for coronary stent procedures, used most often prior to stent deployment and also to improve stent diameter postdeployment. Currently, only about 5% of percutaneous revascularization procedures involve balloon angioplasty alone, so-called plain old balloon angioplasty (POBA).

4. Complications

The types and frequency of complications related to POBA are well known (Table 4-1) and the reduction in acute complications represents the evolutionary improvements in technique and equipment as the procedure has matured.[3]

4.1. Coronary Dissection

Given the mechanism of luminal improvement with balloon angioplasty, it is not surprising that the most

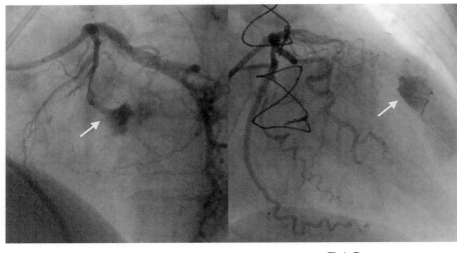

LAO   **RAO**

FIGURE 4-6. Balloon angioplasty resulted in a coronary perforation [arrow, left anterior oblique projection (LAO), left panel] with extensive dye staining [arrow, right anterior oblique projection (RAO), right panel].

TABLE 4-1. Acute complications related to balloon angioplasty.

Complication	Incidence	Treatment options
Coronary dissection	30%–75%	Conservative if Types A, B For Types C–F, prolonged balloon inflation Coronary stenting CABG
Perforation/rupture	0.3%–0.8%	Prolonged balloon inflation Stop anticoagulation Bare-metal stent Covered stent Intravascular coils CABG
No-reflow	0.6%–10%	Variety of vasodilators, including nitroprusside, nitroglycerin, verapamil, adenosine, papaverine, norepinephrine, etc.
Balloon rupture	0.1%–3.6%	Remove catheter Snare if needed CABG
Acute closure	2%–10%	Prolonged balloon inflation Coronary stenting CABG

Abbreviation: CABG, coronary artery bypass graft.

common angiographic complication with this procedure is coronary artery dissection. The incidence of angiographically visible dissection is about 30%–50% of patients undergoing balloon dilatation.[4,5] The incidence of dissection is thought to be related to higher balloon:artery size ratio,[6,7] localized calcium deposits,[8] longer lesions,[7] and the presence of other disease within the target vessel.[7] With the use of intravascular ultrasound to aid in identifying vessel morphology, the incidence of dissection post-PTCA rises to about 75%.[8]

Dissections have been classified by the National Heart, Lung and Blood Institute (NHLBI) according to their angiographic appearance (Table 4-2). Type A is a coronary dissection with only minor radiolucencies within the coronary lumen without a reduction in coronary flow. Type B dissection shows minimal or no dye persistence in the presence of parallel tracts or a double lumen separated by a radiolucent area during contrast injection.

TABLE 4-2. Coronary dissection classification.

Type A	Coronary dissection with only minor radiolucencies within the coronary lumen without a reduction in coronary flow.
Type B	Minimal or no dye persistence in the presence of parallel tracts or a double lumen separated by a radiolucent area during contrast injection.
Type C	Dissection with persistent extraluminal dye after luminal contrast injection.
Type D	Spiral dissection.
Type E	Dissection with new and filling defects.
Type F	This dissection does not fit any of the above types A–E and is associated with impaired flow or total occlusion of the vessel.

Types A and B are thought to be relatively benign whereas types C–F can be important predictors of adverse outcomes, including acute closure requiring require a more aggressive treatment plan.[9]

Type C involves persistent extraluminal dye after luminal contrast injection. Type D is a spiral dissection and Type E involves new persistent filling defects. Type F dissection is one in which the dissection does not fit any of the above types and is associated with impaired flow or total occlusion of the vessel. Types A and B are thought to be relatively benign whereas types C–F can be important predictors of adverse outcomes, including acute closure (see below), and thus require a more aggressive treatment plan.[9]

Before the advent of coronary stents, the treatment of more profound dissections included prolonged balloon inflation at the site of the dissection to help tack up the vessel wall.[10,11] These inflations commonly lasted 30 minutes or more with the use of a specialized perfusion balloon that allowed the passage of about 30% of the normal coronary blood flow while the balloon was inflated. The angiographic success with this technique of prolonged inflation was about 80%.[10,11] For those patients who had persistent dissections with hemodynamic compromise, emergency coronary artery bypass surgery was often performed. In the modern era, stenting has replaced prolonged balloon inflations[12,13] as well as emergency coronary artery bypass graft (CABG)[14]; the use of a stent to tack up dissection planes is now relatively common and considered standard-of-care for more malevolent dissections.

4.2. Vessel Perforation/Rupture

This rare but dreaded complication usually occurs with overaggressive balloon dilatation,[15] although it can occur with guidewires and stenting, as well. The incidence is thankfully quite low with POBA and acute management ranging from a conservative strategy of monitoring to prolonged balloon inflations, (covered) stents, and surgery.

In a recent analysis of the incidence and treatment of coronary artery perforations,[16] the overall incidence was 0.8%. About half of these patients were managed conservatively, with the cessation of antithrombotic and antiplatelet medications and close hemodynamic monitoring. In the remaining patients, significant bleeding into the pericardium and tamponade resulted, requiring emergency pericardiocentesis. In the 10 patients who had received the platelet glycoprotein IIb/IIIa receptor antagonist, abciximab, 9 required urgent pericardiocentesis, suggesting that the additional platelet inhibition allowed for greater bleeding into the pericardial space. Prolonged balloon inflation at the site of the perforation was performed in all patients; 2 patients received covered stents and 8 patients were sent for emergency surgery. The outcome of this event is notable in that, of the 24 patients who required aggressive management, 6 died in-hospital, including 3 postsurgery.

In another retrospective study from 1990 to 1999 of coronary artery perforations,[17] Gruberg and colleagues found an incidence of 0.29%. In this extensive analysis, 10% (8/84) of the patients eventually died. Balloon angioplasty as part of the percutaneous coronary intervention (PCI) procedure was involved in 31% of the 84 cases. Roughly half of the cases were related to atherectomy or laser devices with the other half (52%) related to angioplasty and stenting. The treatment strategies once the perforation was recognized included referral for emergency surgery (39.3%), prolonged balloon inflation (36%), stenting (9%), pericardiocentesis alone (4.3%), and pericardial window (4.3%). Three percent underwent a bypass operation with a pericardial window and 1.1% underwent coil embolization. Overall, the clinical outcomes related to the perforation included death in 10%, tamponade in 31%, myocardial infarction in 34%, repeat coronary angioplasty in 6%, and emergency surgery in 39%. Of the 33 patients who underwent emergency surgery, 6 died (18%), as did 2 in the group who did not go to surgery (4%).

As noted in the above series, prolonged balloon inflation with perfusion balloons to mechanically seal the perforation has been for many years the standard of acute and immediate treatment for significant perforation, along with immediate reversal of anticoagulation. Similar to the experience with vessel dissection, the utility of prolonged balloon inflation for perforation and rupture has been established, with success rates (defined as the avoidance of requiring emergency surgery) ranging from 44% to 90%,[18] and this success rate is dependent upon the extent of the perforation.

Stenting has been another modality employed for the acute treatment of a coronary artery perforation. Bare-metal stents[19] and covered stents with saphenous vein graft[20,21] or polytetrafluoroethylene[22,23] have been used. A recent development in the acute treatment of vessel perforation is the Food and Drug Administration's approval of a polytetrafluoroethylene (PTFE)-covered stent for the specific purpose of bail-out for a vessel perforation/rupture. These stents are composed of a bare-metal skeleton covered with a PTFE sleeve. This sleeve is designed to seal off the primary area of the perforation and allow the vessel to heal. There are some concerns regarding the potential for late thrombosis with the PTFE-covered stents[24]; thus, prolonged dual antiplatelet therapy is recommended for thrombosis prophylaxis.

Intravascular coils, composed of platinum and other materials that promote local thrombosis, have also been employed in the acute treatment of perforation.[25-27] In this technique, the site of the perforation is crossed with a delivery catheter containing the coils; the coils are then delivered across the perforation site and the site is sealed. It may take several coils to complete the closure. While this results in occlusion of the distal vessel with likely infarction, urgent coronary bypass surgery can be averted.

For any extensive perforation, the cardiovascular surgeon should be contacted immediately. If the acute treatments (including pericardiocentesis) within the catheterization laboratory fail, the patient should be sent to emergency surgery, where the perforation can be repaired and the pericardium evacuated. Depending on the status of the vessels and the remainder of the coronary anatomy, bypass grafts may also be placed. As noted above, the mortality risk in these high-risk emergency situations for surgery is high.[16,17] Because of the improvements in PCI techniques and equipment, primarily the widespread use of coronary stents, the need for emergency CABG has decreased significantly.[14]

4.3. The No-Reflow Phenomenon

The no-reflow phenomenon is discussed elsewhere in detail (see Chapter 8).

4.4. Balloon Rupture

Percutaneous transluminal coronary angioplasty balloons are composed of polymer materials that can be graded as compliant, semicompliant, or noncompliant. There is a small but real risk of balloon tears and ruptures that is dependent on both the compliance of the balloon material as well as the target lesion plaque composition.

In the early days of PTCA, the risk of balloon rupture with PTCA was relatively high (up to 3.6%[28]) and related to lesion morphology, most often the presence of calcific plaque. Intravascular ultrasound may be a useful modality to investigate the potential lesion morphology associated with balloon rupture.[29] As the evolution of balloon materials and design has matured, the incidence of balloon tears and rupture and their unintended adverse sequelae appears to be decreasing.[30]

The management of balloon catheter rupture is dependent upon the degree of equipment failure and its sequelae. For balloon tears, recognition involves the unexpected appearance of dye into the target vessel with attempts during balloon inflation. The balloon can be safely removed in the large majority of cases with no sequelae. On rare occasions, pinhole leaks have been described,[31–33] leading to a high-pressure jet of contrast which may dissect and/or perforate the target vessel. In this scenario, the balloon should be immediately removed and the appropriate treatment for the complication initiated.

Rarer still is embolization of balloon material. In this scenario, the balloon material is actually torn and embolized distally. This may cause no-reflow and acute closure of the target vessel. The embolized material may be retrieved with a snare[34] or by placing a buddy-wire with balloon capture on retrieval.[35]

4.5. Acute Closure

Acute or threatened closure is a dreaded complication of PTCA with an incidence of 2%–10%.[36] As noted above, balloon-induced vascular injury typically results in a localized dissection or even rupture which may lead to threatened or complete closure of the target vessel. In a 1988 retrospective analysis by Ellis and colleagues of 140 (2.9%) acute closure cases out of a database of 4772 coronary angioplasty procedures,[37] six important predictors of acute closure were identified: (1) post-PTCA residual stenosis; (2) intimal tear or dissection; (3) use of a prolonged heparin infusion; (4) branch-point target lesion; (5) target stenosis at a angle greater than 45°, and (6) additional PTCA performed within the same target vessel. In a separate analysis, Lincoff and his co-investigators examined another PTCA dataset of 1319 patients and found an acute closure incidence of 8.3%.[38] This dataset included a significant number of patients presenting with acute or recent myocardial infarction (50% of the patients analyzed), which may explain the higher incidence than in the Ellis study. In Lincoff's analysis, 48% of the patients with acute closure had evidence of dissection or thrombus, with an additional 7% harboring both.

The treatments for acute closure have been described above; coronary stents provide a mechanical scaffold for treatment of lesion recoil after PTCA as well as tacking up any local dissection planes. In the modern era, stenting has been very successful for the immediate treatment of acute closure and has become the standard

of care.[12,13,39–42] In rare cases of refractory or worsened closure poststenting, CABG may also be needed.[14]

5. Summary

In the early days of angioplasty, balloon dilatation was the primary treatment option for patients with obstructive coronary artery disease. The complication rate was generally low but these events were somewhat hazardous, given the relatively crude techniques in treating acute problems within the catheterization laboratory. As the angioplasty era has now evolved into the modern stent era, the utility of angioplasty remains, despite the reduction in the total number of POBA interventions. The evolution of materials and techniques has further refined balloon angioplasty and this has contributed to an improvement in outcomes with an associated decline in morbidity and mortality related to angioplasty complications and a willingness to tackle previously undilatable lesions. The incidence and treatment of acute complications has been improved, resulting in an improvement in patient outcomes.

References

1. Grüntzig A. Transluminal dilation of coronary-artery stenosis. Lancet. 1977;1:263.
2. Landau C, Lange RA, Hillis LD. Percutaneous transluminal coronary angioplasty. New Engl J Med. 1994;89:2190–2197.
3. Laskey WK, Williams DO, Vlachos HA, et al. Dynamic Registry Investigators. Changes in the practice of percutaneous coronary intervention: a comparison of enrollment waves in the National Heart, Lung, and Blood Institute (NHLBI) Dynamic Registry. Am J Cardiol. 2001;87:964–969, A3–A4.
4. Holmes DR, Vlietstra RE, Mock MB, et al. Angiographic changes produced by percutaneous transluminal coronary angioplasty. Am J Cardiol. 1983;51:676–683.
5. Matthews BJ, Ewels CJ, Kent KM. Coronary dissection: a predictor of restenosis? Am Heart J. 1988;115:547–554.
6. Nichols AB, Smith R, Berke AD, et al. Importance of balloon size in coronary angioplasty. J Am Coll Cardiol. 1989;13:1094–1100.
7. Sharma SK, Israel DH, Kamean JL, et al. Clinical, angiographic, and procedural determinants of major and minor coronary dissection during angioplasty. Am Heart J. 1993;126:39–47.
8. Fitzgerald PJ, Ports TA, Tock PG. Contribution of localized calcium deposits to dissection after angioplasty. An observational study using intravascular ultrasound. Circulation. 1992;86:64–70.
9. Huber MS, Mooney JF, Madison J, Mooney MR. Use of a morphologic classification to predict clinical outcome after dissection from coronary angioplasty. Am J Cardiol. 1991;68:467–471.
10. Jackman JD Jr, Zidar JP, Tcheng JE, et al. Outcome after prolonged balloon inflations of greater than 20 minutes for

initially unsuccessful percutaneous transluminal coronary angioplasty. Am J Cardiol. 1992;69:1417–1421.

11. Leitschuh ML, Mills RM Jr, Jacobs AK, et al. Outcome after major dissection during coronary angioplasty using the perfusion balloon catheter. Am J Cardiol. 1991;67: 1056–1060.

12. Fischman DL, Savage MP, Leon MB, et al. Effect of intracoronary stenting on intimal dissection after balloon angioplasty: results of quantitative and qualitative coronary analysis. J Am Coll Cardiol. 1991;18:1445–1451.

13. George BS, Voorhees WD, Roubin GS. Multicenter investigation of coronary stenting to treat acute or threatened closure after percutaneous transluminal coronary angioplasty: clinical and angiographic outcomes. J Am Coll Cardiol. 1993;8:135–143.

14. Seshadri N, Whitlow PL, Acharya N, et al. Emergency coronary artery bypass surgery in the contemporary percutaneous coronary intervention era. Circulation. 2002;106: 2346–2350.

15. Nassar H, Hasin Y, Gotsman MS. Cardiac tamponade following coronary arterial rupture during coronary angioplasty. Catheter Cardiovasc Diagn. 1991;23:177–179.

16. Gunning MG, Williams IL, Jewitt DE, et al. Coronary artery perforation during percutaneous intervention: incidence and outcome. Heart. 2002;88:495–498.

17. Gruberg L, Pinnow E, Flood R, et al. Incidence, management, and outcome of coronary artery perforation during percutaneous coronary intervention. Am J Cardiol. 2000; 86:680–682.

18. Ellis SG, Ajluni S, Arnold AZ, et al. Increased coronary perforation in the new device era. Incidence, classification, management, and outcome. Circulation. 1994;90:2725–2730.

19. Thomas MR, Wainwright RJ. Use of an intracoronary stent to control intrapericardial bleeding during coronary artery rupture complicating coronary angioplasty. Catheter Cardiovasc Diagn. 1993;30:169–172.

20. Colombo A, Itoh A, DiMario C. Successful closure of a cornary vessel rupture with a vein graft stent: a case report. Catheter Cardiovasc Diagn. 1996;38:172–174.

21. Caputo RP, Amin N, Marvasti M. Successful treatment of a saphenous vein graft perforation with an autologous vein-covered stent. Catheter Cardiovasc Interv. 1999;48: 382–386.

22. Mulvihill NT, Boccalatte M, Sousa P, et al. Rapid sealing of coronary perforations using polytetrafluoroethylene-covered stents. Am J Cardiol. 2003;91:343–346.

23. Elsner M, Auch-Schwelk W, Britten M. Coronary stent graft covered by polytetrafluoroethylene membrane. Am J Cardiol. 1999;84:335–338.

24. Kwok OH, Ng W, Chow WH. Late stent thrombosis after successful repair of a major coronary artery rupture with a PTFE covered stent. J Invasive Cardiol. 2001;13:391–394.

25. Gaxiola E, Browne KF. Coronary artery perforation repair using microcoil embolization. Catheter Cardiovasc Diagn. 1998;43:474–476.

26. Dorros G, Jain A, Kumar K. Management of coronary artery rupture: covered stent or microcoil embolization. Catheter Cardiovasc Diagn. 1995;36:148–154.

27. Assali AR, Moustapha A, Sdringola S, et al. Successful treatment of coronary artery perforation in an abciximab-treated patient by microcoil embolization. Catheter Cardiovasc Interv. 2000;51:487–489.

28. Simpfendorfer CC, Dimas AP, Zaidi A, et al. Balloon rupture during coronary angioplasty. Angiology. 1986;37: 828–831.

29. Zellner C, Sweeney JP, Ko E, et al. Use of intravascular ultrasound in evaluating repeated balloon rupture during coronary stenting. Catheter Cardiovasc Diagn. 1997;40: 52–54.

30. Chan AW, Rabinowitz A, Webb JG, et al. Adverse events associated with balloon rupture during percutaneous coronary intervention. Can J Cardiol. 1999;15:962–966.

31. Kahn JK, Hartzler GO. Balloon rupture due to lesion morphology during coronary angioplasty. Catheter Cardiovasc Diagn. 1990;21:89–91.

32. Dev V, Kaul U, Mathur A. Pin hole balloon rupture during coronary angioplasty causing dissection and occlusion of the coronary artery. Indian Heart J. 1991;43:393–394.

33. LeMay MR, Beanlands DS. Pinhole balloon rupture during coronary angioplasty causing rupture of the coronary artery. Catheter Cardiovasc Diagn. 1990;19:91–92.

34. Kirsch MJ, Ellwood RA. Removal of a ruptured angioplasty balloon catheter with use of a nitinol goose neck snare. J Vasc Interv Radiol. 1995;6:537–538.

35. Trehan V, Mukhopadhyay S, Yusuf J, et al. Intracoronary fracture and embolization of a coronary angioplasty balloon catheter: retrieval by a simple technique. Catheter Cardiovasc Interv. 2003;58:473–477.

36. Bates ER. Ischemic complications after percutaneous transluminal coronary angioplasty. Am J Med. 2000;108: 309–316.

37. Ellis SG, Roubin GS, King SB 3rd, et al. Angiographic and clinical predictors of acute closure after native vessel coronary angioplasty. Circulation. 1988;77:372–379.

38. Lincoff AM, Popma JJ, Ellis SG, et al. Abrupt vessel closure complicating coronary angioplasty: clinical, angiographic and therapeutic profile. J Am Coll Cardiol. 1992;19: 926–935.

39. Scott NA, Weintraub WS, Carlin SF, et al. Recent changes in the management and outcome of acute closure after percutaneous transluminal coronary angioplasty. Am J Cardiol. 1993;71:1159–1163.

40. Hearn JA, King SB 3rd, Douglas JS Jr, et al. Clinical and angiographic outcomes after coronary artery stenting for acute or threatened closure after percutaneous transluminal coronary angioplasty. Initial results with a balloon-expandable, stainless steel design. Circulation. 1993;88: 2086–2096.

41. Maiello L, Colombo A, Gianrossi R, et al. Coronary stenting for treatment of acute or threatened closure following dissection after coronary balloon angioplasty. Am Heart J. 1993;125:1570–1575.

42. Antoniucci D, Santoro GM, Bolognese L, et al. Bailout Palmaz-Schatz coronary stenting in 39 patients with occlusive dissection complicating conventional angioplasty. Catheter Cardiovasc Diagn. 1995;35:204–209.

5
Coronary Guidewire Complications

Antonio J. Chamoun and Barry F. Uretsky

An 86-year-old male presented with unstable angina. Angiography demonstrated a nondominant right coronary artery (RCA), mild obstruction in the left anterior descending (LAD) coronary artery, several lesions of the mid and distal portions of the left circumflex coronary artery (LCX) as well as a lesion in the ostium of a large first obtuse marginal (OM1) branch.[1]

Heparin and abciximab were administered and a two-wire technique was used with balloon angioplasty followed by stenting performed on the LCX. After predilatation, a 3.0 × 16-mm length NIR stent (Boston Scientific, Inc., Maple Grove, MN) was implanted distally. A 3.5 × 15-mm length Crown stent (Cordis, Inc., Miami Lakes, FL) was placed more proximally in the true LCX. A PT Graphix™ (Boston Scientific) wire was used to cross the lesion in the obtuse marginal branch. After predilatation, a 2.75 × 15-mm length MiniCrown stent was placed in the OM1 ostium. Stent deployment caused some plaque shifting into the main LCX leading to kissing balloon dilatation of the OM1 and the LCX with a satisfactory angiographic result. However, during the dual kissing balloon dilatation, the distal tip of the PT Graphix™ wire was noted to have separated from its core and embolized into the terminal portion of OM1 (Figure 5-1A).

Shortly thereafter, the patient complained of chest discomfort and a distal guidewire-induced coronary perforation was identified (Figure 5-1A). A 2.5-mm diameter dilatation catheter was advanced to the distal OM and inflated at 0.5 atm. Angiography confirmed that this obstructed distal flow and prevented any further contrast leak. To seal the perforation, the balloon was inflated for 25 minutes while intravenous protamine was given, abciximab was discontinued, and a platelet transfusion ordered. Urgent transthoracic echocardiography confirmed the presence of a small pericardial effusion without evidence of tamponade. However, deflation of the balloon after 25 minutes revealed a persistent contrast leak for which the balloon was reinflated at low pressure. Topical thrombin was mixed with normal saline and diluted loversol (Optiray®, Mallinckrodt Inc., St. Louis, MO) to achieve a thrombin concentration of 50 IU/mL. The guidewire was withdrawn from the inflated balloon, which was still inflated in the distal OM. After careful aspiration of the central balloon lumen, 2 mL of the thrombin mixture (100 IU) was slowly injected in that lumen in an attempt to thrombose the tertiary OM branch vessel. The balloon was inflated for 10 minutes after thrombin instillation. Angiography over the next 10 minutes demonstrated complete and persistent occlusion of the distal branch with obliteration of the contrast leak (Figure 5-1B). The patient was subsequently discharged within 48 hours.

Over the past three decades, coronary guidewire (CGW) engineering has resulted in significant refinements to meet the needs of increasingly complex percutaneous coronary interventions (PCI). Gruentzig's fixed guidewire balloon has evolved into a myriad of steerable and independent CGWs paralleling the growing versatile armamentarium of interventional devices. It became clear early on in this process that engineering an ideal, all-purpose CGW would likely be unattainable. Atherosclerosis, a diffuse disease, impacts the coronary lumen in a spectrum of ways from a focal napkin-ring lesion to diffuse long stenoses, concentric lesions to eccentric lesions, soft nonhemodynamically critical plaque to calcified near-occlusive lesions to chronically totally occlusive lesions. These lesions frequently result in very tortuous calcified paths starting at coronary ostia and leading oftentimes to tight lesions in side-branch vessels. The driving goal of engineering CGWs is thus twofold: first, crossing the lesion and second, providing the support and delivery rail for therapeutic devices. Although desirable, a given CGW need not fulfill both purposes. Sometimes, certain design characteristics make a CGW both a tool for a specific purpose, as well as a possibly dangerous tool with potentially fatal complications.

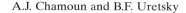

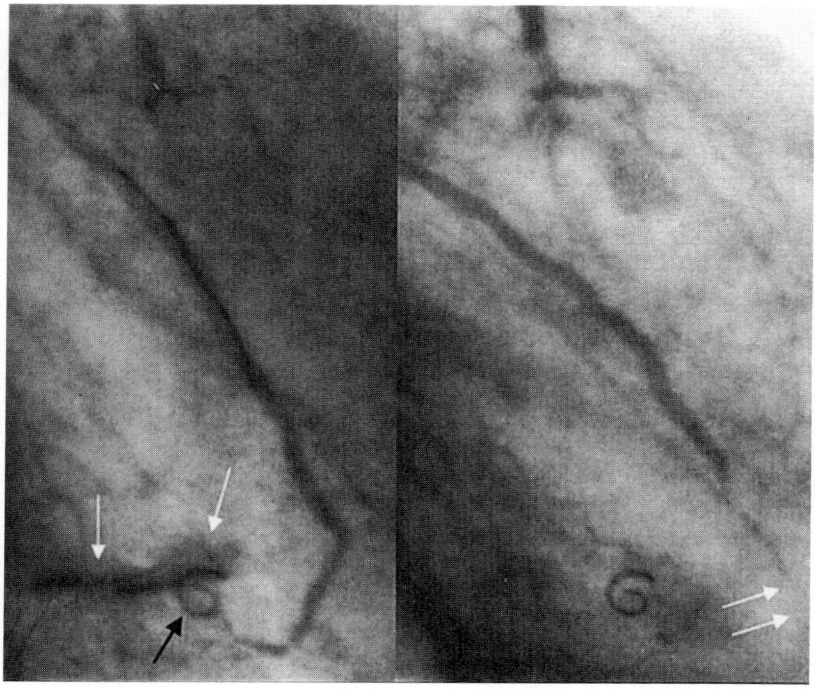

FIGURE 5-1. (A) The distal tip of the PT Graphix™ wire has separated from its core and embolized into the terminal portion of OM1. Extravasation of dye in the pericardium due to distal guidewire-induced coronary perforation is noted. (B) Final angiography demonstrated complete and persistent occlusion of the distal branch with obliteration of the contrast leak. (From Fischell et al.[1] Copyright ©2003. This material is used by permission of Wiley-Liss, Inc., a subsidiary of John Wiley & Sons, Inc.)

After a brief overview of the basic structure and characteristics of CGWs, specific potential and reported complications will be reviewed. The bulk of our knowledge in this regard comes from case reports in the interventional cardiology literature as well as from the experience of individual operators.

1. Guidewire Structure and Characteristics

The majority of current CGWs have a 0.014-inch diameter, although 0.016-, 0.018-, and 0.021-inch wires are still available to provide greater vessel straightening, better torque control, and more support for delivery of PCI devices. The basic structure of a guidewire consists of a central core, a distal flexible spring coil, and a coating. The central core (or shaft) may be either stainless steel, nitinol, or a combination (a stainless-steel proximal shaft with a nitinol distal core). Nitinol is kink resistant and maintains better wire integrity, especially in tortuous anatomy. The central core distal end tapers in varying steps up to three tapers. The less tapering steps and the more distal the tapering starts, the greater the support and possible torque control. The distal core may terminate in a shaping ribbon or continue to the tip (core-to-tip design). This latter design enhances torque response and decreases wire prolapse and may provide different degrees of tip stiffness depending on the terminal core

taper diameter and length. Shaping ribbon designs usually constitute soft tips. In either case wires may have a straight tip requiring shaping or be preshaped, usually as a J (45°).

The distal core, often as it starts tapering, is surrounded by a flexible spring coil made of either tungsten or, more frequently, platinum, providing radiopacity to the tip. These are most often manufactured as short tips (2–3 cm) interfering minimally with assessment of fine luminal details or less often as long tips (25–40 cm). The flexible spring coil terminates in a distal tip weld, minimizing the risk of vessel perforation. Polytetrafluoroethylene (PTFE) may be used as a polymer cover to increase the lubricity of the proximal shaft. The flexible spring coil crossing tip is usually coated with silicon, PTFE, a hydrophobic coating [e.g., Microglide™ (hydroxyapatite)] or a hydrophilic coating [e.g., Hydrocoat (epoxy)] (Tables 5-1 and 5-2, and Figure 5-2).

2. Coronary Perforation by Guidewire

2.1. Mechanism

Coronary perforation ranges from vessel puncture by the CGW, manifested as minimal dye staining without adverse hemodynamic consequences, to wire exit with rapid build-up of a pericardial effusion leading to tamponade, to vessel rupture with brisk extravasation of

TABLE 5-1. Examples of coronary guidewires: classification by support provided.

	Cordis	Guidant	Boston Scientific	Medtronic AVE	Jomed/Abbott
High Support	Stabilizer XS	Iron Man	Platinum Plus Mailman	AVE Standard	Confianza Grand Slam
	Stabilizer Plus	All Star X S'port Balance HW	Choice XS Trooper XS ChoICE PT® XS	GT1 Support	Standard
	Stabilizer BP Stabilizer MW	HTFII XS Wiggle Cross-IT wires	Patriot	GT2 Fusion	Miraclebros12 Miraclebros6 Medium
	ATW MW Shinobi	BMW Pilot wires	PT Graphix™ Intermediate Luge PT2 MS ChoICE PT®	GT1 Direct	Miraclebros4.5 Miraclebros3 Prowater
Light Support	Wizdom Wizdom ST	HTFII Balance Whisper MS	Choice Floppy Trooper Floppy	GT1 Floppy Hyperflex Silk	Soft Light

blood into the pericardial space, tamponade, and abrupt hemodynamic collapse[2] (Figure 5-3).

Coronary perforation during PCI occurs with an incidence of 0.2% to 0.8% with higher incidences reported since the advent of stenting and atherectomy devices.[3–10] Half of those cases may lead to tamponade, hemodynamic collapse, emergent surgery, or death.[3,4,7] Moreover, short of a timely adequate therapeutic intervention, the outcome of a CGW-induced perforation is particularly serious when glycoprotein IIb/IIIa inhibitors (GPI) are used.[3,4,7] Most of these cases are manifest during PCI although a delayed presentation, as late as 16 hours post-PCI, has been reported.[11] In a large series reviewing outcomes of coronary artery perforation during PCI, 90% of perforations where abciximab had been administered led to the development of pericardial tamponade.[3] On the other hand, prior cardiac surgery may confer some protection against tamponade and hemodynamic collapse due to postsurgical mediastinal adhesions and absence of a true pericardial space at risk.[12] Eccentricity, tortuosity, and lesion length greater than 10 mm have been associated with an increased risk of this complication.[13] Coronary guidewire–induced perforations are believed to account for about 20%–40% of all perforations.[1,3,10,14] The majority of these are distal small end-of-vessel perforations except when the culprit is a chronically occluded vessel. Seventeen percent of all perforations and 25% of those leading to clinical sequelae occur in cases of chronic

TABLE 5-2. Examples of coronary guidewires: classification by tip stiffness.

	Cordis	Guidant	Boston Scientific	Medtronic AVE	Jomed/Abbott
Extra stiff tip	Shinobi	Cross-IT 300XT Cross-IT 200XT Pilot 200 Pilot 150	Platinum Plus Crosswire Choice Standard		Confianza Miraclebros12
	Wizdom Supersoft Stabilizer BP Supersoft Wizdom Soft Stabilizer BP Soft	Cross-IT 100XT X S'port Pilot 50 Balance HW Whisper MS	PT2 MS Choice Intermediate ChoICE PT® Choice XS Trooper Intermediate Mailman Luge Choice Floppy	AVE Standard	Standard Miraclebros6 Miraclebros4.5 Medium Miraclebros3 Prowater
	Wizdom ST ATW MW	Iron Man All Star BMW Balance HTFII XS, HTFII	Patriot Trooper Floppy	GT1 Support GT1 Direct GT2 Fusion GT1 Floppy Hyperflex Silk	Grand Slam Soft Light
Soft tip					

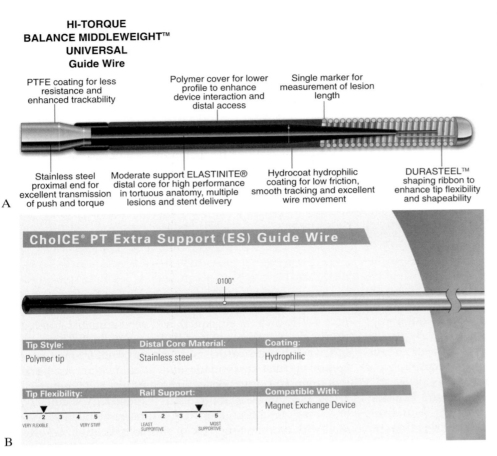

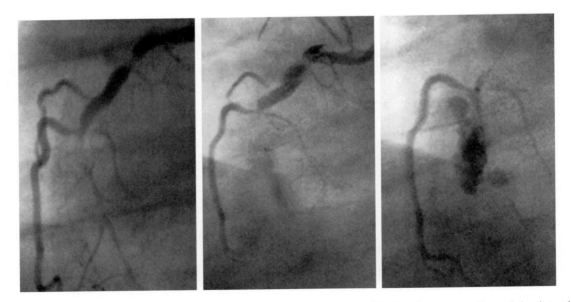

FIGURE 5-2. Examples of coronary guidewire construction. (A) HI-TORQUE Balance Middleweight UNIVERSAL™ Guide Wire (from Guidant Corporation). (B) ChoICE® PT Extra Support Guide Wire (from Boston Scientific Corporation).

occlusions.[3] Increased lubricity and stiffness are probably the most important intrinsic CGW properties increasing the risk of coronary perforation. Reports abound in the literature on wires—such as the ChoICE PT® (Boston Scientific, Maple Grove, MN), a lubricious, moderately stiff older generation wire—in causing coronary perforations.[1,15–19] Such wires are both particularly useful and dangerous in cases of chronic total occlusions.

FIGURE 5-3. Perforation after failure to cross a chronic total occlusion of the RCA. Frank extravasation of dye into the pericardial space is consistent with a type III perforation. (http://www.tctmd.com.)

2.2. Prevention and Management

The majority of proximal mid-epicardial vessel perforation occurs secondary to therapeutic coronary devices or during treatment of chronic total occlusions.[2,3,14,20–22] These particular scenarios are discussed separately in corresponding chapters of this text. We will limit this discussion to CGW end-vessel–induced perforation. As it is the current practice of most interventionists treating chronic total occlusions, we suggest withholding GPI administration until very complex (tortuous, long, and eccentric) lesions are crossed especially when stiff-tip or lubricious CGWs such as a ChoICE PT® are being used. In such lesions an over-the-wire (OTW) system should be considered to allow exchange of the highly lubricious CGW to a possibly safer nonhydrophilic-coated CGW as soon as the OTW balloon or exchange catheter can be positioned securely to permit the exchange. Allowing the hydrophilic CGW to form a loop at its tip to avoid trauma to the end-vessel may not confer greater safety as the slippery tip may migrate unnoticed into a distal branch causing perforation during device exchanges.[15]

If, despite meticulous care, a distal perforation occurs, a stepwise approach should be taken. A small-diameter short balloon should be inflated at low pressure after being advanced as distal as possible in the culprit vessel to minimize the amount of ischemic myocardium. A cine-fluoroscopic dye injection should verify the integrity of the seal. Concomitantly, reversal of heparin anticoagulation with intravenous protamine may be done. At least 10 to 15 minutes of balloon inflation should be allowed before testing for a successful seal of the perforation. Meanwhile, an emergent transthoracic echocardiogram should be obtained to assess the amount of pericardial effusion. A pericardiocentesis tray should be readily available and a cardiothoracic surgeon made aware of the situation. If the perforation persists, a longer balloon inflation of 25 to 30 minutes may be attempted. Concurrent analgesia may be required during these long inflation times to alleviate ischemic pain. If a GPI had been used, the infusion should be stopped. Platelets should also be transfused if abciximab is the GPI administered.[20]

If the perforation occurs in a small branch of the proximal or middle segments of a main epicardial vessel, deploying a short covered stent in the main vessel to occlude the ostium of the branch may be successful in stopping the extravasation.[23–27] Although this may be accomplished relatively easily, infarction of all the myocardium supplied by this branch is likely and potential future morbidity of a covered stent implantation (i.e., edge restenosis, stent thrombosis, and target vessel revascularization) is possible.[23–26,28–35] When all other measures have failed, percutaneous sealing of the perforation by coronary occlusion may still be attempted before emergent surgery is performed. Organized thrombus from autologous blood,[36] gelfoam sponge,[37] microcoil,[19] polyvinyl alcohol,[16] and thrombin[1] have all been employed successfully. An OTW system is necessary to perform any of these procedures. Autologous clotted blood injection through a balloon catheter central lumen may be challenging and multiple attempts may be required.[36] Gelfoam sponge is made of gelatine that is able to absorb and hold within its interstices multiple times its weight in blood. When soaked in a sclerosing agent it may provide permanent vessel occlusion. In one report, two sponges of 2-mm diameter soaked in contrast for 20 seconds and delivered through a 3.0 Fr Transit catheter (Cordis) positioned 1 cm proximal to the perforation site achieved a successful seal.[37] Gelfoam seems to hasten clot formation and provide support for thrombus formation. In a distal coronary bed it provides long enough vessel occlusion to allow the perforation site to permanently thrombose and seal. In another report, a perforated distal coronary artery was embolized successfully with a single helical platinum microcoil delivered in a fairly similar fashion through a Tracker catheter (Target Therapeutics, Fremont, CA).[19] Polyvinyl alcohol (PVA) form (COUNTOUR emboli, CE 6003, ITC, San Francisco, CA) suspended solution as a 3-mL mixture (approximately quarter vial of 355–500 μm) with contrast agent was injected slowly over 3 minutes through an OTW balloon catheter positioned as distal as possible and inflated at low pressure in a case of distal coronary perforation.[16] In this report, PVA injection achieved a successful seal without reversal of heparin anticoagulation with protamine. In another report, lyophilized topical thrombin powder was mixed with normal saline and dilute contrast to achieve a concentration of 50 or 100 IU/mL. One hundred international units and 300 IU were injected slowly over 5 minutes through an inflated balloon catheter after protamine was administered and platelets were transfused to reverse heparin and abciximab effects in two patients, respectively, sealing successfully the distal coronary perforations with the balloon left inflated in place for 10 to 15 minutes[1] (Table 5-3, Figures 5-4–5-8).

TABLE 5-3. Classification of coronary perforation.

Perforation class	Definition	Risk of tamponade (%)
I	Extraluminal crater without contrast agent extravasation	8
II	Pericardial or myocardial blush without contrast agent jetting	13
III	Contrast agent jetting through a frank (≥ 1 mm) perforation	63
CS (cavity spilling)	Perforation into a cardiac chamber or the coronary sinus	0

Source: Modified from Ellis et al.[2]

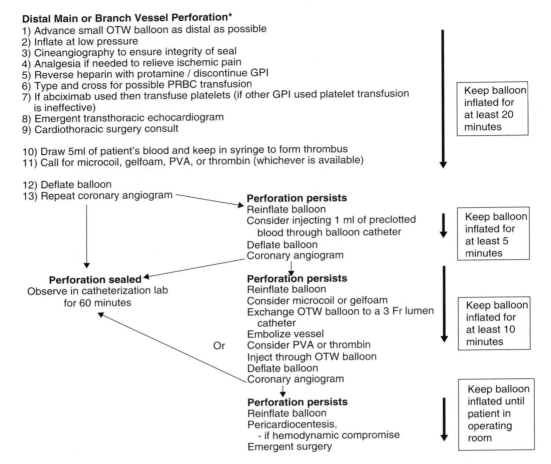

Distal Main or Branch Vessel Perforation*
1) Advance small OTW balloon as distal as possible
2) Inflate at low pressure
3) Cineangiography to ensure integrity of seal
4) Analgesia if needed to relieve ischemic pain
5) Reverse heparin with protamine / discontinue GPI
6) Type and cross for possible PRBC transfusion
7) If abciximab used then transfuse platelets (if other GPI used platelet transfusion
   is ineffective)
8) Emergent transthoracic echocardiogram
9) Cardiothoracic surgery consult

10) Draw 5ml of patient's blood and keep in syringe to form thrombus
11) Call for microcoil, gelfoam, PVA, or thrombin (whichever is available)

12) Deflate balloon
13) Repeat coronary angiogram

> Keep balloon inflated for at least 20 minutes

Perforation persists
Reinflate balloon
Consider injecting 1 ml of preclotted
   blood through balloon catheter
Deflate balloon
Coronary angiogram

> Keep balloon inflated for at least 5 minutes

Perforation sealed
Observe in catheterization lab
for 60 minutes

Perforation persists
Reinflate balloon
Consider microcoil or gelfoam
Exchange OTW balloon to a 3 Fr lumen
   catheter
Embolize vessel
Or   Consider PVA or thrombin
Inject through OTW balloon
Deflate balloon
Coronary angiogram

> Keep balloon inflated for at least 10 minutes

Perforation persists
Reinflate balloon
Pericardiocentesis,
   - if hemodynamic compromise
Emergent surgery

> Keep balloon inflated until patient in operating room

FIGURE 5-4. Algorithm for Distal Coronary Artery Perforation Management (see text for details). *If the perforation occurs in a small branch of the proximal or middle segments of a main epicardial vessel, deploying a short covered stent in the main vessel to occlude the ostium of the branch is an alternative solution.

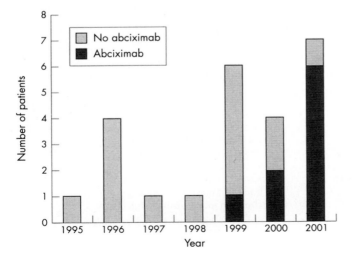

FIGURE 5-5. Number of patients where coronary vessel perforation resulted in hemodynamically significant pericardial effusion per year in a series of 6245 patients. A progressive increase in the relative number of hemodynamically significant pericardial effusions associated with the increasing use of abciximab is noted since its introduction to the cardiac catheterization laboratory. (Reprinted from Gunning et al.,[3] Heart 2002; 88:495–498, with permission from the BMJ Publishing Group.)

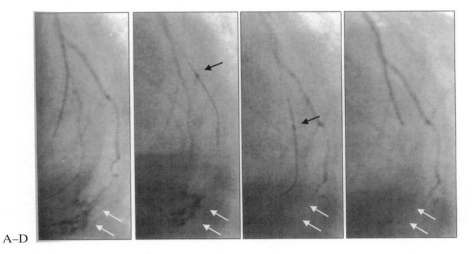

A–D

FIGURE 5-6. Angiography demonstrating successful treatment of distal coronary artery perforation with thrombin. (A) White arrows highlight area of contrast extravasation at perforation site. (B) The small balloon (black arrow) is inflated in the posterior branch, which was initially felt to be the perforation site. Contrast injection demonstrates persistent leak arising from the more anterior branch (white arrows in B). This site of perfora-tion is confirmed by the lack of contrast extravasation during injection with the balloon inflated (black arrow) in the anterior branch (C). Finally, in (D), there is no further communication of contrast into distal perforation site after local injection of 300 IU of thrombin (white arrows). (From Fischell et al.[1] Copyright 2003. This material is used by permission of Wiley-Liss, Inc., a subsidiary of John Wiley & Sons, Inc.)

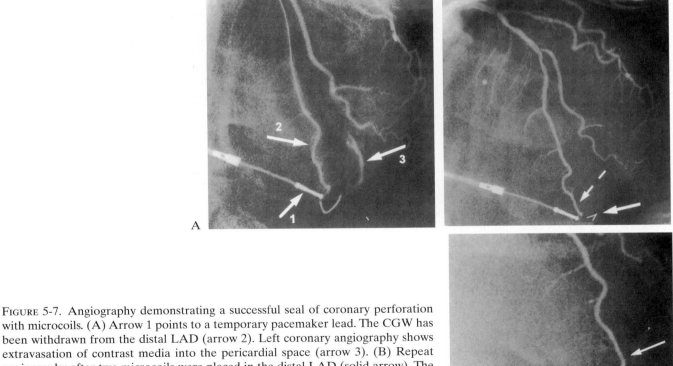

FIGURE 5-7. Angiography demonstrating a successful seal of coronary perforation with microcoils. (A) Arrow 1 points to a temporary pacemaker lead. The CGW has been withdrawn from the distal LAD (arrow 2). Left coronary angiography shows extravasation of contrast media into the pericardial space (arrow 3). (B) Repeat angiography after two microcoils were placed in the distal LAD (solid arrow). The distal LAD (broken arrow) is occluded and contrast extravasation is no longer visible. (C) Repeat left coronary arteriography after 48 hours shows the microcoils to be in place (broken arrow) and the distal LAD remains occluded (solid arrow). (From Gaxiola and Browne.[19] This material is used by permission of Wiley-LISS, Inco, a subsidiary of John Wiley & Sons, Inc.)

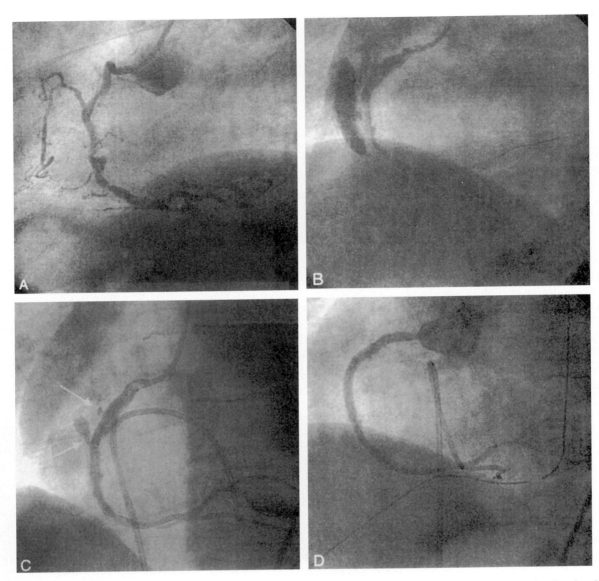

FIGURE 5-8. Angiography showing successful treatment of coronary perforation using a covered stent. (A) Left anterior oblique cranial projection demonstrating diffuse right coronary artery atheroma and a severe stenosis in the midsegment of the vessel. (B) Contrast leakage into the pericardium after high-pressure stent deployment in the mid right coronary artery with decreased anterograde flow. (C) Angiogram revealing 2 separate sites of vessel perforation (arrows) in the proximal and mid right coronary artery after a 3-minute balloon inflation over the rupture sites. (D) Final angiographic result after implantation of two Jomed stent grafts, one in the proximal and one in the mid right coronary artery. The patient required urgent pericardial drainage; a drain is in place in the pericardium, as well as a Swan-Ganz catheter in the right ventricle. (Reprinted from American Journal of Cardiology 91, Mulvihill et al. "Rapid sealing of coronary performations," 343–346, copyright 2003, with permission from the Excerpta Medica Inc.)

3. Pseudolesions

3.1. Mechanism

Artefactual lesions appearing during the course of PCI have been termed *pseudolesions, pseudostenoses, crumpled coronary, accordion, intussusception,* or *concertina* effect.[38–48] This phenomenon is mostly observed in tortu-ous vessels and is believed to result from mechanical invagination of the coronary arterial wall at different sites as a result of the straightening effect of CGWs, mostly those with a stiff distal core. Most cases have been reported in tortuous right coronary arteries (RCA) although left anterior descending (LAD), left circumflex (LCX), and left internal thoracic artery graft (LITA) pseudostenoses have been described with an overall quoted incidence of about 0.4%.[39–48] These lesions may very well become flow limiting, causing angina or even hemodynamic compromise.[44,49] The differential diagnosis of such neolesions includes dissection, spasm, embolization, and thrombus.

3.2. Prevention and Management

A high index of suspicion is essential in recognizing pseudolesions, especially when stiff CGWs are used. An erroneous diagnosis of a true new lesion might call for an unwarranted intervention at the site with its attendant potential risks. Intracoronary nitroglycerin will not disinvaginate the arterial wall but may help distinguish these lesions from true spasm.

If a monorail system is being used, the CGW may be cautiously withdrawn to where the floppy segment of the distal tip lies equally on either side of the lesion. Advancing the balloon beyond the lesion while pulling back the CGW may also be attempted although extra care should be taken to avoid overwithdrawal of the CGW and possible wire exit when a monorail system is in place. These maneuvers usually allow the vessel to reconform to its true anatomy as the arterial wall disinvaginates in case of an accordion effect while maintaining safe CGW access beyond the lesion, if this is a true lesion such as a dissection.

An OTW system allows safer negotiation of pseudolesions. Although a simple CGW pull-back up to the floppy tip may be performed as described above, this may not be the optimal approach because renegotiating proximal tortuosities to the lesion in severely diseased vessels may be more difficult than anticipated, resulting occasionally in wire prolapse as a result of lost support even when the floppy end is across the lesion. Moreover, multiple pseudostenoses may be induced along a long segment, rendering a partial wire pull-back insufficient to assess the full vessel length. Therefore, the safest approach would be to advance the balloon as distal as possible to the most distal neolesion and completely withdraw the CGW from the coronary system into the guiding catheter to allow the artery to reconform to its prior curvature. If doubt still persists after this maneuver, one should carefully remove the wire and balloon to study the coronary segment in question. Alternatively, intravascular ultrasound (IVUS) may be performed to clarify the nature of the lesion. In case of a pseudolesion, a localized elliptic-shaped lumen narrowing or severe lumen asymmetry with absence of severe atherosclerosis is demonstrated.[38] A pathognomonic image of a flattened, three-layered wall overlying a hypoechogenic space may also be visualized, representing a partial coronary intussusception.[38] If the need for a stiff CGW is no longer warranted, wire exchange to a softer CGW should be strongly considered to prevent untoward hemodynamic consequences of pseudostenoses.[44] Finally, using a pressure wire for physiological guidance of stent deployment may be misleading in presence of pseudolesions[49] (Figures 5-9–5-13).

4. Treating In-Stent Lesions: Guidewire Passage through Stent Struts

4.1. Mechanism

A rare but potentially serious complication encountered while treating in-stent lesions, that is, in-stent restenosis or stent thrombosis, is wire passage through the stent struts. Stent design, length, or multiplicity are not believed to be predisposing factors.[50] After 1 month of deployment, complete endothelialization is expected.[51,52] However, neointimal hyperplasia causing in-stent restenosis within the stent may be uneven and a loose interface between the vessel wall and the stent struts sometimes exits. This interface might present little resistance to wire passage, especially hydrophilic CGWs. Downstream beyond the stent or even within long stents the wire may easily be redirected into the true lumen depending on tissue resistance. Another potential mechanism in cases of stent thrombosis or in-stent restenosis is wire passage through an isolated stent strut in the vessel lumen in malapposed stents or ones with disrupted architecture during initial stent deployment technique. A situation where this complication is of particular concern is in treating in-stent main vessel ostial lesions, where stent struts may be protruding in the aorta or stent architecture may have been distorted by guiding catheter manipulations. Most often, wire passage through the stent struts and redirection into the true lumen is not recognized because a dissection is not usually visible. Stent avulsion with total vessel occlusion and balloon entrapment may result if balloon passage and inflation are performed.[50]

4.2. Prevention and Management

A sharp J bend to the tip of the CGW so as to form a leading loop while crossing the stent might be of some help in preventing erratic wire passage through stent struts. A high index of suspicion should raise this possibility while treating in-stent lesions when unexplained significant resistance to balloon advancement is encountered. When suspected, wire position in relation to the stent should be carefully analyzed in orthogonal views. A tangential or eccentric orientation of the wire should strongly suggest this problem when unexplained obstruction to the balloon is felt.[50] A different CGW with different tracking properties may be used to cross the in-stent lesion, preferably while leaving either the initial

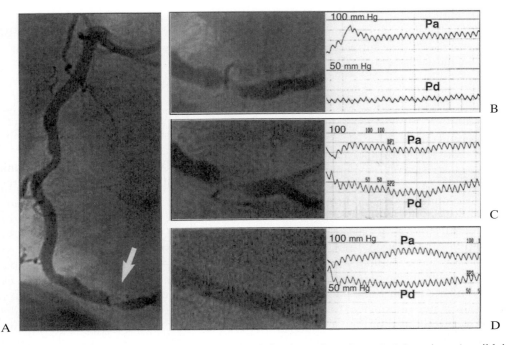

FIGURE 5-9. (A) Baseline coronary angiography of the right coronary artery showing moderate tortuosity in the proximal and mid segments, and a severe stenosis in its distal segment. (B, C) Angiographic and physiological findings before angioplasty (A, B), immediately after predilatation with a 2.5-mm balloon (C), and following stent implantation (D). The pressure tracings in (B) demonstrate a fully exhausted vasodilatory reserve, without modification of the translesional gradient following adenosine administration. A mild improvement is evident after predilatation (C), with still a marked residual stenosis and a suboptimal functional result (FFR 0.56.). In spite of achieving a good angiographic result after stent implantation (D), a persistent, suboptimal functional result (FFR 0.62) is noted. (From Escaned et al.[49] Copyright ©2000. This material is used by permission of Wiley-Liss, Inc., a subsidiary of John Wiley & Sons, Inc.)

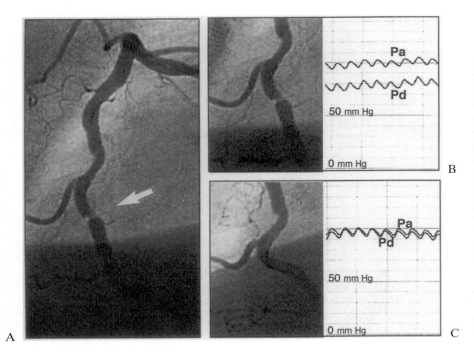

FIGURE 5-10. (A) Left lateral view of the right coronary artery while the pressure guidewire is positioned through the stented site. A marked narrowing distal to one of the preexisting bends, suggesting pseudostenosis, is noted in the mid segment of the vessel. Withdrawal of the pressure guidewire through the stent revealed persistence of the pressure gradient and the referred pseudorestenosis (B). However, crossing the vessel bend with the pressure sensor was immediately followed by complete resolution of the pressure gradient, with angiographic disappearance of the pseudostenosis when the floppy tip allowed the vessel to return to its original configuration (C). (From Escaned et al.[49] Copyright ©2000. This material is used by permission of Wiley-Liss, Inc., a subsidiary of John Wiley & Sons, Inc.)

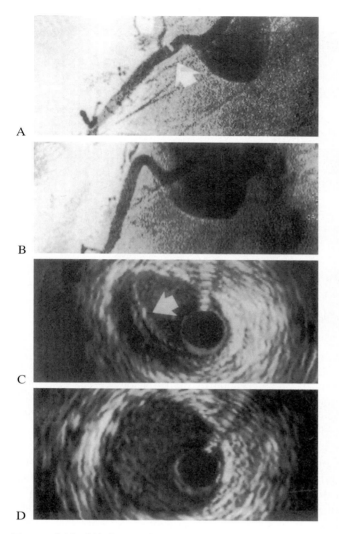

FIGURE 5-11. (A) Severe focal angiographic narrowing of the proximal right coronary artery (arrow). (B) After removing the guidewire the artery reassumes its normal curvature and the image of stenosis (pseudostenosis) disappears. (C) Intravascular ultrasound image at the site of pseudostenosis disclosing an elliptic lumen narrowing with a flattened wall showing a three-layered appearance (arrow) and a posterior hypoechogenic space (the hallmark of coronary intussusception). (D) Distal reference segment revealing a healthy vessel with larger total vessel area (demonstrating vessel shrinkage at the site of pseudostenosis). (From Alfonso et al.[38] Copyright ©1999. This material is used by permission of Wiley-Liss, Inc., a subsidiary of John Wiley & Sons, Inc.)

wire in place or even the deflated balloon at the site to block the false lumen as an attempt to cross the true lumen is being carried out.[53] Alternatively, the smallest balloon with radiopaque markers at either end should be used for initial dilatation. A noncoaxial marker position should dictate, if any, a very low pressure inflation[50] (Figure 5-14).

5. Wire Kinking, Entanglement, and Entrapment

5.1. Mechanism

Wire kinking, entanglement, and entrapment are rare complications during coronary intervention.[54–56] Kinking may result from overtorquing and forceful advancement of a CGW across complex lesions.[57] In theory, nitinol single-core CGWs are less likely to kink as nitinol is a kink-resistant material and torque transmission from

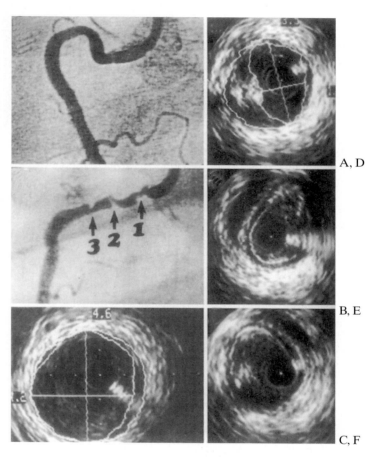

FIGURE 5-12. (A) Shepherd's crook configuration of the proximal right coronary artery. (B) After the advancement of a stiff guidewire, multiple, complex stenoses could be visualized. (D) Lumen narrowing caused by plaque protrusion detected by intravascular ultrasound. (E) Focal, severe angiographic stenosis that on intravascular imaging proved to be a wrinkle without significant plaque burden. (F) Moderate stenosis showing again the typical image of flattened intimal thickening associated with a posterior echo-free space highly suggestive of intussusception. (C) Intravascular imaging of the distal reference segment showing mild intimal thickening and a larger total vessel area. (From Alfonso.[38] Copyright ©1999. This material is used by permission of Wiley-Liss, Inc., a subsidiary of John Wiley & Sons, Inc.)

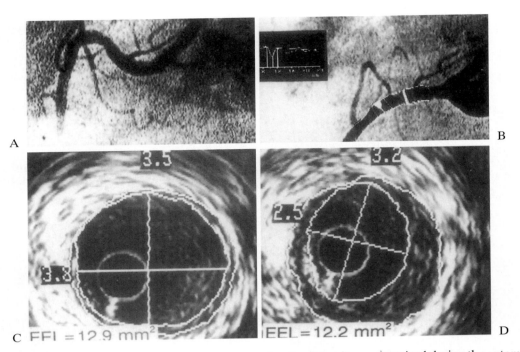

FIGURE 5-13. Coronary angiogram of the right coronary artery before intervention (A), and after the advancement of a stiff guidewire, showing the appearance of a coronary narrowing (B). Intravascular ultrasound image of the distal reference coronary segment (C). At the stenotic site, a hypoechogenic semilunar image was visualized (D). This image was so faint and localized that it was unnoticed during the automatic motorized pullback. However, it could be recognized after careful manual ultrasonic interrogation of the suspicious coronary segment. *Abbreviation*: EEL, external elastic lamina. (From Alfonso.[38] Copyright ©1999. This material is used by permission of Wiley-Liss, Inc., a subsidiary of John Wiley & Sons, Inc.)

shaft to wire tip with a single-core design is a one-to-one angle phenomenon. Entanglement and entrapment usually occur on a kinked CGW as forceful advancement or improper coronary device manipulation is performed on such wires.[56,57] Rarely, a CGW may intentionally be jailed in a side branch for ostial protection while stenting the main vessel in bifurcating lesions.[58]

Coronary guidewire entrapment has been reported during IVUS catheter manipulations.[55,59] Particular caution should be exercised when using a pressure wire to perform an IVUS study, a practice that has become popular in some centers to gather and correlate hemodynamic with two-dimensional ultrasonographic lesional data before and after PCI in a rapid fashion.[60–65] The

FIGURE 5-14. In-stent lesion treatment complication. (A) Right coronary angiogram in LAO view showing an in-stent restenosis. The long stented area extends from mid right coronary segment to the proximal segment of the posterior left ventricular branch distal to crux (see also Figure 5-2). (B) Right coronary angiogram in LAO view showing a 3 × 30-mm Omnipass balloon obstruction in the mid portion of the stented area. The long stented segment is well seen. The stenosis does not seem to be critically severe so as to make the passage of a conventional balloon difficult. (C) The image shows tangential, eccentric, noncoaxial lie of a 3 × 20-mm balloon within the stent. The proximal radiopaque marker is peripheral and appears to be outside the stent compared to the distal marker, which is central and probably intraluminal. The balloon seems to have exited from the stent in mid region and re-entered the lumen after a short distance forward. (D) Right coronary angiogram in LAO view after first balloon inflation. Two lumens are created. The inner true lumen is defined by the limits of the stent, while the outer false lumen houses the wire and the balloon. The stent has avulsed from the wall and outlines the inner true lumen. (E) The image shows looped distal end of the guidewire for facilitated antegrade passage. The wire should preferably be straightened after crossing the stent. This angiogram was in fact taken after pulling out the first wire and balloon and giving the tip a simulated loop, but is deliberately sequenced before (D) for purposes of better comprehension and clarity. (F) The image shows two guidewires separated in the mid stented region. The inner one is the intraluminal second wire. The first wire, which is the outer one with the balloon over it, is outside the stent in this region. (G) The image shows a 3 × 20-mm Adante (Scimed) balloon positioned across the double lumen. The lie of the balloon within the true lumen needs to be emphasized. Compared to (C), the position, as suggested by the radiopaque markers, is more central and coaxial. (H) Right coronary angiogram in LAO view showing a good final angioplasty result. The stent is completely expanded. (From Jain et al.[50] Copyright ©2001. This material is used by permission of Wiley-Liss, Inc., a subsidiary of John Wiley & Sons, Inc.)

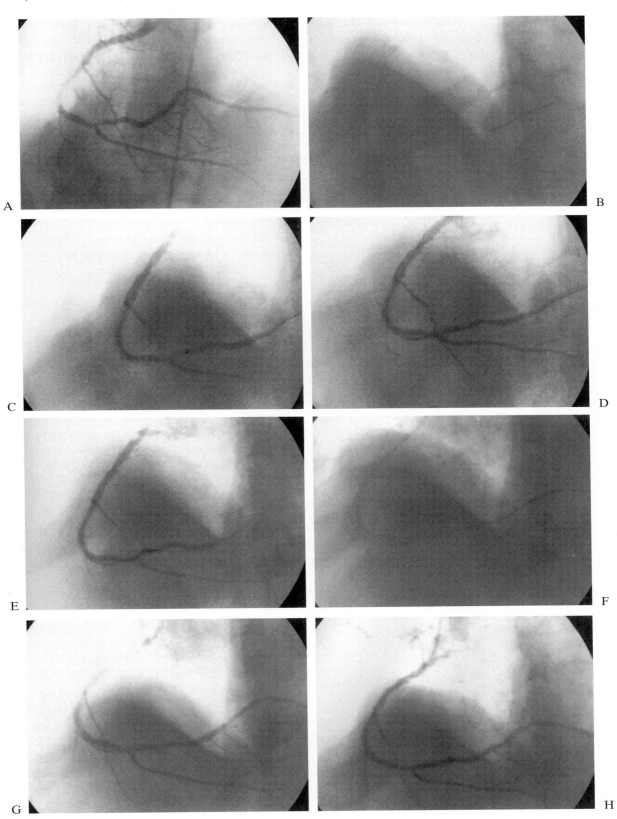

intrinsic characteristics of the pressure wire, in conjunction with the short monorail segment of standard IVUS catheters, likely predisposes this tool to this complication in complex lesions.

5.2. Prevention and Management

As is true for most complications, lesion severity, complexity, calcification, and proximal tortuosity are factors that may predispose to CGW kinking, entanglement, and entrapment. Left circumflex lesions may be prone to such complications due to the already tortuous path requiring careful manipulation of CGWs. Another situation that is particularly permissive to CGW kinking, entanglement, and entrapment is during treatment of bifurcation or trifurcation lesions. Thoughtful assessment of such lesions includes weighing the risk and benefits of a conservative approach versus PCI. Operator skill in planning, organizing, and choosing the appropriate equipment is paramount to lessen the likelihood of such complications. An OTW single-core nitinol CGW with an OTW coronary device might decrease this risk in theory because the wire and device will always tend to torque or move as a unit if overtorquing or forceful maneuvers are performed. When treating bifurcation or trifurcation lesions, using at least one OTW system and preloading devices up to the coronary ostia before negotiating the coronary anatomy may decrease the risk of entanglement. When wire kinking leads to entanglement and entrapment, the safest approach is to remove the CGW and coronary diagnostic or therapeutic device as a unit. Removing the guiding catheter as part of the assembly without trying to pull the coronary equipment into the guiding catheter is further advised because extra strain may lead to CGW fracture and loss if such maneuver is attempted[54,55,57] (Figures 5-15 and 5-16).

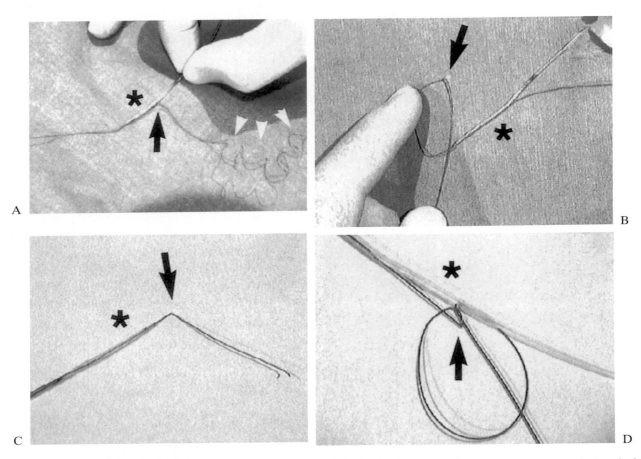

FIGURE 5-15. Pressure wire–IVUS catheter entrapment. Direct visual inspection of the two systems performed in 4 patients, revealing the kinked part of the pressure wire (black arrows) and the distal tip of the IVUS catheter (asterisks). (A) The kinked part of the pressure wire was stuck at the entrance of the monorail segment of the IVUS catheter. Its unraveled part formed a large ribbon (white arrowheads). (B) The most kinked part of the pressure wire was clearly identified within the loop. (C) The kinked part of the pressure wire had already been slightly displaced from the distal part of the imaging catheter. (D) A complex looping of the pressure wire is demonstrated. The wire encircled its most kinked part which, in turn, entangled the monorail segment of the IVUS catheter. (From Alfonso et al.[55] Copyright ©2000. This material is used by permission of Wiley-Liss, Inc., a subsidiary of John Wiley & Sons, Inc.)

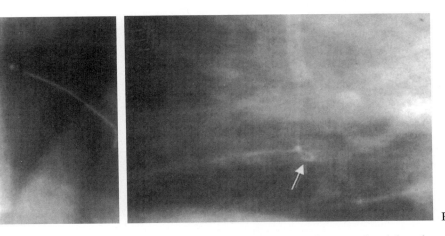

A   B

FIGURE 5-16. Pressure wire–IVUS catheter entrapment. (A) A large loop of the pressure wire (arrows) was visualized in the aortic root when resistance to the retrieval of the imaging catheter was felt. (B) The pressure wire entrapped the imaging catheter. The guiding catheter was disengaged and then the wire catheter assembly had to be removed as a unit. (From Alfonso et al.[55] Copyright ©2000. This material is used by permission of Wiley-Liss, Inc., a subsidiary of John Wiley & Sons, Inc.)

6. Coronary Guidewire Fracture

6.1. Mechanism

Although very rare, CGW breakage may result during wire manipulation while attempting to cross complex lesions.[17,54–57,66–72] This may especially follow CGW entanglement, entrapment, or kinking in the coronary circulation with different therapeutic or diagnostic coronary devices such as IVUS catheters.[17,55,59,69–71] As mentioned above, if inadvertent force is applied to advance the IVUS catheter across tortuous, calcified, and highly stenotic vessels, wire kinking, entrapment, and subsequent fracture may ensue. Another theoretical concern with CGW breakage is during pull-back of a CGW left in a side branch for ostial protection while stenting the main vessel, a so-called bifurcation treatment jailing technique.[58] Although unproven, non–single-core CGWs would seem to be at higher risk for such complication.

6.2. Prevention and Management

As in prevention of any other complication, operator skill in wire manipulation and proper use of coronary devices is paramount. A possibly helpful tip while negotiating tortuous, calcified, severely stenotic lesions is not to torque a CGW greater than 360° in any direction at one time. Keeping constant hold of the torquer device at all times while crossing a lesion usually makes it difficult to impose such extreme torque on the CGW without a conscious effort to do so.

If the CGW broken fragment remains partly within the guiding catheter, a balloon may be advanced over a wire carefully past the proximal part of the broken fragment and then inflated to trap it between the outer wall of the balloon and the inner wall of the catheter before the whole assembly is removed as a unit.[68] Alternatively, a simple balloon such as a Trapper™ may be used for the same purpose. Another approach is to deploy a stent within the guiding catheter to jail the wire fragment prior to removal of the assembly.[73] If the broken wire fragment is lost outside the guiding catheter with its proximal part outside the coronary circulation, a snaring device is needed to retrieve the fragment.[74,75] If the broken wire is lost entirely within the coronary circulation, snaring or surgical removal may be the only available option.[57] Alternatively, a short CGW fragment that has embolized distally in a main vessel or is trapped in its entirety in a small branch may be left in place while the patient is on chronic antiplatelet therapy.[54] When a short fractured CGW fragment is stuck on a plaque in a proximal or middle segment of a main vessel, stenting along the length of the fragment, although unreported previously, may be considered if the risk of acute vessel thrombosis is thought to be higher than expected for a stent in that segment (Figures 5-17 and 5-18).

7. Coronary Guidewire–Induced Dissection

7.1. Mechanism

Significant coronary dissections may occasionally be due to CGWs. The majority of severe dissections usually follow use of balloons, stents, atherectomy devices, or specialized wires (e.g., laser wire) in severely tortuous vessels with complex calcified lesions.[76–78] Attempts at PCI of chronic total occlusions (CTO) requiring stiffer lubri-

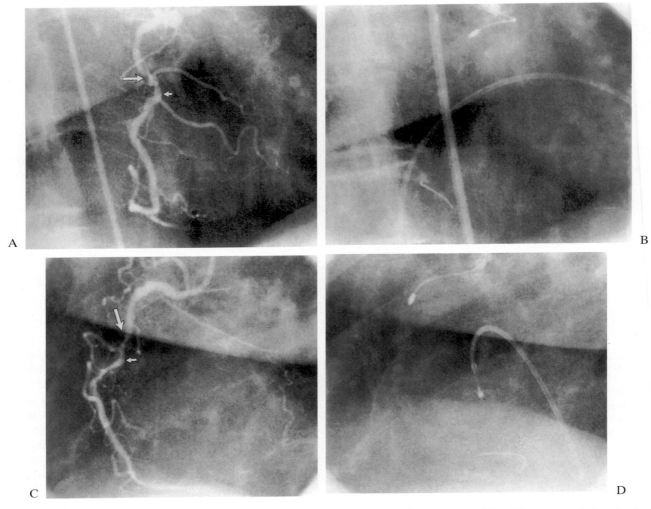

FIGURE 5-17. Floppy Rotawire (SCIMED, Maple Grove, MN) fracture during rotablation leading to coronary perforation and tamponade due to a free moving burr. (A) RAO and (B) LAO end-diastolic views of the tortuous and severely calcified mid-RCA lesion (large arrow). The 90° exit angulation is clearly seen in both views. (C) RAO and (D) LAO views of the fractured guidewire in the distal RCA and rotablator burr proximal to the lesion. (*Source*: Woodfield et al.[17])

cious CGWs may result in dissections as the wire enters the occluding lesion eccentrically at the interface of the vessel wall and the fibrotic hard lesion. The presence of an unrecognized healed chronic dissection following prior coronary manipulation would also significantly increase the risk of dissection extension if the CGW is forcefully advanced into the false lumen. Another situation is the production of an acute dissection during PCI, loss of wire position, and propagation of dissection during reinsertion and advancement of wire into false lumen rather than true lumen. Finally, in the setting of an acute coronary syndrome where plaque rupture is usually causative, wire passage beneath the ruptured plaque and into the vessel wall may cause a dissection.

7.2. Prevention and Management

Operator skill and experience is paramount in preventing CGW-induced dissection especially in high-risk situations or CTO that facilitate this complication. Developing a tactile feel to wire resistance and avoiding wrinkling of the tip while advancing the CGW usually ensures a free tip that can be safely advanced. Extra care should certainly be exercised when lubricious stiff CGWs are being used. Moreover, a careful study of the coronary lesion anatomy in multiple orthogonal views, even of what appears to be a simple lesion, should be done prior to proceeding with PCI. After crossing the lesion, meticulous review of CGW position in relation to the vessel

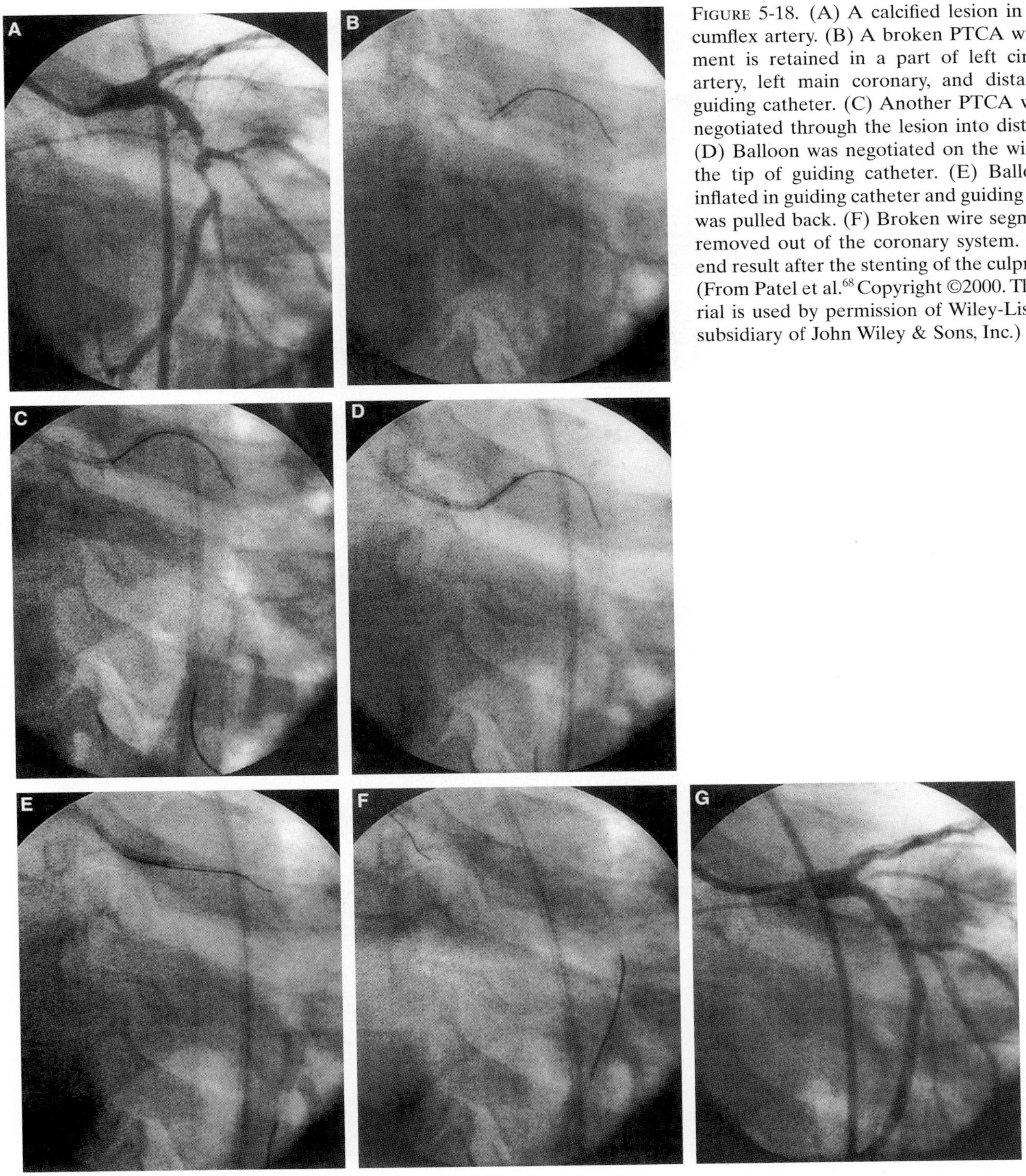

FIGURE 5-18. (A) A calcified lesion in left circumflex artery. (B) A broken PTCA wire fragment is retained in a part of left circumflex artery, left main coronary, and distal tip of guiding catheter. (C) Another PTCA wire was negotiated through the lesion into distal LCX. (D) Balloon was negotiated on the wire up to the tip of guiding catheter. (E) Balloon was inflated in guiding catheter and guiding catheter was pulled back. (F) Broken wire segment was removed out of the coronary system. (G) The end result after the stenting of the culprit block. (From Patel et al.[68] Copyright ©2000. This material is used by permission of Wiley-Liss, Inc., a subsidiary of John Wiley & Sons, Inc.)

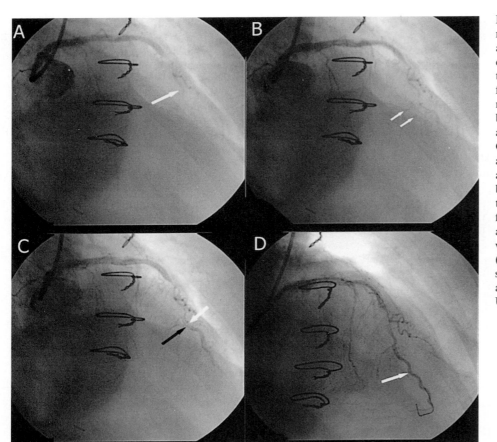

Figure 5-19. Spiral dissection of the mid distal LAD in a highly calcified and tortuous vessel following stent deployment in a high-grade lesion of the mid LAD. A careful frame-by-frame review of the angiogram was necessary to identify the true lumen before CGW reinsertion and advancement after loss of initial CGW position. (A) Initial dye propagation into the true lumen (white arrow). (B) Filling of septal branches (white arrows) as dye fills the true lumen. (C) Retrograde filling of the false lumen (black arrow points to false lumen and white arrow points to true lumen). (D) Coronary guidewire positioned successfully in the true lumen (white arrow). (Courtesy of Barry F. Uretsky, M.D.)

wall in orthogonal cineangiographic views to ensure an intraluminal position may be helpful. A tangential position along the vessel wall all the way to the CGW tip with straightening or wrinkling of the tip should raise suspicions about a subintimal wire position. At times, a careful IVUS catheter advancement may be helpful, if doubt still persists as to the lesion anatomy and its relation to guidewire position.

Most importantly, if it is decided to proceed with PCI, any unexpected intracoronary resistance to balloon advancement should raise suspicion of such a complication. A wise approach is to leave the uninflated balloon over its wire where resistance is met to obstruct the possible false lumen while an attempt at recrossing the lesion with another wire is carried out. In case of a CTO, one cannot overemphasize the importance of recognizing the lesion's nose cone or nipple if present as a relatively safe spot for wire advancement. An equally crucial point is identifying the true lumen of a chronic dissection or that of an acute dissection following device manipulation prior to any attempt at wire manipulation. In the latter scenario, maintaining a safe distal wire position is of utmost importance. However, if the wire is inadvertently pulled back or a chronic dissection is being primarily

crossed, a frame-by-frame review of the diagnostic cineangiogram to study dye progression through the true lumen and into the branching vessels is paramount to establish a safe CGW road map. When successful intraluminal wire position is assured, treatment of the dissection should generally follow the conventionally accepted approach regardless of its etiology. A distal to proximal bail-out stenting strategy is strongly advocated when coronary flow is impaired or severe luminal narrowing is present[78-84] (Figure 5-19).

8. Conclusions

Knowledge of wire characteristics (i.e., tip and body lubricity and stiffness) is paramount for safe handling of CGWs in complex PCI. Avoidance of very aggressive wire manipulations and upstream glycoprotein IIb/IIIa inhibitors in cases such as chronic total occlusions may prevent serious perforations leading to tamponade. Availability of at least one of the suggested rescue methods described in the text is recommended before attempting such PCI. Careful attention to the CGW straightening effect on baseline tortuosities should prevent unwarranted treatment of wire-induced pseudolesions. A high index of suspicion while treating in-stent lesions is essential to avoid subintimal or sub-stent advancement of balloons and subsequent dilatation causing stent avulsion. When treating bifurcation or tri-furcation lesions, using at least one OTW system and pre-loading devices to the coronary ostia before negotiating complex coronary anatomy may decrease the risk of entanglement, kinking, and potential wire fracture. Although practiced by some, we still recommend avoid-ance of intentional wire jailing that may lead to CGW tip breakage and loss in the side branch on pull-back attempts. The majority of severe dissections occur during alternative therapeutic device use. In such cases, main-taining a stable distal CGW position is crucial and if inadvertently lost, careful frame-by-frame study of the angiogram is invaluable in identifying a safe road map to advance the CGW into the true lumen.

Despite our growing experience in complex PCI, inter-ventionists may still fall victims to CGW complications. Some of these complications are preventable and when, despite careful planning, they do occur, good judgment, experience, and adherence to the above recommended steps may avert catastrophic consequences.

References

1. Fischell TA, Korban EH, Lauer MA. Successful treatment of distal coronary guidewire-induced perforation with balloon catheter delivery of intracoronary thrombin. Catheter Cardiovasc Interv. 2003;58:370–374.
2. Ellis SG, Ajluni S, Arnold AZ, et al. Increased coronary perforation in the new device era. Incidence, classification, management, and outcome. Circulation. 1994;90:2725–2730.
3. Gunning MG, Williams IL, Jewitt DE, et al. Coronary artery perforation during percutaneous intervention: incidence and outcome. Heart. 2002;88:495–498.
4. Von Sohsten R, Kopistansky C, Cohen M, Kussmaul WG 3rd. Cardiac tamponade in the "new device" era: evaluation of 6999 consecutive percutaneous coronary interventions. Am Heart J. 2000;140:279–283.
5. Kimbiris D, Iskandrian AS, Goel I, et al. Transluminal coro-nary angioplasty complicated by coronary artery perfora-tion. Catheter Cardiovasc Diagn. 1982;8:481–487.
6. Grollier G, Bories H, Commeau P, Foucault JP, Potier JC. Coronary artery perforation during coronary angioplasty. Clin Cardiol. 1986;9:27–29.
7. Gruberg L, Pinnow E, Flood R, et al. Incidence, manage-ment, and outcome of coronary artery perforation during percutaneous coronary intervention. Am J Cardiol. 2000; 86:680–682, A8.
8. Topaz O, Cowley MJ, Vetrovec GW. Coronary perforation during angioplasty: angiographic detection and demonstra-tion of complete healing. Catheter Cardiovasc Diagn. 1992; 27:284–288.
9. Nassar H, Hasin Y, Gotsman MS. Cardiac tamponade following coronary arterial rupture during coronary angioplasty. Catheter Cardiovasc Diagn. 1991;23:177–179.
10. Fukutomi T, Suzuki T, Popma JJ, et al. Early and late clini-cal outcomes following coronary perforation in patients undergoing percutaneous coronary intervention. Circ J. 2002;66:349–356.
11. Abhyankar AD, England D, Bernstein L, Harris PJ. Delayed appearance of distal coronary perforation follow-ing stent implantation. Catheter Cardiovasc Diagn. 1998; 43:311–312.
12. Seshadri N, Whitlow PL, Acharya N, et al. Emergency coro-nary artery bypass surgery in the contemporary percuta-neous coronary intervention era. Circulation. 2002;106: 2346–2350.
13. Flood RD, Popma JJ, Chuang YC, et al. Incidence, angio-graphic predictors and clinical significance of coronary per-foration occurring after new device angioplasty. J Am Coll Cardiol. 1994;23:301.
14. Ajluni SC, Glazier S, Blankenship L, et al. Perforations after percutaneous coronary interventions: clinical, angiographic, and therapeutic observations. Catheter Cardiovasc Diagn. 1994;32:206–212.
15. Wong CM, Kwong Mak GY, Chung DT. Distal coronary artery perforation resulting from the use of hydrophilic coated guidewire in tortuous vessels. Catheter Cardiovasc Diagn. 1998;44:93–96.
16. Yoo BS, Yoon J, Lee SH, et al. Guidewire-induced coronary artery perforation treated with transcatheter injection of polyvinyl alcohol form. Catheter Cardiovasc Interv. 2001; 52:231–234.
17. Woodfield SL, Lopez A, Heuser RR. Fracture of coronary guidewire during rotational atherectomy with coronary perforation and tamponade. Catheter Cardiovasc Diagn. 1998;44:220–223.
18. Aslam MS, Messersmith RN, Gilbert J, Lakier JB. Success-ful management of coronary artery perforation with helical platinum microcoil embolization. Catheter Cardiovasc Interv. 2000;51:320–322.
19. Gaxiola E, Browne KF. Coronary artery perforation repair using microcoil embolization. Catheter Cardiovasc Diagn. 1998;43:474–476.
20. Dippel EJ, Kereiakes DJ, Tramuta DA, et al. Coronary per-foration during percutaneous coronary intervention in the era of abciximab platelet glycoprotein IIb/IIIa blockade: an algorithm for percutaneous management. Catheter Cardio-vasc Interv. 2001;52:279–286.
21. Hamburger JN, Serruys PW, Scabra-Gomes R, et al. Recanalization of total coronary occlusions using a laser guidewire (the European TOTAL Surveillance Study). Am J Cardiol. 1997;80:1419–1423.
22. Stone GW, Rutherford BD, McConahay DR, et al. Proce-dural outcome of angioplasty for total coronary artery occlusion: an analysis of 971 lesions in 905 patients. J Am Coll Cardiol. 1990;15:849–856.
23. Casella G, Werner F, Klauss VV, Mudra H. Successful treat-ment of coronary artery perforation during angioplasty using a new membrane-coated stent. J Invasive Cardiol. 1999;11:622–626.

24. Albiero R, Nishida T, Corvaja N, et al. Left internal mammary artery graft perforation repair using polytetrafluoroethylene-covered stents. Catheter Cardiovasc Interv. 2000;51:78–82.

25. Briguori C, Nishida T, Anzuini A, et al. Emergency polytetrafluoroethylene-covered stent implantation to treat coronary ruptures. Circulation. 2000;102:3028–3031.

26. Campbell PG, Hall JA, Harcombe AA, de Belder MA. The Jomed Covered Stent Graft for coronary artery aneurysms and acute perforation: a successful device which needs careful deployment and may not reduce restenosis. J Invasive Cardiol. 2000;12:272–276.

27. Mulvihill NT, Boccalatte M, Sousa P, et al. Rapid sealing of coronary perforations using polytetrafluoroethylene-covered stents. Am J Cardiol. 2003;91:343–346.

28. Silver KH, Bauman WB, Berkovitz KE. Dual-catheter covered stenting: a novel approach to the treatment of large coronary artery perforations. J Invasive Cardiol. 2003;15: 348–350.

29. Gyenes G, Lazzam C, Feindel C, Roth SL. Successful treatment of a saphenous vein graft pseudoaneurysm with PTFE-covered JoStents. Can J Cardiol. 2003;19: 569–571.

30. Yilmaz H, Demir I, Sancaktar O, Basarici I. Successful management of osteal perforation of left anterior descending artery with coated stent. Int J Cardiol. 2003;88:293–296.

31. Salwan R, Mathur A, Jhamb DK, Seth A. Deep intubation of 8 Fr guiding catheter to deliver coronary stent graft to seal coronary perforation: a case report. Catheter Cardiovasc Interv. 2001;54:59–62.

32. Ruiz-Nodar JM, Mainar V, Bordes P, Jordan A. [Repair of saphenous vein perforation with covered stent during angioplastic]. Rev Esp Cardiol. 2001;54:120–122.

33. Caputo RP, Amin N, Marvasti M, et al. Successful treatment of a saphenous vein graft perforation with an autologous vein-covered stent. Catheter Cardiovasc Interv. 1999;48: 382–386.

34. Welge D, Haude M, von Birgelen C, et al. [Management of coronary perforation after percutaneous balloon angioplasty with a new membrane stent]. Z Kardiol. 1998;87: 948–953.

35. Ramsdale DR, Mushahwar SS, Morris JL. Repair of coronary artery perforation after rotastenting by implantation of the JoStent covered stent. Catheter Cardiovasc Diagn. 1998;45:310–313.

36. Cordero H, Gupta N, Underwood PL, Gogte ST, Heuser RR. Intracoronary autologous blood to seal a coronary perforation. Herz. 2001;26:157–160.

37. Dixon SR, Webster MW, Ormiston JA, et al. Gelfoam embolization of a distal coronary artery guidewire perforation. Catheter Cardiovasc Interv. 2000;49:214–217.

38. Alfonso F, Delgado A, Magalhaes D, et al. Value of intravascular ultrasound in the assessment of coronary pseudostenosis during coronary interventions. Catheter Cardiovasc Interv. 1999;46:327–332.

39. Alvarez JA, Leiva G, Manavella B, Cosentino JJ. Left main crumpling during left anterior descending angioplasty: hitherto unreported location for the "accordion effect." Catheter Cardiovasc Interv. 2001;52:363–367.

40. Asakura Y, Ishikawa S, Asakura K, et al. Successful stenting on tortuous coronary artery with accordion phenomenon: strategy—a case report. Angiology. 1999;50: 765–770.

41. Deligonul U, Tatineni S, Johnson R, Kern MJ. Accordion right coronary artery: an unusual complication of PTCA guidewire entrapment. Catheter Cardiovasc Diagn. 1991; 23:111–113.

42. Goel PK, Agarwal A, Kapoor A. "Concertina" effect during angioplasty of tortuous right and left coronary arteries and importance of using over-the-wire system: a case report. Indian Heart J. 2001;53:87–90.

43. Gouveia D, Escudero J, Domingo E, Anivarro I, Angel J, Soler JS. [De-novo reversible stenoses in tortuous arteries during coronary angioplasty due to the accordion effect. A clinical case and review of the literature]. Rev Port Cardiol. 1997;16:1037–1042, 957.

44. Oyama N, Urasawa K, Sakai H, Kitabatake A. A case of accordion phenomenon accompanied by severe transmural myocardial ischemia. Jpn Heart J. 2002;43:49–54.

45. Premchand RK, Loubeyre C, Lefevre T, et al. Tortuous internal mammary artery angioplasty: accordion effect with limitation of flow. J Invasive Cardiol. 1999;11:372–374.

46. Rauh RA, Ninneman RW, Joseph D, et al. Accordion effect in tortuous right coronary arteries during percutaneous transluminal coronary angioplasty. Catheter Cardiovasc Diagn. 1991;23:107–110.

47. Shea PJ. Mechanical coronary artery shortening with vessel wall deformity during directional coronary atherectomy: first reported case involving the left anterior descending artery. Catheter Cardiovasc Diagn. 1994;33:241–244.

48. Tomai F, Sciarra L, Gioffre PA. Accordion effect of left anterior descending coronary artery after successful stent implantation. G Ital Cardiol. 1999;29:803–804.

49. Escaned J, Flores A, Garcia P, et al. Guidewire-induced coronary pseudostenosis as a source of error during physiological guidance of stent deployment. Catheter Cardiovasc Interv. 2000;51:91–94.

50. Jain D, Kurowski V, Katus HA, Richardt G. A unique pitfall in percutaneous coronary angioplasty of in-stent restenosis: guidewire passage out of the stent. Catheter Cardiovasc Interv. 2001;53:229–233.

51. Schneider DB, Dichek DA. Intravascular stent endothelialization. A goal worth pursuing? Circulation. 1997;95: 308–310.

52. Van Belle E, Tio FO, Couffinhal T, et al. Stent endothelialization. Time course, impact of local catheter delivery, feasibility of recombinant protein administration, and response to cytokine expedition. Circulation. 1997;95:438–448.

53. Abernethy WB 3rd, Choo JK, Oesterle SN, Jang IK. Balloon deflection technique: a method to facilitate entry of a balloon catheter into a deployed stent. Catheter Cardiovasc Interv. 2000;51:312–313.

54. Lotan C, Hasin Y, Stone D, et al. Guide wire entrapment during PTCA: a potentially dangerous complication. Catheter Cardiovasc Diagn. 1987;13:309–312.

55. Alfonso F, Flores A, Escaned J, et al. Pressure wire kinking, entanglement, and entrapment during intravascular ultra-

sound studies: a potentially dangerous complication. Catheter Cardiovasc Interv. 2000;50:221–225.

56. Reith S, Volk O, Klues HG. [Mobilization and retrieval of an entrapped guidewire in the righ coronary artery]. Z Kardiol. 2002;91:58–61.

57. Arce-Gonzalez JM, Schwartz L, Ganassin L, et al. Complications associated with the guide wire in percutaneous transluminal coronary angioplasty. J Am Coll Cardiol. 1987;10:218–221.

58. Lefevre T, Louvard Y, Morice MC, et al. Stenting of bifurcation lesions: a rational approach. J Interv Cardiol. 2001;14:573–585.

59. Batkoff BW, Linker DT. Safety of intracoronary ultrasound: data from a Multicenter European Registry. Catheter Cardiovasc Diagn. 1996;38:238–241.

60. Bech GJ, Pijls NH, De Bruyne B, et al. Usefulness of fractional flow reserve to predict clinical outcome after balloon angioplasty. Circulation. 1999;99:883–888.

61. Pijls NH, De Bruyne B, Peels K, et al. Measurement of fractional flow reserve to assess the functional severity of coronary-artery stenoses. N Engl J Med. 1996;334:1703–1708.

62. Pijls NH, Van Gelder B, Van der Voort P, et al. Fractional flow reserve. A useful index to evaluate the influence of an epicardial coronary stenosis on myocardial blood flow. Circulation. 1995;92:3183–3193.

63. Serruys PW, de Bruyne B, Carlier S, et al. Randomized comparison of primary stenting and provisional balloon angioplasty guided by flow velocity measurement. Doppler Endpoints Balloon Angioplasty Trial Europe (DEBATE) II Study Group. Circulation. 2000;102:2930–2937.

64. Serruys PW, di Mario C, Piek J, et al. Prognostic value of intracoronary flow velocity and diameter stenosis in assessing the short- and long-term outcomes of coronary balloon angioplasty: the DEBATE Study (Doppler Endpoints Balloon Angioplasty Trial Europe). Circulation. 1997;96:3369–3977.

65. Di Mario C, Gil R, de Feyter PJ, et al. Utilization of translesional hemodynamics: comparison of pressure and flow methods in stenosis assessment in patients with coronary artery disease. Catheter Cardiovasc Diagn. 1996;38:189–201.

66. Foster-Smith K, Garratt KN, Holmes DR Jr. Guidewire transection during rotational coronary atherectomy due to guide catheter dislodgement and wire kinking. Catheter Cardiovasc Diagn. 1995;35:224–227.

67. Mintz GS, Bemis CE, Unwala AA, et al. An alternative method for transcatheter retrieval of intracoronary angioplasty equipment fragments. Catheter Cardiovasc Diagn. 1990;20:247–250.

68. Patel T, Shah S, Pandya R, et al. Broken guidewire fragment: a simplified retrieval technique. Catheter Cardiovasc Interv. 2000;51:483–486.

69. Keltai M, Bartek I, Biro V. Guidewire snap causing left main coronary occlusion during coronary angioplasty. Catheter Cardiovasc Diagn. 1986;12:324–326.

70. Hwang MH, Hsieh AA, Silverman P, Loeb HS. The fracture, dislodgement and retrieval of a probe III balloon-on-a-wire catheter. J Invasive Cardiol. 1994;6:154–156.

71. Stellin G, Ramondo A, Bortolotti U. Guidewire fracture: an unusual complication of percutaneous transluminal coronary angioplasty. Int J Cardiol. 1987;17:339–342.

72. Dias AR, Garcia DP, Arie S, et al. [Fracture and intracoronary retention of a guidewire catheter in percutaneous transluminal angioplasty. A case report]. Arq Bras Cardiol. 1989;53:165–166.

73. Prasan A, Brieger D, Adams MR, Bailey B. Stent deployment within a guide catheter aids removal of a fractured buddy wire. Catheter Cardiovasc Interv. 2002;56:212–214.

74. Eggebrecht H, Haude M, von Birgelen C, et al. Nonsurgical retrieval of embolized coronary stents. Catheter Cardiovasc Interv. 2000;51:432–440.

75. Pande AK, Doucet S. Percutaneous retrieval of transsected rotablator coronary guidewire using Amplatz "Goose-Neck snare." Indian Heart J. 1998;50:439–442.

76. Cequier A, Mauri J, Gomez-Hospital JA, et al. [Intracoronary stents in the treatment of angioplasty complications]. Rev Esp Cardiol. 1997;50(suppl 2):21–30.

77. Eeckhout E, Wijns W, Meier B, Goy JJ. Indications for intracoronary stent placement: the European view. Working Group on Coronary Circulation of the European Society of Cardiology. Eur Heart J. 1999;20:1014–1019.

78. Bonnet JL, Avran A, Quilici J, et al. [Acute complications of coronary angioplasty: prevention and management]. Arch Mal Coeur Vaiss. 1999;92:1571–1578.

79. Rath PC, Tripathy MP. Management of coronary artery dissection and perforation following coronary angioplasty by intra coronary stent. J Invasive Cardiol. 1997;9:197–199.

80. Hanratty CG, McKeown PP, O'Keeffe DB. Coronary stenting in the setting of spontaneous coronary artery dissection. Int J Cardiol. 1998;67:197–199.

81. Levin TN, Carroll JD, Feldman T. Bail-out stenting for flow limiting dissections after rotational atherectomy in complex coronary lesions. Catheter Cardiovasc Diagn. 1996;37:300–304.

82. Schomig A, Kastrati A, Mudra H, et al. Four-year experience with Palmaz-Schatz stenting in coronary angioplasty complicated by dissection with threatened or present vessel closure. Circulation. 1994;90:2716–2724.

83. Alfonso F, Hernandez R, Goicolea J, et al. Coronary stenting for acute coronary dissection after coronary angioplasty: implications of residual dissection. J Am Coll Cardiol. 1994;24:989–995.

84. Haude M, Erbel R, Straub U, et al. Results of intracoronary stents for management of coronary dissection after balloon angioplasty. Am J Cardiol. 1991;67:691–696.

6
Complications Related to Coronary Stenting

Samuel M. Butman

1. Case

A 70-year-old woman was referred for possible coronary intervention for an ostial right coronary stenosis discovered during a workup for chest pain where an abnormal nuclear stress study had revealed inferior wall ischemia (Figure 6-1). The coronary intervention was performed using a 7 French Judkins right guiding catheter with predilatation of the area, followed by subsequent stent implantation of a 4.0 = 18-mm stent (Figure 6-2). An additional inflation was performed at 14 atm with a short balloon to assure good stent deployment. The patient left the laboratory without any complaints, but 3 hours later, she developed some moderate chest discomfort, unlike her previous angina. She was given sublingual nitroglycerin, and subsequently developed sinus bradycardia and mild hypotension. An electrocardiogram obtained during that time was normal. She was given intravenous fluids with some response, but soon developed progressive hypotension and bradycardia. Cardiopulmonary resuscitation was begun when she lost both pulse and consciousness. Urgent echocardiography followed by bedside surgical subxyphoid exploration confirmed the suspected hemopericardium. Dissection of the ascending aorta was confirmed at urgent aortography and coronary angiography (Figure 6-3). The latter revealed no evidence of flow compromise to the right coronary artery despite the aortic dissection. The patient made a modest recovery in the hospital without surgical intervention after the hemopericardium was drained, but did not return to her previous state of health.

2. Introduction

Complications, fortunately uncommon, may occur during any one or more of the many steps involved in properly delivering the coronary stent to the area of need, be it placement of the guide catheter, advancement of the guidewire, or during preparatory balloon or device use, as described in previous chapters (Table 6-1). Furthermore, additional complications can occur after the stent and its delivery balloon are being or have been removed. This chapter focuses on the complications reported to date with regard to the coronary stent and its delivery platform.

Proper stenting is the mainstay of the majority of percutaneous coronary interventions today and will be for the foreseeable future. Over 1,000,000 coronary angioplasty procedures are performed annually in the United States with 1 in 1500 Americans having a coated stent implanted by the end of 2003.[1] The number continues to increase with expanding indications, improved design, and better long-term outcomes with the development of stents with various coatings to reduce the incidence of restenosis.[2] The incidence of significant complications is very low.[3-6] In one study of 3340 patients with native coronary artery and saphenous vein graft disease who were treated with new devices, major in-hospital ischemic complications (death, Q-wave myocardial infarction, or emergency coronary artery bypass surgery) occurred in 2.7% of the planned and 9.9% of the unplanned procedures.[4] Multivariate analysis revealed several predictors of major ischemic complications, which included post–myocardial infarction (MI) angina, severe concomitant noncardiac disease, multivessel disease, and de novo lesions. In saphenous vein graft lesions, the independent predictors of major complications for planned procedures included age, high surgical risk [odds ratio (OR) = 4.34], and presence of thrombus (OR = 2.62).

The factors responsible for the occurrence of in-hospital complications and prolonged hospital stay after coronary stent intervention were reported by an Italian consortium, the Registro Impianto Stent Endocoronarico (RISE Study Group).[5] Consecutive patients undergoing coronary stent implantation at 16 medical centers in Italy were prospectively enrolled in the registry. Major

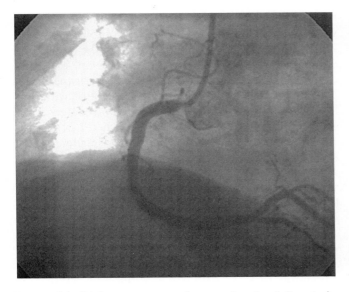

FIGURE 6-1. Right coronary angiogram showing left anterior oblique projection. There is a significant lesion at the ostium, confirmed by nonselective injections and not relieved by intracoronary nitroglycerin.

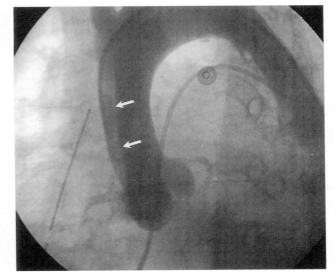

FIGURE 6-3. Aortography reveals a false lumen (arrows) that was not seen to obstruct flow to the right coronary artery.

ischemic complications were defined as death, Q-wave MI, or a need for emergency bypass surgery and emergency repeat angioplasty. The study group consisted of 939 patients in whom 1392 stents were implanted in 1006 lesions. During hospitalization, there were 45 major ischemic complications in 39 patients (4.2%), with 13 events related to acute or subacute thrombosis (1.4%). On multivariate logistic regression analysis, the following factors were predictive of in-hospital complications: increasing age [OR 2.19, 95% confidence interval (CI), 1.18–4.07], unplanned stenting (OR 3.46, 95% CI, 1.65–7.23), and maximal inflation pressure (OR 0.83, 95% CI, 0.75–0.93). Mean hospital stay after stent implantation was 4.1 ± 4.4 days, and a prolonged hospital stay, important in this age of cost containment, was related by multivariate regression analysis to female sex ($P = 0.0001$), prior bypass surgery ($P = 0.03$), nonelective stenting ($P = 0.0001$), use of periprocedural anticoagulation ($P = 0.0001$), and development of major ischemic com-

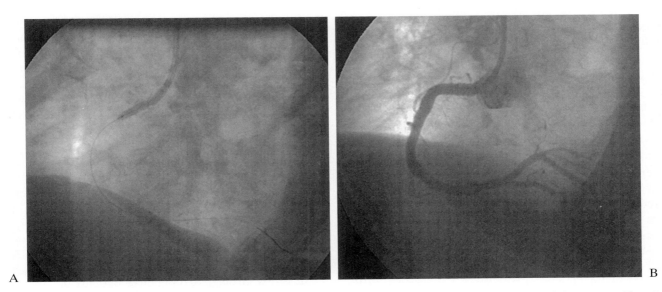

FIGURE 6-2. (A) Balloon angioplasty was performed without incident followed by stent deployment and high-pressure dilatation with a short balloon. (B) Final angiogram after stent implantation.

TABLE 6-1. Complications of the coronary stenting procedure.

Complication	Guide catheter	Guidewire	Stent delivery
Stent loss			X
Stent damage	X		X
Stent migration			X
Balloon rupture			X
Balloon shaft fracture			X
Coronary artery damage	X	X	X
Device entrapment		X	X

plications ($P = 0.0001$). This registry revealed that in an unselected population of patients undergoing coronary stenting, major ischemic complications occur at a relatively low rate (4.2%) and that thrombotic events can be kept at 1.4%.

After the initial introduction and the quick and eager acceptance of coronary stents, the reports were more focused on comparisons to the present era and comparison with other devices (primarily, rotational or directional atherectomy), and there were few reports of complications related to the stent itself.[6-8]

The introduction of coronary stenting for the treatment of acute vessel closure vastly improved the safety of PCI. Data is available regarding angioplasty complication rates when bail-out stenting was made available.[6] Major complications occurred in 4.1% of patients before stent availability and 2.0% afterwards ($P \leq 0.01$). The reduction in complications included in-hospital death (1.1% present vs. 0.7% poststent), Q-wave MI (0.5% present vs. 0.3% poststent), and emergency bypass surgery (2.9% present vs. 1.1% poststent). Furthermore, the introduction of coronary stents has been associated with a 50% reduction in major complications despite greater patient acuity. In this chapter, we will review some of the more unusual reported complications, in addition to those better known.

2. The Early Problems

2.1. Stent Loss

The introduction of the Palmaz-Schatz (Cordis Corporation, Miami, FL) stent, with its delivery sheath, made all interventional cardiologists worry about potential stent loss during delivery, be it in the coronary or peripheral circulations. Reports were not few, but the rate of stent loss was low and adverse effects were fortunately minimal.[9]

Although rarely associated with any clinical sequelae, and despite the majority of contemporary stents now being sheathless, care is still important to prevent this possibility, especially in patients with unfavorable anatomic characteristics. The latter includes lesions in the left circumflex artery, at bend points, and in calcified vessels. Adverse outcomes or more complicated procedures can arise from distal migration of the stent in the coronary or peripheral circulation when full expansion cannot be obtained.[10,11] In one of our earlier experiences, a stent was dislodged from its delivery balloon within the left main/circumflex artery junction.[12] Fortunately, it was still on the guidewire and could be pushed by the delivery balloon into the desired position. A smaller, compliant balloon was then successfully used to reenter the undeployed stent within the lesion and prepare for what was a surprisingly easy and successful deployment (Figures 6-4 and 6-5).

Embolization of coronary stents before deployment is a rare but challenging complication of coronary stenting with a variety of methods for nonsurgical stent retrieval available. In one report, there were 20 cases (0.90%) of intracoronary stent embolization among 2211 patients who underwent implantation of 4066 stents.[13] Twelve of 1147 manually crimped stents (1.04%) and 8 of 2919 premounted stents were lost (0.27%, $P < 0.01$) during retraction of the delivery system because the target lesion could not be either reached or crossed. Percutaneous retrieval was successfully carried out in 10 of 14 patients in whom retrieval was attempted. In 10 patients, stent retrieval was tried with 1.5-mm low-profile angioplasty balloon catheters (success in 7/10) and in 7 cases with myocardial biopsy forceps or a gooseneck snare (success in 3/7). Three patients (15%) underwent urgent coronary artery bypass surgery after failed percutaneous retrieval, but their outcomes were fatal. In two other patients, the stents were compressed against the vessel wall by another stent, without compromising coronary blood flow. In two patients, a stent was lost to the periphery without clinical side effects; treatment was conservative in these cases. Stent retrieval from the coronary circulation with low-profile angioplasty balloon catheters remains a readily available and technically familiar approach that has a relatively high success rate. While embolization of stents before deployment is rare, it is a serious complication of coronary stenting. Fortunately, manual mounting of stents, previously associated with a significantly higher risk of stent embolization, is now rarely necessary.

2.2. Stent Damage

When not lost or retrieved, the stent can be inadvertently damaged, as well. Damage to the stent may occur before, during, or after delivery to the coronary lesion. It may be damaged during the manufacturing process, during packaging, during its preparation outside the patient, during its course through a guiding catheter, and finally during attempts at placement in a diseased coronary vessel. Furthermore, the stent can be damaged after delivery, as well. An example of the latter occurred when avulsion of

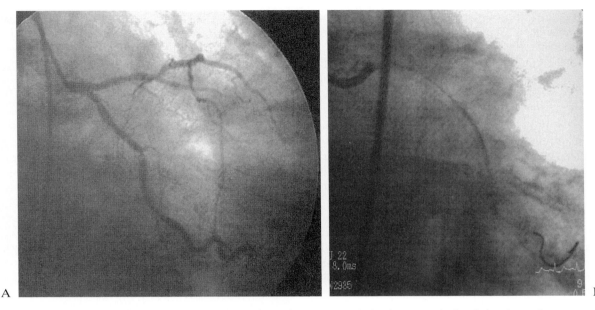

A   B

FIGURE 6-4. (A) Right anterior oblique coronary artery (RAO) caudal view of proximal left circumflex artery focal stenosis. (B) Similar view with 7 French guiding catheter. The undeployed stent has been pushed from its more proximal location to the desired area of the left circumflex artery. (From Butman.[12] Copyright ©2000, reprinted with permission of Wiley-Liss, Inc., a subsidiary of John Wiley & Sons, Inc.)

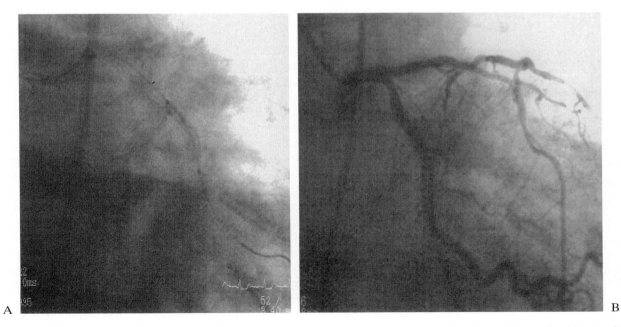

A   B

FIGURE 6-5. (A) Same view. The undeployed stent has been recrossed and predilatated with a low-profile 2.0-mm compliant balloon. The markers of a 3.0-mm semicompliant balloon are lined up for a successful stent expansion. (B) The final angiogram reveals a good angiographic result without evidence of dissection, or trauma to the vessel. (From Butman.[12] Copyright ©2000, reprinted with permission of Wiley-Liss, Inc., a subsidiary of John Wiley & Sons, Inc.)

one or more stent struts occurred when a cutting balloon was used during therapy of an aorto-ostial in-stent restenosis lesion[14] (Figure 6-6, see color plate).

In one of the earlier designs of a coronary stent delivery system, additional stents were required to successfully seal a coronary dissection caused by an articulation stent strut extension during attempts to deploy a stent in a tortuous, calcified right coronary artery (Figure 6-7).[15] In this instance, manipulation of the stent sheath in a tortuous calcified artery produced serial dissections. While less commonly used today, caution should still be the rule when employing rigid sheathed stent systems through tortuous vessels.

When not damaged itself, the stent or our efforts to deliver it may lead to complications, as well. Coronary dissection and even rupture may occur before or during high-pressure balloon expansion of a delivered stent.[16] Severe hemodynamic compromise may occur after saphenous vein graft rupture during high-pressure coronary stent deployment.[17] Immediate balloon inflation followed by implantation of a polytetrafluoroethylene-covered stent can be lifesaving.

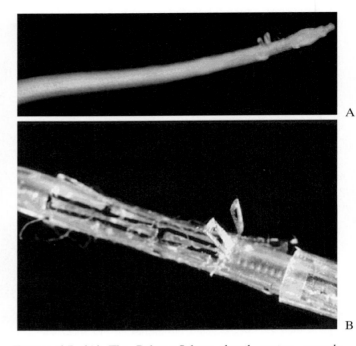

FIGURE 6-7. (A) The Palmaz-Schatz sheath system reveals protrusion of the articulation stent struts despite not being deployed. (B) Close-up view of the articulation stent struts reveals severe bends at a right angle from the sheath–stent system. (From Craig et al.[15] Copyright ©1997, reprinted with permission of Wiley-Liss, Inc., a subsidiary of John Wiley & Sons, Inc.)

3. Issues with Stent Delivery

3.1. Multiple Stents

Because the average number of stents delivered per patient is between 1.5 and 2, a question of whether there is a greater risk when multiple stents are placed was raised. Initial reports had suggested higher procedural and long-term complications among patients treated with multiple stents for diffuse lesions and/or long dissections. Procedural success, major complications, and clinical outcomes in a consecutive series of 1790 patients treated with either multiple (≥3) contiguous stents in single lesions or with only one or two stents were compared.[18] Multiple stents were implanted more often in larger vessels, in the right coronary artery, or in a saphenous vein graft, and for unfavorable lesion characteristics, including long (≥20 mm), calcified, ulcerated, thrombotic, and/or flow-obstructing lesions. Procedural success was similar whether 1 or 2 or ≥3 stents were used. However, non–Q-wave MI was more frequent in the multiple stent group (22.8% vs. 13.4%, $P = 0.005$). Target lesion revascularization was not different between the two groups and overall cardiac event-free survival was similar during follow-up.

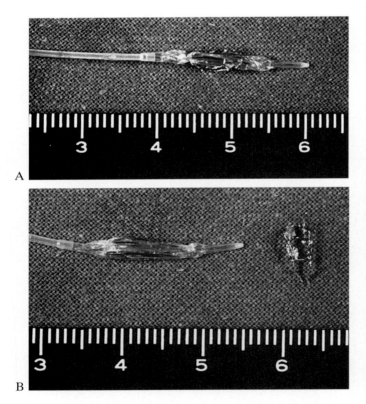

FIGURE 6-6. (A) Close-up image of the avulsed Be Bravo stent struts wrapping around the cutting balloon. (B) After manual removal from the cutting balloon, the avulsed and distorted stent struts are seen on the right. (From Wang et al.[14] Copyright ©2002, reprinted with permission of Wiley-Liss, Inc., a subsidiary of John Wiley & Sons, Inc.) (See color plate.)

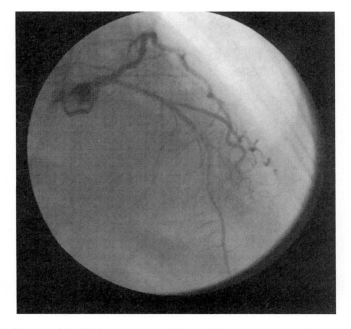

FIGURE 6-8. Right anterior oblique left coronary angiogram reveals an ulcerated lesion in the mid left anterior descending artery. (From Sasseen et al.[22] Copyright ©2002, reprinted with permission of Wiley-Liss, Inc., a subsidiary of John Wiley & Sons, Inc.)

3.2. Stent Migration and Damage

With balloon-expandable stents and stent delivery systems now lower in profile, if the stent struts are not firmly embedded into the arterial wall after initial deployment, stent migration may occur during subsequent passage of a balloon into the stent for high-pressure balloon dilatation.[19] Even when we try to use more sophisticated methods to improve on outcomes, there are hidden risks. Intravascular ultrasound, while not universally used, is generally regarded as helpful in complex or uncertain cases.[20] However, even here the stent may be damaged or dislodged during intracoronary ultrasound imaging and surgical or other intervention may be required.[21] Another complication reported requiring definitive therapy has been ultrasound catheter tip entrapment within the stent (Figures 6-8 and 6-9).[22]

Stent embolization is a rare but acknowledged complication of coronary stenting (Figure 6-10).[23] In this report, with the guidewire still within the embolized stent, the device could be deployed, albeit not in its originally intended target area. Embolization, while typically evident at the time of the loss, may on occasion only be realized later at a follow-up angiogram or intervention.

3.3. Side Branch Intervention Risks

As stent use continues to increase, interventional cardiologists are increasingly faced with patients that require procedures in the vicinity of previously deployed stents.

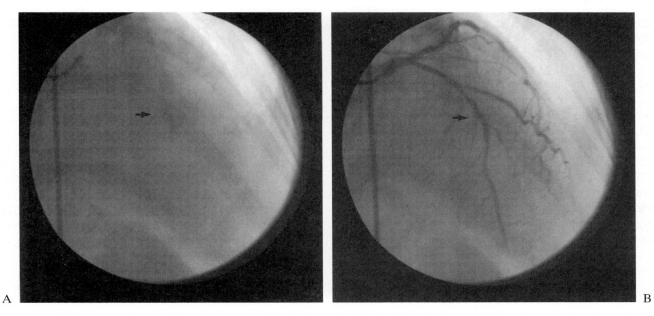

A B

FIGURE 6-9. (A) During intravascular ultrasound pull-back, the most distal aspect of the sheath remained fixed on a stent strut leaving the catheter tip fixed within the stent. (B) After final balloon inflations within the stent, there was TIMI 3 flow despite having the intravascular ultrasound catheter lodged within the stent. (From Sasseen et al.[22] Copyright ©2002, reprinted with permission of Wiley-Liss, Inc., a subsidiary of John Wiley & Sons, Inc.)

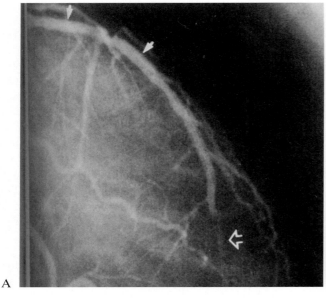 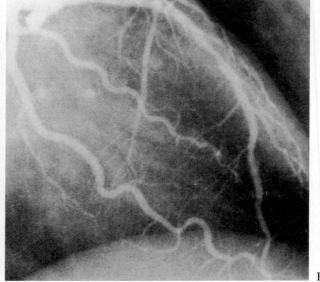

A   B

FIGURE 6-10. (A) The guidewire can be seen passing through the embolized, unexpanded half-stent (open arrow) in the distal left anterior descending coronary artery (LAD). The sites of the two full stents are indicated by the closed arrows. (B) Follow- ing deployment of the embolized half-stent in the distal LAD, flow has improved and the lumen is patent. (From Kirk and Herzog.[23] Copyright ©1997, reprinted with permission of Wiley-Liss, Inc., a subsidiary of John Wiley & Sons, Inc.)

Interventions involving side branches may lead to inadvertent and often unexpected complications as well. In one report, when devices were trapped by the stent, traction on the device resulted in stent dislodgment.[24] The stents were successfully extracted, however, and replaced without complications.

Protection of a side branch and its treatment are a continuing source of creative ways to treat complex anatomy. One method to protect a side branch involves leaving a wire in place while a stent is delivered to the parent vessel. The risk of this approach is fixation of the protective wire in the side branch by the newly delivered stent. The guidewire may become unraveled after positioning an undeployed stent. However, its successful retrieval by removal of the undeployed stent may still be possible.[25] Although side branch protection and placement of a stent with the guidewire left in place is commonly performed without complication, it should be realized that this practice is not without hazard because of the unusual, but serious consequences that could ensue if the entrapped wire were to unravel.

3.4. Balloon Rupture

Balloon rupture occurred in 6% of consecutive patients in one series during coronary stenting.[26] This uncommon event usually does not have clinical or angiographic sequelae, but in some cases, it may induce a new coronary dissection, which may need to be treated. If limited, these can be managed with low-pressure balloon inflations or additional stenting, but further complications may still occur. A ruptured balloon, with or without its broken catheter, can be further complicated by being trapped in an incompletely opened stent.[27] Urgent coronary bypass surgery is usually the only method of salvage in such an event.

3.5. Fracture of the Delivery Balloon Shaft

Fracture of the balloon catheter shaft, particularly when metal reinforced, may occur proximal to the haemostatic Y-adapter.[28] In one report, while attempting to push the stent–balloon assembly through a tortuous vessel, the delivery system carrying the stent had a stainless-steel hypotube constituting the proximal stiff portion of the shaft. The authors suggested that it would probably be prudent to change the catheter or the dilatation strategy once the shaft shows any buckling.

4. Damage to the Coronary Artery

Localized or extensive native coronary or bypass graft dissection caused by balloon rupture at any pressure during stent deployment is fortunately uncommon. However, the diseased and now damaged coronary artery

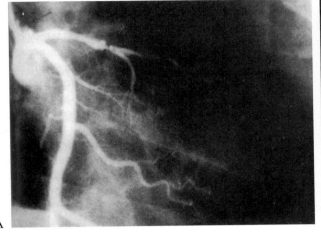

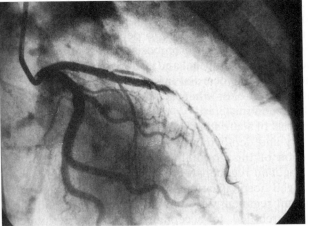

A

B

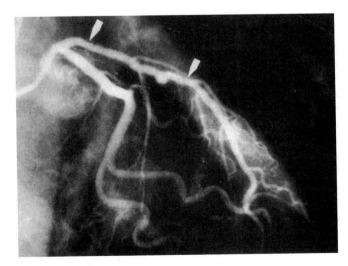

FIGURE 6-11. (A) Severe proximal LAD stenosis. (B) After successful primary stent implantation, there is no residual stenosis and excellent distal flow. (From Nisanci et al.[30] Copyright ©1997, reprinted with permission of Wiley-Liss, Inc., a subsidiary of John Wiley & Sons, Inc.)

may lead to pseudoaneurysmal or true aneurysm formation, fistula formation, or frank perforation with ensuing cardiac tamponade.

4.1. Coronary Artery Aneurysm, Rupture

Pseudoaneurysm formation after either recognized or unrecognized dissection and perforation may also occur. In one report, a giant pseudoaneurysm in a stented coronary segment occurred after stent placement for chronic total occlusion.[29] The aneurysm was treated successfully with the deployment of a covered stent. Aneurysmatic dilation of a coronary artery detected months after successful primary stent implantation has been reported as well (Figures 6-11 and 6-12).[30] In this particular report, the development of an aneurysm occurred in the absence of angiographically visible dissection or other possible causative factors.

4.2. Coronary Artery Fistula Formation

Four months following the placement of a stent in a high-grade, complex lesion of the proximal right coronary artery, restenosis, and contrast spill with rapid clearance into the right atrial space were evident on coronary angiography in one report.[31] Fortunately for the patient, the calculated shunt fraction of the coronary to right atrial fistula was trivial and hemodynamically insignificant.

4.3. Device Entrapment

Overzealous, inappropriate, or unnecessary use of novel or higher profile devices may also lead to complications. Entrapment of a cutting balloon within a deployed stent,

discussed earlier with a favorable outcome, can also result in acute occlusion of the coronary artery and actual extraction of the stent on withdrawal as well.[32] Removal of the cutting balloon in this case resulted in acute occlusion of the coronary artery. While commonly used, application of a cutting balloon for in-stent restenosis still mandates caution given its higher profile.

4.4. Acute and Subacute Stent Thrombosis

Subacute stent thrombosis is a rare complication, associated with a 40%–60% risk of myocardial infarction, and

FIGURE 6-12. Six months later, as part of routine surveillance, an angiogram revealed a discrete saccular aneurismal dilatation. The arrows indicate the proximal and distal margins of the implanted stent. (From Nisanci et al.[30] Copyright ©1997, reprinted with permission of Wiley-Liss, Inc., a subsidiary of John Wiley & Sons, Inc.)

22. Sasseen BM, Burke JA, Shah R, et al. Intravascular ultrasound catheter entrapment after coronary artery stenting. Catheter Cardiovasc Interv. 2002;57:229–233.

23. Kirk MM, Herzog WR. Deployment of a previously embolized, unexpanded, and disarticulated Palmaz-Schatz stent. Catheter Cardiovasc Diagn. 1997;42:331–334.

24. Grantham JA, Tiede D, Holmes DR. Technical considerations when intervening with coronary device catheters in the vicinity of previously deployed stents. Catheter Cardiovasc Interv. 2001;52:214–217.

25. Thew ST, Klein LW. Report of an undeployed stent causing the unraveling of a coronary artery guidewire being used for sidebranch protection. J Invasive Cardiol. 2002;14: 106–107.

26. Alfonso F, Perez-Vizcayno MJ, Hernandez R, et al. Clinical and angiographic implications of balloon rupture during coronary stenting. Am J Cardiol. 1997;80:1077–1080.

27. Cheng LC, Lee J, Chiu SW. A rare complication of PTCS: ruptured balloon with retained broken catheter. Ann Thorac Cardiovasc Surg. 2000;6:266–267.

28. Jain D, Hartmann F, Katus HA, Richardt G. An unusual complication of metallic balloon shaft fracture during coronary angioplasty. J Invasive Cardiol. 2001;13:314–316.

29. Kishi K, Hiasa Y, Takahashi T. Delayed development of a giant coronary pseudoaneurysm after stent placement for chronic total occlusion. J Invasive Cardiol. 2003;15:273–276.

30. Nisanci Y, Coskun I, Oncul A, Umman S. Coronary artery aneurysm development after successful primary stent implantation. Catheter Cardiovasc Diagn. 1997;42:420–422.

31. Karim MA. Coronary artery aneurysmal fistula: a late complication of stent deployment. Int J Cardiol. 1996; 57:207–209.

32. Kawamura A, Asakura Y, Ishikawa S, et al. Extraction of previously deployed stent by an entrapped cutting balloon due to the blade fracture. Catheter Cardiovasc Interv. 2002;57:239–243.

33. Virmani R, Guagliumi G, Farb A, et al. Localized hypersensitivity and late coronary thrombosis secondary to a sirolimus-eluting stent: should we be cautious? Circulation. 2004;109:701–705.

34. Liistro F, Colombo A. Late acute thrombosis after paclitaxel eluting stent implantation. Heart. 2001;86:262–264.

35. Schomig A, Neumann FJ, Kastrati A, et al. A randomized comparison of antiplatelet and anticoagulant therapy after the placement of coronary-artery stents. N Engl J Med. 1996;334:1084–1089.

36. Schuhlen H, Hadamitzky M, Walter H, et al. Major benefit from antiplatelet therapy for patients at high risk for adverse cardiac events after coronary Palmaz-Schatz stent placement: analysis of a prospective risk stratification protocol in the Intracoronary Stenting and Antithrombotic Regimen (ISAR) trial. Circulation. 1997;95:2015–2021.

37. Alfonso F, Garcia-Touchard A, Lopez-Meneses M, et al. Ticlopidine pretreatment before coronary stenting is associated with sustained decrease in adverse events. Data from the Evaluation of Platelets IIb/IIIa Inhibitor for Stenting (EPISTENT) Trial. Ital Heart J Suppl. 2001;(2):805–806.

38. Silva JA, White CJ, Ramee SR, et al. Treatment of coronary stent thrombosis with rheolytic thrombectomy: results from a multicenter experience. Catheter Cardiovasc Interv. 2003;58:11–17.

39. Smith SC, Winters KJ, Lasala JM. Stent thrombosis in a patient receiving chemotherapy. Catheter Cardiovasc Diagn. 1997;40:383–386.

40. Danenberg HD, Lotan C, Hasin Y, et al. Acute myocardial infarction—a late complication of intracoronary stent placement. Clin Cardiol. 2000;23:376–378.

41. Tolerico PH, McKendall GR. Femoral endarteritis as a complication of percutaneous coronary intervention. J Invasive Cardiol. 2000;12:155–157.

42. Bouchart F, Dubar A, Bessou JP, et al. Pseudomonas aeruginosa coronary stent infection. Ann Thorac Surg. 1997;64:1810–1813.

43. Amin H, Munt B, Ignaszewski A. Staphylococcus aureus pericarditis with tamponade complicating coronary angioplasty and stenting. Can J Cardiol. 1998;14:1148–1150.

44. Dieter RS. Coronary artery stent infection. Clin Cardiol. 2000;23:808–810.

45. Liu JC, Cziperle DJ, Kleinman B, Loeb H. Coronary abscess: a complication of stenting. Catheter Cardiovasc Interv. 2003;58:69–71.

46. Bottner RK, Hardigan KR. Cardiac tamponade following stent implantation with adjuvant platelet IIb/IIIa receptor inhibitor administration. Catheter Cardiovasc Diagn. 1997; 40:380–382.

47. Foster-Smith KW, Garratt KN, Higano ST, Holmes DR. Retrieval techniques for managing flexible intracoronary stent misplacement. Catheter Cardiovasc Diagn. 1993;30: 63–68.

48. Cishek MB, Laslett L, Gershony G. Balloon catheter retrieval of dislodged coronary artery stents: a novel technique. Catheter Cardiovasc Diagn. 1995;34:350–352.

49. Berder V, Bedossa M, Gras D, et al. Retrieval of a lost coronary stent from the descending aorta using a PTCA balloon and biopsy forceps. Catheter Cardiovasc Diagn. 1993;28: 351–353.

50. Patel TM, Shah SC, Gupta AK, Ranjan A. Successful retrieval of transradially delivered unexpanded coronary stent from the left main coronary artery. Indian Heart J. 2002;54:715–716.

51. Kaluza GL, Joseph J, Lee JR, et al. Catastrophic outcomes of noncardiac surgery soon after coronary stenting. J Am Coll Cardiol. 2000;35:1288–1294.

52. Wilson SH, Fasseas P, Orford JL, et al. Clinical outcome of patients undergoing non-cardiac surgery in the two months following coronary stenting. J Am Coll Cardiol. 2003;42: 234–240.

7
Complications of Atherectomy Devices

Gurpreet Baweja, Ashish Pershad, Richard R. Heuser, and Samuel M. Butman

1. Case

An 83-year-old male underwent coronary angiography, which revealed a heavily calcified, completely occluded proximal left anterior descending artery (LAD), a 60%–70% stenosis of the proximal left circumflex, and significant disease in the distal dominant right coronary artery. Percutaneous revascularization of the LAD was attempted.

A 7 Fr guiding catheter was placed into the ostium of the left main artery. After numerous failed attempts to cross the lesion with balloon catheters, it was decided to perform rotational atherectomy. A rotational atherectomy guidewire was advanced into the distal LAD. A 1.25-mm diameter rotational atherectomy burr was then advanced to the lesion and atherectomy was performed at 150,000 rpm, with passage through the calcified area into the mid-LAD. Following this, attempt to retract the burr from the LAD failed (Figure 7-1A). It would freely advance distally, but would not come back through the original calcified lesion. Intracoronary nitroglycerin did not resolve the problem.

The guiding catheter was then withdrawn approximately 1 cm from the ostium of the left main, leaving the Rotablator burr and wire across the lesion. A second guiding catheter was then placed into the left main artery via the left femoral approach. A 2-mm diameter Ace Balloon (Scimed, Maple Grove, MN) was then passed into the LAD. The guidewire was advanced distally into a septal branch just beyond the original calcified lesion but proximal to the entrapped Rotablator burr (Figure 7-1B). Balloon dilatation was then performed at the site of the calcified area, with near-full expansion occurring at 8 atm of pressure. After the dilatation, the burr was easily removed. Angiography revealed flow into the distal LAD without evidence of coronary dissection or perforation (Figure 7-1C).

2. Introduction

A variety of interventional devices are available for percutaneous coronary interventions. The most widely used devices are balloons for angioplasty and stents for additional support and long-term benefit. Atherectomy devices are niche devices that ablate, score, or extract plaque and are either used as a stand-alone technique or in combination with balloon angioplasty and stent placement for the treatment of coronary lesions. Atherectomy devices, initially viewed as competitive technology to angioplasty with balloons, are now considered complimentary to balloon angioplasty and stenting.

There have been several different types of atherectomy devices and methods available, including: (i) cutting balloon atherectomy, (ii) rotational atherectomy, (iii) directional atherectomy, (iv) transluminal extraction atherectomy, and (v) several types of laser atherectomy devices, including holmium, Nd:Yag, and excimer lasers. The use of directional atherectomy, transluminal extraction, and laser atherectomy has fallen out of favor in the United States but may still have a role in specific lesion subsets. We will describe the techniques and some of the known and reported complications associated with each.

Cutting balloon angioplasty and rotational atherectomy are the most commonly used atherectomy tools today. Atherectomy devices have been associated with a higher complication rate than procedures simply utilizing balloon angioplasty and stents.[1] The lesions necessitating the use of these devices are typically more complex, typically American College of Cardiology/American Heart Association (ACC/AHA) class B1–B2 or C lesions. In addition, these devices are associated with device-specific complications that add to the degree of difficulty of the procedure, thereby making the incidence of complications with their use higher than with conventional angioplasty balloons and stents. Finally, the devices have a

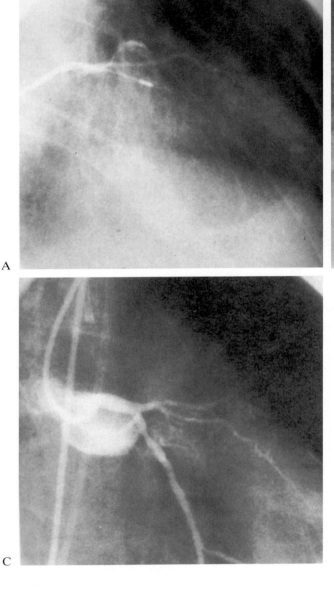

FIGURE 7-1. (A) Area of entrapment of the rotational atherectomy burr (1.25-mm diameter) in the proximal left anterior descending artery (LAD). (B) Balloon dilation of the calcified area in the LAD, proximal to the entrapped burr. Note the distal wire tip in a septal perforator branch. (C) Final angiography after the burr was removed. No evidence of perforation or dissection. (Reproduced with permission from Grise et al.[22])

higher profile and require specific, typically stiffer guiding catheters, and larger arterial sheaths for access.

3. Cutting Balloon Atherectomy

Cutting balloon angioplasty (CBA) combines conventional angioplasty with microsurgical technology in an attempt to minimize vessel trauma and injury during balloon dilatation of coronary stenoses. Cutting balloon angioplasty consists of microsurgical blades or atherotomes mounted longitudinally on the outer surface of a noncompliant polyethylene terephthalate (PET) balloon. These unique atherotomes score the plaque at the lesion site and accomplish dilatation of the target lesion at lower inflation pressures than a conventional balloon. Acute gain is achieved primarily via plaque compression and, to a lesser extent, vessel wall expansion, thereby reducing elastic recoil.

Because the device is a hybrid between an atherectomy catheter and a balloon angioplasty (BA) catheter, the risks of complications are higher than BA, but lower than other atherectomy devices. The incidence of angiographically significant dissections and coronary perforations has been reported to be 3.6% and 0.9%, respectively.[2] In the Global Randomized Trial of the CB, the rates of dissection and perforation as a complication of this device were in the 0.5%–1% range. Risk factors for dissection are lesion length and angiographic severity of stenosis; however, minor dissections do not appear to negatively impact clinical event or restenosis rates.[3]

When CBA is used to treat ostial side branch disease a potential complication is the retention of the device in the side branch, if care is not taken to have a portion of the balloon within the parent vessel. This is of particular concern when treating side branches through stent struts in the parent vessel. The deflated profile of the CBA is larger than a standard balloon catheter due to both the fixed metal atherotomes and the noncompliant balloon material that is used (Table 7-1).

Complications unique to CBA include acute dissection, delayed presentation of perforation, and focal coronary aneurysms. Case reports of perforations presenting 4 days after the index coronary intervention have been described.[4] Follow-up angiography has identified coronary aneurysms at the site of CBA as early as 4 weeks following intervention and as late as 6 months later.[5] The hypothesis for the etiology of the aneurysms is that the injury created by the atherotomes at the lesion site extends to the subintimal tissue, leading to gradual thinning of the vessel wall with subsequent aneurismal change. These complications are typically seen with aggressive oversizing of the balloon in eccentric lesions or in calcified vessels at higher inflation pressures (Figure 7-2).

Another rare but unique complication of CBA is the inadvertent dislodgement and/or extraction of mature stents after the device is trapped in the vicinity of stents.[6–8] The mechanism of this complication is that either the initial wire passage was through a stent strut or, more rarely, the actual constraint and distortion of the cutting balloon blade by the stent strut results in entrapment. In case of entrapment, attempts to detach the blade from the stent strut by sequentially inflating and deflating the balloon or referral for surgery may be the only management options. Careful attention to inflation pressure guidelines and appropriate sizing of the device appear to be the two critical steps in minimizing the possibility of this complication occurring.

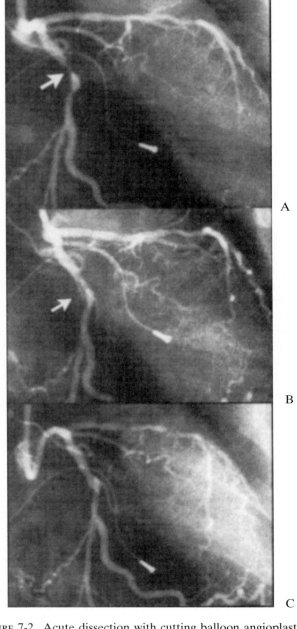

A

B

C

FIGURE 7-2. Acute dissection with cutting balloon angioplasty. (A) Angiography demonstrates a stenosis in the proximal left circumflex artery (arrow). (B) A type C dissection is noted following cutting balloon angioplasty. (C) No evidence of angiographic restenosis in the 6-month follow-up angiogram. (Reprinted from American Journal of Cardiology 81 (11), Marti et al.[3] Copyright 1998, with permission from Excerpta Medica, Inc.)

TABLE 7-1. Cutting balloon: comparison of the first-generation devices and second-generation devices.

First-generation device	Ultra 2
Rigid atherotomes making tortuous vessel negotiation difficult.	Longer T notches in atherotome base to increase flexibility of device.
Catheter without hydrophilic coating and therefore less lubricious.	Smaller catheter shaft (2Fr) with Bioslide hydrophilic coating to improve crossability and smaller catheter tip to improve deliverability.

4. Rotational Atherectomy

A major limitation of BA is the inability to dilate heavily calcified lesions and the immediate elastic recoil noted in ostial lesions whereby the initial satisfactory result may lack durability. This failure rate of BA has been reported to be as high as 4.7%.[9] Rotational atherectomy (RA) uses differential cutting and orthogonal displacement of plaque to cause plaque abrasion and thereby improve luminal diameter.

There are two general approaches to lumen enlargement with RA. The first is a technique that relies on small burr sizes and modification of lesion compliance prior to conventional angioplasty and stent placement. The burr: artery ratio in this strategy is 0.5–0.6. This approach facilitates lumen enlargement by angioplasty rather than lesion debulking. An alternate strategy involves using relatively large burr sizes to achieve greater lesion debulking and therefore lumen enlargement. The burr:artery ratio in this instance is approximately 0.8. The application of the aggressive debulking strategy is limited by failure to access some lesions due to excessive tortuosity, dissections, and severe bradycardia. The immediate and long-term results, however, are similar with either strategy with regard to late target vessel revascularization and clinical restenosis.[10,11]

The risk of non–Q-wave myocardial infarction (MI) is reported at 6%–11%, depending on the series studied.[12–14] Clinical complications are similar to those reported following BA. Death, Q-wave MI, and urgent coronary artery bypass graft surgery (CABG) occur in 0.8%, 0.9%, and 1.6% of patients, respectively.[15] The use of potent antiplatelet agents, such as abciximab and clopidogrel, combined with lower rotational speeds have contributed to refinement of the technique and a decline in the incidence of non–ST-segment elevation MI following RA.[16]

The periprocedural complications of the RA device are somewhat unique and can vary in acute versus stable coronary syndrome. Diffuse spasm at the site of atherectomy is common and can be minimized with prophylactic administration of large doses of intracoronary vasodilators. The angiographic complications include dissection (7.5%–10.4%), abrupt closure (2.5%–2.6%), slow flow or no-reflow phenomenon (2.9%–9.1%), and perforation (0.6%–1.5%).[12,17]

The incidence of the no-reflow phenomenon following percutaneous coronary intervention has been reported to be highest following RA.[12] The common denominator of no-reflow is inadequately perfused myocardium without evidence of persistent mechanical epicardial obstruction, usually with concomitant myocardial ischemia.[18] While perhaps intuitively obvious, potential mechanisms for no-reflow during RA include microvascular dysfunction due to alpha constriction and vasospasm, distal embolization of thrombus and debris, capillary plugging by red blood cells and activated neutrophils, endothelial cell dysfunction with loss of capillary integrity, interstitial cell dysfunction, and increased angiotensin II receptor density.[19] A suggested strategy for prevention of no-reflow follow-

ing RA is the routine use of abciximab, intracoronary adenosine, and a drug cocktail in the flush solution including nitrates, verapamil, and heparin.[16,20,21] Nonetheless, elevation of cardiac markers of myocardial injury has been the rule rather than the exception with this device.

Coronary perforation and subsequent tamponade is a rare complication of coronary interventions, but RA has had relatively high reported rates.[12,22,23] Once recognized, the treatment involves prolonged balloon inflation and reversal of anticoagulation for distal perforations, and ideally implantation of a covered stent for proximal or midvessel perforation.[24] The burr:artery ratio is the major determinant in periprocedural complications. The incidence of immediate serious angiographic complications was 5.1% when the burr:artery ratio was less than 0.7, but more than doubled to 12.7% when the ratio was greater than 0.7.[25]

Due to the unique mechanism of plaque debulking, a few other complications are also specific to this device. These include guidewire bias, fracture of the drive shaft, and burr entrapment.[26–28] Burr entrapment, as described in the case example at the beginning of this chapter, typically occurs with smaller burr sizes and a tight stenosis where the burr is able to cross the lesion, but does not ablate sufficient plaque to be able to return to a neutral position. This has been called the Kokesi phenomenon.[29] A Kokesi doll is a Japanese wooden doll made of a separate head and body. The head has a bulb-shaped neck and the body has a hole. The hole in the body is smaller than the bulb-shaped neck. When the neck is inserted into the hole of the body, the body is rotated at high speeds and the neck is pushed into the body. Once inside the hole, the head of the doll can be rotated but not pulled out of the body. This phenomenon occurs because the frictional heat generated enlarges the orifice and the coefficient of friction is lower than the coefficient of friction at rest. The entrapment of the burr is an analogous situation to that described with the Kokesi doll. The management of this uncomfortable situation involves exclusion of coronary vasospasm, followed by balloon dilatation at the site of the original stenosis, thereby permitting retraction of the burr.[22]

The risk of access-site bleeding with atherectomy devices in earlier trials was higher than with angioplasty alone because of the large sheath sizes necessary and more aggressive anticoagulation regimens used with these newer devices. Bleeding risk was reported to be between 1% and 7%, with need for surgical repair in 2% of cases in an early series of patients.[30]

The availability of large lumen but smaller French sized guiding catheters now allows for the use of 6F guiding catheters for burr sizes up to 1.5 mm and 7F guiding catheters for burr sizes up to 2 mm. The need for a 9F guiding catheter, which was commonplace in the early days of RA, is now rare. The predictors of groin complications in patients undergoing atherectomy are older age, female gender, obesity, hypertension, prolonged heparin administration, and presentation with unstable anginal syndromes.[30]

The predictors of an overall adverse outcome in patients undergoing RA include higher degree ACC/AHA lesion score, diffuse disease, female gender, right coronary artery lesions, and more severe stenosis angulation.[12,31,32] For the device to be used successfully in high-risk patients, elective use of the intraaortic balloon pump favors procedural hemodynamic stability and successful outcomes as well.[33]

The occurrence of a significant creatine kinase–MB (CPK-MB) or troponin leak following percutaneous coronary intervention is associated with a poorer prognosis. As discussed above, one expects a higher incidence of CPK-MB leak following RA, given that the plaque is pulverized and distal embolization almost expected. While the incidence of CPK-MB elevation during RA is reported to be higher than with BA, it initially was reported to be lower than with stand-alone stenting.[34] Changes in RA technique and concomitant medical therapy, including the use of intravenous antiplatelet agents and intracoronary calcium channel blockers in combination with slow burr advancement, short ablation times, multiple burr approaches, and avoidance of hypotension during ablation have contributed favorably in reducing the incidence of CPK-MB leaks during RA.[10]

5. Directional Atherectomy

The directional atherectomy catheter, an over-the-wire cutting and retrieval system, is designed to remove obstructive atheroma with directional control. Angiographic studies reveal that the method of lumen enlargement is one-third due to excision of atherosclerotic tissue and two-thirds the result of stretching of the vessel wall.[35,36] However, intravascular studies suggest that 50%–70% of the acute lumen gain is actually due to plaque excision.[37] Whichever the method, this rigid and relatively large device is now less commonly used due to the ease and safety of coronary stenting and the lack of competitive scientific data to support its widespread use.

While the incidence of complications following directional coronary atherectomy (DCA) was reported to be similar to that following balloon angioplasty, in randomized studies the incidence of severe coronary dissection leading to abrupt closure of the vessel was 7%.[38–40] Dissection may be caused by deep seating of the special and unique guiding catheters, the nose cone of the atherectomy device itself, and, rarely, the guide wire. The difference in the incidence of dissections in the BOAT (Balloon vs. Optimal Atherectomy Trial) and the CAVEAT (Coronary Angioplasty Versus Excisional Atherectomy Trial) trials have been attributed to the experience of the investigators using the device and operator technique.[39,40]

The principal mechanism of abrupt closure following BA is dissection, whereas the most common cause following directional atherectomy is thrombosis.[41] Although angiography is not sensitive for thrombus detection, it is thought to complicate 2% of atherectomy procedures.[42,43]

Distal embolization and no-reflow may complicate up to 13.4% of atherectomy procedures, being more frequent in vein grafts and in thrombus-laden lesions. Dislodgement of thrombus or friable plaque from the target lesion or from incomplete capture of tissue stored in the nosecone collection chamber appear to be the causes. An unusual complication of dislodgement of nosecone itself has also been described (Figures 7-3 and 7-4).

The incidence of perforation with directional atherectomy is 1%. Occasionally a perforation is related to attempts to snip the dissection flap in the setting of acute abrupt closure.[44] The management of perforations in the setting of directional atherectomy is no different than following angioplasty. However, the site of a contained perforation managed conservatively may lead to focal ectasia, pseudoaneurysm, and restenosis[45–47] (Figures 7-5 and 7-6).

Although initially thought of as an acceptable strategy in the management of bifurcation lesions, the incidence of side branch occlusion and major adverse cardiac events was noted to be high with the use of directional atherectomy in the CAVEAT I trial.[45] Directional atherectomy is no longer a preferred method in the management of coronary bifurcations.

While the incidence of death, Q-wave MI, or CABG or vascular complications was no higher with DCA when compared to angioplasty, the incidence of non–Q-wave MI is higher with directional atherectomy when compared to angioplasty in the major trials.[39,40] Creatine kinase–MB leak may possibly be mitigated with the concurrent use of glycoprotein IIb/IIIa platelet receptor antagonists, but still may confer a worse long-term outcome when a significant leak occurs.[46,47] Risk factors predictive of complications following directional coronary atherectomy include operator inexperience and lesion angulation.[48]

Clinical trials with directional atherectomy have not fulfilled the initial goal and hope of reduced restenosis rates compared to an angioplasty/stent strategy.[1] While vascular remodeling accounts for the majority of the late loss after an atherectomy procedure, intravascular ultrasound studies suggest that intimal proliferation is the major mechanism for restenosis.[49,50]

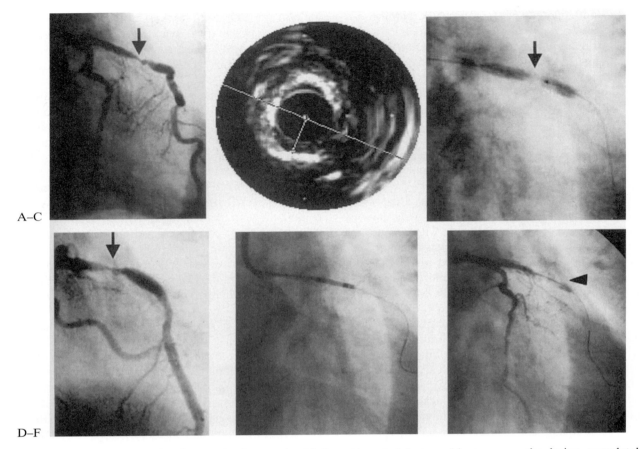

A–C

D–F

FIGURE 7-3. A high-grade lesion is seen in the proximal left anterior descending (LAD) artery (upper left, A). Intravascular ultrasound imaging demonstrates a fibrocalcific plaque (upper middle, B). High-pressure balloon inflation was ineffective (upper right, C) and mild haziness was visible after the inflation (lower left, D). Directional atherectomy was attempted but unable to cross the lesion completely. The nosecone (arrowhead) to LAD can be seen now detached from the catheter (lower middle and right, E and F). Also note the dissection extending back to the origin of the LAD. (Reproduced with permission from Suguta M, et al. Catheter Cardiovasc Interv. 2001;54:526–530.)

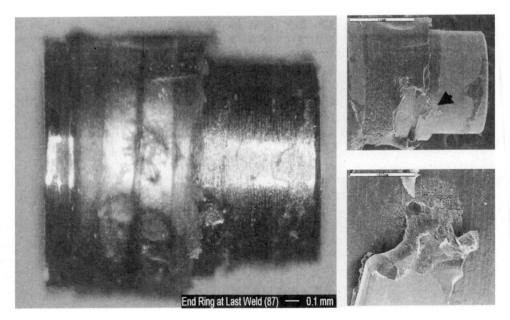

FIGURE 7-4. Photo of damaged directional atherectomy catheter (left). Electron micrographs show dimple sign (arrowhead). (Reproduced with permission from Suguta M, et al. Catheter Cardiovasc Interv. 2001;54:526–530.)

End Ring at Last Weld (87) ——— 0.1 mm

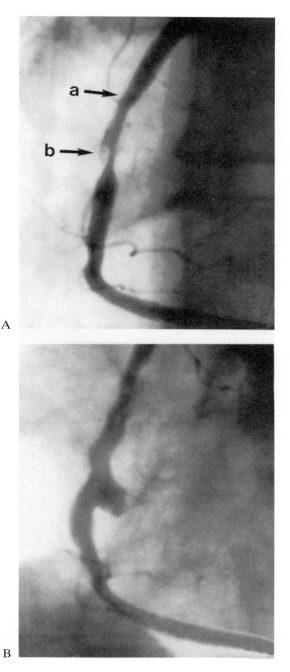

A

B

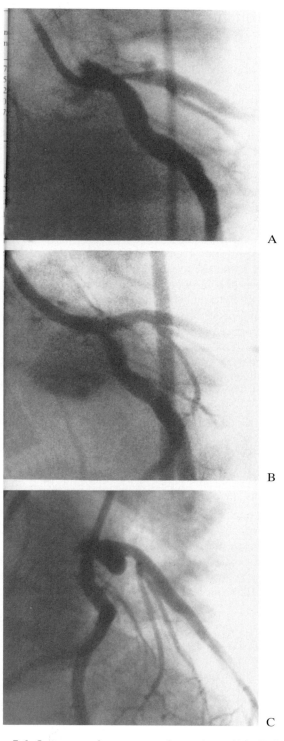

A

B

C

FIGURE 7-5. Acute pseudoaneurysm formation. (A) Balloon angioplasty performed in the proximal segment of right coronary artery caused significant dissection (arrows a and b). (B) A large pseudoaneurysm formed following adjuvant directional coronary atherectomy. Inspection during emergency bypass surgery revealed a significant hematoma in the right coronary artery without any blood in pericardium. (Reproduced with permission from Hinohara T, et al. Catheter Cardiovasc Diagn. 1993;(suppl 1):61–71.)

FIGURE 7-6. Late pseudoaneurysm formation. (A) Before directional atherectomy (DCA) a significant ostial left anterior descending artery lesion is evident. (B) Post-DCA the result appears excellent except for mild irregularity at the site. (C) Three months later a large pseudoaneurysm is noted at the atherectomy site. (Reproduced with permission from Hinohara T, et al. Catheter Cardiovasc Diagn. 1993;(suppl 1):61–71.)

6. Transluminal Extractional Atherectomy

The role of transluminal extraction atherectomy (TEC) in the current armentarium of interventional devices is controversial. It primarily served as an adjunct to stenting in thrombotic/degenerated bypass vein grafts. Its use in native coronary arteries is less certain. Transluminal extractional atherectomy is an over-the-wire cutting and aspiration system with two stainless-steel blades attached to a flexible hollow torque tube whose proximal end is attached to a vacuum bottle for aspiration of excised atheroma, thrombus, and debris. A warmed lactated Ringer's solution is infused under pressure to create a slurry of blood and tissue which facilitates aspiration. Transluminal extractional atherectomy guiding catheters are typically stiffer, and over rotation and deep seating increase the risk of ostial injury. Additionally, due to the stiff guidewires needed, temporary but confusing psuedolesions are frequent within the vessel.

Angiographic complications after vein graft TEC, similar to those with conventional BA, include distal embolization, no reflow, and abrupt closure. As with any mechanical device, unusual complications can be seen. Detachment of TEC cutter head from the shaft while in a graft has been reported (Figure 7-7). Distal embolization is more likely to occur in grafts with filling defects and in old degenerated grafts.[51] The use of abciximab or other glycoprotein inhibitors did not impact the incidence of CPK-MB elevation after transluminal extraction atherectomy in high-risk vein grafts when compared to historical controls.[52]

The explanation of the lack of effect of glycoprotein inhibitors in vein grafts is unknown, but it has been hypothesized that the major mechanism leading to CPK-MB elevation is from distal embolization of soft acellular atheromatous material found under the fibrous cap rather than the thrombus per se.[52]

7. Laser Angioplasty

Although BA and coronary stenting are now the mainstay of mechanical revascularization, there were and still are several potential advantages in the use of laser angioplasty in treating lesions not well suited for conventional BA. These include an avid absorption of laser energy within both thrombus and atherosclerotic plaques, thereby facilitating the rapid removal of clot while simultaneously debulking underlying plaque. Finally, and perhaps more interesting, is the potential for vaporization of harmful vasoactive and procoagulant substances as well.[53,54] The laser angioplasty technique

has improved considerably over the years with a more optimal wavelength selection, a greater availability of multifiber catheters, and the wisdom of technique advancements including saline flush and slow advancement, and there has been significantly reduction in the number of adverse events associated with the laser technique.[55,56]

Despite potential advantages and technical advancements, the larger issue of whether laser ablation is the optimal means of treating atherosclerosis is unresolved. Like other ablative techniques, this technique has not improved clinical outcomes nor has it lowered restenosis rates in randomized clinical trials.[57,58] In a recent meta-analysis of three major comparative trials between balloon angioplasty and laser angioplasty (excimer or holmium),[1] there was no difference in 30-day mortality among groups, and 30-day major adverse cardiac events, angiographic restenosis, and cumulative revascularization (up to 360 days) favored balloon angioplasty.

The feasibility and safety of excimer laser angioplasty in the acute myocardial infarction setting were reported in CARAMEL (Cohort of Acute Revascularization in Myocardial Infarction with Excimer Laser) study.[59] Overall procedural success was 91% with establishment of thrombolysis in myocardial infarction (TIMI) grade 3 flow and initial reduction of stenosis from 83% to 52%, down to 20% after stenting. Death occurred in 4% of patients (all presented with cardiogenic shock). Complications included perforation (0.6%), dissection (5% major and 3% minor), acute closure (0.6%), distal embolization (2%), no reflow (0.6%), late thrombosis (1.4%), and bleeding (3%). Figure 7-8 shows a case of laser angioplasty–related perforation of the right coronary artery.

Laser angioplasty has also been found useful as an adjunct to treat in-stent restenosis by reducing the amount of hyperplastic tissue within the stent and allowing more effective balloon dilatation. The data from Laser Angioplasty for Restenotic Stents (LARS) multicenter registry demonstrated a high procedural success rate (98.9%) and a low rate of complications (1.1%), as well as a trend towards better angiographic result compared with BA alone.[60] Major complications, including death, MI, or urgent revascularization, were comparable to BA, and minor complications, including repeat BA or catheterization, recurrent angina, renarrowing of more than 50%, and vascular or bleeding events, also occurred with similar frequencies in both groups. However, because this was not a randomized trial, the advent of drug-eluting stents, and the additional risks with this treatment, further studies to assess the benefit of laser angioplasty over conventional angioplasty in this setting are not likely.

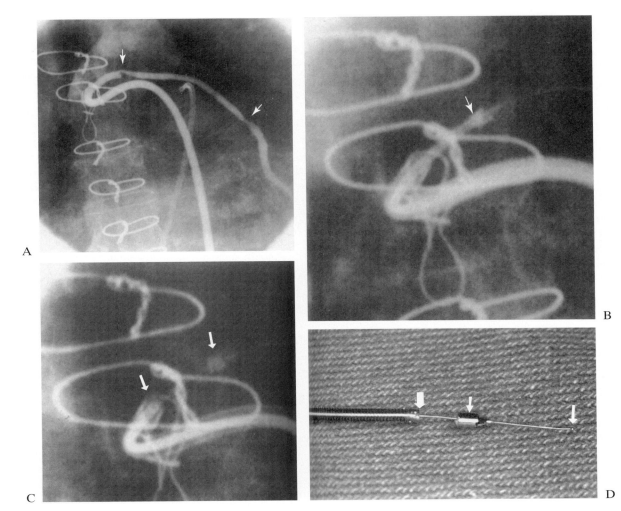

FIGURE 7-7. Detachment of transluminal extraction catheter (TEC) cutter head from shaft. (A) Saphenous vein bypass graft to obtuse marginal branch with significant proximal and distal stenosis (arrowheads). (B) A TEC catheter in the proximal portion of the saphenous graft. Note the discontinuity between torque-tube shaft (arrow) and TEC cutter. (C) Dislodgement of TEC cutter (arrow) in proximal saphenous graft. End of torque-tube shaft is seen within guiding catheter (arrow). (D) Detached cutter (middle arrow) from torque-tube shaft (wide arrow) and guidewire (arrow). (Reproduced with permission from Mishra JP, et al. Catheter Cardiovasc Diagn. 1997; 42:325–327.)

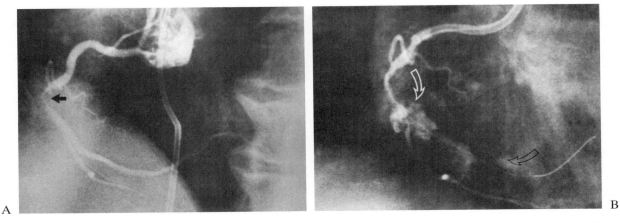

FIGURE 7-8. (A) A 95% eccentric stenosis (arrow) is evident in the mid portion of the right coronary artery. (B) After laser angioplasty, a large collection of contrast is seen adjacent to the course of right coronary artery indicative of perforation (arrows). Little flow is seen distally due to compression by the hematoma. (Reproduced with permission from Parker JD, et al. Catheter Cardiovasc Diagn. 1991;22:118–123.)

8. Conclusions

Atherectomy devices remain important niche devices in the interventional arena. They are no longer competing technologies to angioplasty/stents but are complimentary. Each of the atherectomy devices has device-specific complications related to their mechanism of action. Recognizing the correct indications and inherent limitations in the use of various atherectomy devices and diligence to good angioplasty technique serve to keep these at the minimum. The concepts of plaque excision, modification, and debulking still remain attractive in this new era of drug-eluting stents. Further modifications, or, hopefully, newer devices, may still bring the concept back into a more accepted and wider role in the treatment of atherosclerotic lesions.

References

1. Bittl JA, Chew DP, Topol EJ, et al. Meta-analysis of randomized trials of percutaneous transluminal coronary angioplasty versus atherectomy, cutting balloon athertomy, or laser angioplasty. J Am Coll Cardiol. 2004;43:936–942.
2. Kondo T, Kawaguchi K, Awaji Y, Mochizuki M. Immediate and chronic results of cutting balloon angioplasty: a matched comparison with conventional angioplasty. Clin Cardiol. 1997;20:459–463.
3. Marti U, Martin V, Garcia J, et al. Significance of angiographic coronary dissection after cutting balloon angioplasty. Am J Cardiol. 1998;81:1349–1352.
4. Maruo T, Yasuda S, Miyazaki S. Delayed appearance of coronary artery perforation following cutting balloon angioplasty. Catheter Cardiovasc Interv. 2002;57:529–531.
5. Bertrand OF, Mongraim R, Soulami, et al. Development of coronary artery aneurysm after cutting balloon angioplasty. Catheter Cardiovasc Interv. 1998;44:449–452.
6. Harb TS, Ling FS. Inadvertent stent extraction six months after implantation by an entrapped cutting balloon. Catheter Cardiovasc Interv. 2001;53:415–419.
7. Grantham JA, Tiede DJ, Holmes DR Jr. Technical considerations when intervening with coronary device catheters in the vicinity of previously deployed stents. Catheter Cardiovasc Interv. 2001;52:214–217.
8. Kawamura A, Asakura Y, Ishikawa S, et al. Extraction of previously deployed stent by an entrapped cutting balloon due to the blade fracture. Catheter Cardiovasc Interv. 2002;57:239–243.
9. Myler RK, Shaw RE, Stertzer SH, et al. Lesion morphology and coronary angioplasty: current experience and analysis. J Am Coll Cardiol. 1992;19:1641–1652.
10. Kini A, Marmur J, Duvvuri S, et al. Rotational atherectomy: Improved procedural outcome with evolution of technique and equipment. Catheter Cardiovasc Interv. 1999;46:305–311.
11. Bass TA, Williams DO, Ho KKL, et al. Is an aggressive rotablator strategy preferable to a standard Rotablator strategy in patients with heavily calcified coronary lesions? A report from the STRATAS trial. J Am Coll Cardiol. 1998;31:378A.
12. Ellis SG, Popma JJ, Buchbinder M, et al. Relation of clinical presentation, stenosis morphology, and operator technique to the procedural results of rotational atherectomy facilitated angioplasty. Circulation. 1994;89:882–892.
13. Kobayashi Y, De Gregorio J, Kobayashi N, et al. Lower restenosis rate with stenting following aggressive versus less aggressive rotational atherectomy. Catheter Cardiovasc Interv. 1999;46:406–414.
14. Brown DL, George CJ, Steenkiste AR, et al. High-speed rotational atherectomy of human coronary stenoses: acute and one-year outcomes from the New Approaches to Coronary Intervention (NACI) registry. Am J Cardiol. 1997; 80:60K–67K.
15. Warth DC, Leon MB, O'Neill W, et al. Rotational atherectomy multicenter registry: acute results, complications and 6-month angiographic follow-up in 709 patients. J Am Coll Cardiol. 1994;24:641–648.
16. Williams MS, Coller BS, Vaananen HJ, et al. Activation of platelets in platelet rich plasma by rotablation is speed dependant and can be inhibited with abciximab. Circulation. 1998;98:742–748.
17. Doshi SN, Kini A, Kim MC, et al. A comparative study of rotational atherectomy in acute and stable coronary syndromes in the modern era. Am J Cardiol. 2003;92: 1404–1408.
18. Kloner RA Ganote CE, Jennings RB. The no-reflow phenomenon after temporary coronary occlusion in the dog. J Clin Invest. 1974;54:1496–1508.
19. Klein LW, Kern MJ, Berger P, et al. Suggested management of the no-reflow phenomenon in the cardiac catheterization laboratory. Catheter Cardiovasc Interv. 2003;60:194–201.
20. Hanna GP, Yhiop P, Fujise K, et al. Intra-coronary adenosine administered during rotational atherectomy of complex lesions in native coronary arteries reduces incidence of no-reflow phenomenon. Catheter Cardiovasc Interv. 1999;48:275–278.
21. Cohen BM, Weber VJ, Blum RR, et al. Cocktail attenuation of rotational ablation flow effects CARAFE pilot study. Catheter Cardiovasc Diagn. 1996;(suppl 3):69–72.
22. Grise MA, Yeager MJ, Tierstein PS. A case of entrapped rotational atherectomy burr. Catheter Cardiovasc Interv. 2002;57:31–33.
23. Von Sohsten R, Kopistansky C, Cohen M. Kussmaul WG 3rd. Cardiac tamponade in the "new device era": evaluation of 6999 consecutive percutaneous coronary interventions. Am Heart J. 2000;140:279–283.
24. Ramsdale DR, Mushawar SS, Morris JL. Repair of coronary artery perforation after rotastenting by implantation of the Jostent covered stent. Catheter Cardiovasc Diagn. 1998;45:310–313.
25. Safian RD, Feldman T, Muller DW, et al. Coronary angioplasty and rotablator atherectomy trial (CARAT): immediate and late results of a prospective multicenter randomized trial. Catheter Cardiovasc Interv. 2001;53: 213–220.
26. Woodfield SL, Lopez A, Heuser RR. Fracture of coronary guidewire during rotational atherectomy with coronary perforation and tamponade. Catheter Cardiovasc Diagn. 1998;44:220–223.

27. Reisman M, Harms V. Guide wire bias: potential sources of complications with rotational atherectomy. Catheter Cardiovasc Diagn. 1996;3(suppl):64–68.

28. Medizinische K. A rare unreported complication during coronary rotational atherectomy. J Invasive Cardiol. 2000;12:428–430.

29. Kaneda H, Saito S, Hosokawa G, et al. Trapped rotablator: Kokesi phenomenon. Catheter Cardiovasc Interv. 2000;49: 82–84.

30. Waksman R, King SB 3rd, Douglas JS, et al. Predictors of groin complications after balloon and new device coronary intervention. Am J Cardiol. 1995;75:886–889.

31. Teirstein PS, Warth DC, Haq N, et al. High speed rotational atherectomy for patients with diffuse coronary disease. J Am Coll Cardiol. 1991;18:1694–1701.

32. Ellis SG, Vandormael MG, Cowley MJ, et al. Coronary angiographic and clinical determinants of procedural outcome with angioplasty for multivessel disease. Implications for patient selection. Multivessel Angioplasty Prognosis Study Group. Circulation. 1990;82:1193–1202.

33. Ryan TJ, Faxon DP, Gunnar RM, et al. Guidelines for percutaneous transluminal coronary angioplasty. A report of the ACC/AHA task force on assessment of diagnostic and therapeutic cardiovascular procedures. J Am Coll Cardiol. 1988;12:529–545.

34. Sharma S, Kini A, Kini S, et al. Creatine kinase MB enzyme elevation after coronary intervention with different devices. J Am Coll Cardiol. 1998;31(suppl A):215A.

35. Penny WF, Schmidt DA, Safian RD, et al. Insights into the mechanism of lumen enlargement after directional coronary atherectomy. Am J Cardiol. 1991;67:435–437.

36. Rowe MH, Robertson GC, Simpson JB, et al. Amount of tissue removed by directional coronary atherectomy. Circulation. 1990;82:III-312.

37. Matar F, Mintz G, Farb A, et al. The contribution of tissue removal to lumen improvement after directional coronary atherectomy. Am J Cardiol. 1994;74:647–650.

38. Fortuna R, Walston D, Hansell H, Schulz GY. Directional coronary atherectomy: experience in 310 patients. J Invasive Cardiol. 1995;7:57–64.

39. Topol E, Leya F, Pinkerton C, et al. A comparison of directional atherectomy with coronary angioplasty in patients with coronary artery disease. N Engl J Med. 1993; 329:221–227.

40. Baim DS, Cutlip DE, Sharma SK, et al. Final results of the balloon versus optimal atherectomy trial (BOAT). Circulation. 1998;329:221–227.

41. Popma J, Topol E, Hinohara T, et al. Abrupt vessel closure after directional coronary atherectomy. J Am Coll Cardiol. 1992;19:1372–1379.

42. Carrozza J, Baim J. Complications of directional coronary atherectomy. Incidence, causes and management. Am J Cardiol. 1993;72:47E–54E.

43. Mehta S, Popma J, Margolis JR, et al. Complications with new angioplasty devices: are these device specific? J Am Coll Cardiol. 1996;27:168A.

44. Selmon MR, Robertson GC, Simpson JB, et al. Retrieval of media and adventitia by directional coronary atherectomy and angiographic correlation. Circulation. 1990;82:III-624.

45. Brener SJ, Leya FS, Apperson-Hansen C, et al. A comparison of debulking versus dilatation of bifurcation coronary arterial narrowings (from the CAVEAT I trial). Am J Cardiol. 1996;78:1039–1041.

46. Cutlip DE, Ho KKL, Senerchia C, et al. Classification of myocardial infarction after directional coronary atherectomy and relation to clinical outcome: results of the OARS trial. Circulation. 1995;92:I–616.

47. Lefkovits J, Blankenship JC, Anderson K, et al. Increased risk of non Q wave MI after directional atherectomy is platelet dependent: evidence from the EPIC trial. J Am Coll Cardiol. 1996;28:849–850.

48. Ellis S, De Cesare N, Pinkerton C, et al. Relation of stenosis morphology and clinical presentation to the procedural results of directional coronary atherectomy. Circulation. 1991;84:644–653.

49. Mintz G, Kent KM, Satler LF, et al. Dimorphic mechanisms of re-stenosis after DCA and stents: a serial intravascular ultrasound study. Circulation. 1995;92:I–546.

50. Mitsuo K, Degawa T, Nakamura S, et al. Serial intravascular ultrasound evaluation of the mechanism of re-stenosis after directional coronary atherectomy. Circulation. 1995; 92:I–149.

51. Hong MK, Popma JJ, Pichard AD, et al. Clinical significance of distal embolization after transluminal extraction atherectomy in diffusely diseased saphenous vein grafts. Am Heart J. 1994;127:1496–1503.

52. Khan MA, Liu MW, Chio FL, et al. Effect of abciximab on cardiac enzyme elevation after TEC in high risk saphenous vein graft lesions: comparison with a historical control group. Catheter Cardiovasc Interv. 2001;52:40–44.

53. Topaz O. Plaque removal and thrombus dissolution with pulsed-wave lasers' photoacoustic energy—biotissue interactions and their clinical manifestations. Cardiology. 1996; 87:384–391.

54. Topaz O, Minisi AJ, Bernardo NL, et al. Alterations of platelet aggregation kinetics with ultraviolet laser emission: the "stunned platelet" phenomenon. Thromb Haemost. 2001;86:1087–1093.

55. Tcheng JE. Saline infusion in excimer laser coronary angioplasty. Semin Interv Cardiol. 1996;1:135–141.

56. Topaz O, Lippincott R, Bellendir J, et al. "Optimally spaced" excimer laser coronary catheters: performance analysis. J Clin Laser Med Surg. 2001;19:9–14.

57. Appelman YE, Piek JJ, Strikwerda S, et al. Randomised trial of excimer laser angioplasty versus balloon angioplasty for treatment of obstructive coronary artery disease. Lancet. 1996;347:79–84.

58. Stone GW, de Marchena E, Dageforde D, et al. Prospective, randomized, multicenter comparison of laser-facilitated balloon angioplasty versus stand-alone balloon angioplasty in patients with obstructive coronary artery disease. The Laser Angioplasty Versus Angioplasty (LAVA) Trial Investigators. J Am Coll Cardiol. 1997;30:1714–1721.

59. Topaz O, Ebersole D, Das T. Excimer laser angioplasty in acute myocardial infarction (the CARMEL multicenter trial). Am J Cardiol. 2004;93:694–701.

60. Giri S, Ito S, Lansky AJ, et al. Clinical and angiographic outcome in the laser angioplasty for restenotic stents (LARS) multicenter registry. Catheter Cardiovasc Interv. 2001;52:24–34.

8
The No-Reflow Phenomenon

H.M. Omar Farouque and David P. Lee

A 53-year-old man presented to the emergency room with an acute inferolateral myocardial infarction (MI) of 2 hours duration. Urgent coronary angiography showed minor obstructive disease in the left coronary system and a 100% thrombotic occlusion in the mid segment of a large right coronary artery (Figure 8-1A). After one inflation with a 3.0 × 15-mm balloon a severe stenosis was apparent (Figure 8-1B), and the patient became profoundly bradycardic and hypotensive. There was thrombolysis in myocardial infarction (TIMI) grade 1 flow into the distal vessel. Temporary pacing and intravenous fluid administration were initiated with an improvement in hemodynamics. Further balloon inflations were performed across the lesion with minimal improvement in coronary flow. An intravenous abciximab infusion was begun. A 3.5 × 18-mm Medtronic AVE S670 stent was deployed across the occluded segment resulting in TIMI grade 1 epicardial flow. There was a hazy filling defect at the proximal stent edge. An overlapping 4.0 × 9-mm Medtronic AVE S7 stent was deployed to cover this area. Angiography revealed minimal residual stenosis, but slow filling of the vessel into the distal main right coronary artery and its branches (Figure 8-1C). Over a 25-minute period, small boluses of intracoronary nitroglycerin (total of 150 μg), and adenosine (total 168 μg) were given through the guiding catheter and an intra-aortic balloon pump was deployed via the contralateral femoral artery. Epicardial coronary flow improved to TIMI grade 2 (Figure 8-1D), but myocardial perfusion was poor with distal occlusion of a posterolateral branch and impaired microvascular flow (Figure 8-1E, F). The blood pressure stabilized, and the patient was transferred to the coronary care unit with mild ongoing chest discomfort and residual ST-segment elevation. The creatine kinase level peaked at 3295 U/L. Intra-aortic balloon pump support was continued for 36 hours. The patient's in-hospital course was complicated by left ventricular failure, but he was discharged from the hospital 5 days after admission.

This case of no-reflow occurring in the context of an acute infarct coronary intervention is illustrative of an infrequent but difficult management problem faced by the interventional cardiologist. In spite of expeditious treatment, normal coronary flow could not be reestablished. The patient went on to sustain a large inferolateral myocardial infarct. In this chapter aspects of coronary no-reflow relevant to the interventional cardiologist are reviewed.

1. Definition and Historical Aspects

The term *no-reflow phenomenon* was coined by Majno and colleagues over three decades ago to describe a process wherein tissue reperfusion was impaired after temporary interruption of cerebral blood flow in rabbits.[1] In fact, the no-reflow phenomenon had previously been described in other organ systems, including the heart.[2] Subsequently, Kloner and colleagues observed persistent no-reflow in canine hearts after 90 minutes of complete coronary occlusion.[3] They undertook detailed electron microscopic studies of the poorly reperfused regions and found evidence of prominent ultrastructural changes within the coronary microvessels. It was apparent from these early studies that the microvasculature was central to the pathophysiology of no-reflow.

Several years after the discovery of coronary no-reflow in animals, Schofer and colleagues provided preliminary data for impaired capillary reperfusion in patients with reperfused acute anterior MI.[4] Subsequently, Bates and colleagues reported a case of angiographic no-reflow after acute anterior infarction treated with thrombolysis.[5] Coronary no-reflow occurring in the setting of percutaneous coronary intervention (PCI) was initially reported by Kitazume and colleagues,[6] and soon afterwards by Wilson and colleagues.[7] The typical features were reduced coronary blood flow as evidenced by poor contrast washout and transient, but severe, myocardial

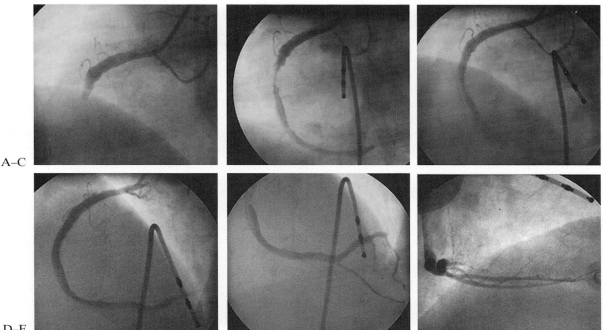

A–C

D–F

FIGURE 8-1. Right coronary angioplasty and stenting complicated by no-reflow in the setting of an acute inferolateral myocardial infarction. Angiographic images are of the right coronary artery in the left anterior oblique projection (A–E), and right anterior oblique projection (F). Refer to the case report in the text for details.

ischemia immediately after balloon dilatation of the culprit lesion in the absence of persisting mechanical obstruction. The coronary flow disturbances were unresponsive to intracoronary nitroglycerin and thrombolytic infusion.[7] After these early reports, a greater awareness of this syndrome was forthcoming.[8–11]

2. Angiographic Diagnosis and Assessment of No-Reflow

The recognition of the no-reflow phenomenon during PCI is usually self-evident. In its most dramatic form, one may see a stagnant column of contrast dye with a slight to-and-fro motion within the epicardial vessel adjacent to the lesion site after angioplasty or stenting. The essential element is a decrease in antegrade epicardial flow in the absence of a mechanical cause. However, there has been no clear consensus regarding its definition. Recently, it has been suggested that reduced antegrade flow (slow flow) or a complete absence of antegrade flow (no flow) represent differing degrees of the same phenomenon, both of which lead to myocardial ischemia.[12] In an effort to simplify the terminology, Eeckhout and Kern recommend that the expression *no-reflow* be used to describe the spectrum of flow disturbances typified by any reduction of antegrade epicardial blood flow.[12]

The TIMI (thrombolysis in myocardial infarction) classification, which was devised to categorize coronary blood flow after thrombolytic therapy for MI, is often used as a convenient qualitative measure of epicardial blood flow (Table 8-1).[13] Using this angiographic classification, no-reflow can be defined as anything less than

TABLE 8-1. Definition of TIMI epicardial blood flow grades.

TIMI flow grade	Definition
Grade 0	No perfusion: no antegrade flow beyond the occlusion.
Grade 1	Penetration without perfusion: contrast dye passes beyond the obstruction but does not opacify the vessel beyond the obstruction for the duration of filming.
Grade 2	Partial perfusion: contrast dye passes beyond the obstruction and opacifies the vessel beyond it. The rate of entry of contrast dye into the vessel distal to the obstruction, or its rate of clearance from the distal vessel, or both, is visibly slower than that of an opposite coronary artery or the coronary bed proximal to the obstruction.
Grade 3	Complete perfusion: flow of contrast dye distal to the obstruction occurs as promptly as flow into the vessel proximal to the obstruction. Clearance of contrast dye from the involved bed is as rapid as clearance of contrast dye from an uninvolved bed in the same artery or an opposite coronary artery.

TIMI grade 3 flow after an otherwise successful PCI. To standardize the assessment of epicardial coronary flow and to enhance its reproducibility, the TIMI flow classification has been further refined to create the corrected TIMI frame count.[14] This measure has been used in angiographic trials, but has little role in assessing no-reflow acutely in the catheterization laboratory. A more useful measurement that can be assessed during PCI is the myocardial blush observed after contrast dye injections.[15] This concept was developed further into the semiquantitative TIMI myocardial perfusion grade classification.[16] Using this angiographic method, one can assess tissue perfusion by examining the filling and clearance of contrast dye from the myocardium itself. This is a reflection of myocardial tissue perfusion and has been shown to be a predictor of mortality after pharmacologic or mechanical reperfusion of MI that is independent of epicardial coronary flow.[15-17] As is the case with TIMI epicardial flow grades, clinical outcomes are better in patients with normal myocardial perfusion grades. Moreover, patients with TIMI grade 3 epicardial flow may be further stratified according to outcome based on myocardial perfusion grades, with the lowest mortality rates seen in the subgroup with normal myocardial perfusion.[16] These findings underscore the importance of tissue-level perfusion in determining outcomes.

An important aspect in the definition of no-reflow is the exclusion of a persisting mechanical etiology for flow reduction. This includes the presence of a significant residual stenosis, epicardial spasm, an obstructive dissection flap, or thrombus. Competitive flow from coronary collaterals may also mimic the appearance of no-reflow. These abnormalities can often be detected during angiography in multiple projections. Intravascular ultrasound may be of use to exclude some of the former when ambiguity persists. Pressure gradient measurements across the epicardial vessel, and distal vessel angiography can also be utilized to elucidate the cause of flow disturbances after angioplasty.[18] The absence of a pressure gradient between the guiding catheter and distal vessel through an infusion catheter suggests that an intervening epicardial obstruction is unlikely. Contrast injection through the infusion catheter can help exclude distal obstruction caused by macroembolism. In the presence of no-reflow, contrast washout remains poor and may reflux into the proximal vessel.

Blood flow characteristics in patients with no-reflow have been studied using intracoronary Doppler flow velocimetry.[19] The typical features include early systolic flow reversal, reduction in systolic antegrade flow velocity, and a rapid deceleration of diastolic flow velocity. The use of a pressure-sensing guidewire may also enable further assessment of the coronary microcirculation.[20] Although these invasive methods have some appeal in instances of diagnostic uncertainty, no-reflow can usually be recognized from clinical and angiographic data leading to prompt initiation of therapy. The additional manipulations required are time-consuming in an emergent setting, and cannot be recommended for routine management of no-reflow.

3. Incidence and Predisposing Factors

Several large retrospective studies have examined the incidence of no-reflow after PCI. Piana and colleagues reviewed the procedural records and angiograms of 1919 patients at a single center.[10] The overall incidence of no-reflow (TIMI flow <3) was 2.0%. This study established that patients having acute infarct and saphenous vein graft PCI are most susceptible. Other factors associated with no-reflow were recanalization of an occluded vessel and angiographic evidence of thrombus. Using a more stringent definition of no-reflow (TIMI flow ≤1), Abbo and colleagues reported their experience in 10,676 coronary interventions, where no-reflow was seen in 0.6% of patients.[11] Factors that were associated with no-reflow included PCI in the setting of MI, and complex lesion morphology (lesion ulceration, calcification, thrombus, total occlusion). This group later highlighted the risk of inducing no-reflow (TIMI flow <3) when intervening on degenerated vein grafts, which was seen in 42% of cases.[21] Similar findings have been reported from a more contemporary series of 4264 patients in which no-reflow (TIMI flow ≤1) was identified in 3.2% of patients.[22] In a multivariate analysis, vein graft PCI, acute infarct PCI, unstable angina, cardiogenic shock, and complex lesion subsets [American Heart Association (AHA) type B2 and C lesions] were associated with a greater likelihood of no-reflow.

Perhaps the highest incidence of no-reflow occurs in degenerated and thrombotic saphenous vein grafts.[23] Sdringola and colleagues found several clinical and angiographic factors to be independent predictors of the occurrence of no-reflow (TIMI flow <3) in saphenous vein grafts, including thrombus [odds ratio (OR) = 6.9], acute coronary syndromes (OR = 6.4), degenerated vein grafts (OR = 5.2), and ulcerated lesions (OR = 3.4).[23] The risk of no-reflow was 1%–10% if no or one factor was present, 20%–40% for two factors, and 60%–90% in the presence of three or more factors. Negative univariate predictors included vein graft age <3 years and interventions at the graft ostium or instent restenotic lesions.

Clinical and angiographic variables that may predict no-reflow in the infarct setting include inferior location, a large infarct-related artery (≥4mm), and evidence of heavy thrombus burden in the infarct-related artery.[24] In this study, no-reflow (TIMI flow ≤2) occurred in 15% of patients during acute infarct PCI. Pre-interventional angiographic features that independently predicted no-reflow included an abrupt cutoff at the occlusion site, thrombus proximal to the occlusion, persistent distal dye staining, and an incomplete obstruction with thrombus having a linear dimension more than three times the reference lumen diameter. Delayed reperfusion was a predictor of no-reflow in this study; however, other studies have not confirmed this finding.[25] Pre-intervention intravascular ultrasound studies indicate that large vessels and atheroma with ultrasound features indicating lipid-rich plaques are independent predictors of no-reflow during infarct PCI, with the likely mechanism being distal embolization of plaque fragments.[26] An intriguing clinical factor associated with no-reflow after acute anterior infarct PCI is the absence of pre-infarction angina.[25,27] The potential mechanism by which prior angina protects against no-reflow is unclear but may be related to ischemic myocardial or microvascular preconditioning.

The occurrence of no-reflow varies according to the type of interventional device used. No-reflow is more frequent in patients having rotational atherectomy (7.7%), extraction atherectomy (4.5%), or directional atherectomy (1.7%), compared to balloon angioplasty (0.3%).[11] Other studies have found an incidence of no-reflow between 1.2% and 15.7% during rotational atherectomy, with the variability due in part to differing definitions of no-reflow.[28–32] Typically no-reflow is observed after a treatment run once the burr has been retracted. The mechanism of no-reflow is believed to be related to the generation of microparticulate debris during plaque ablation and platelet activation with resulting microvascular dysfunction. The formation of microbubbles may also play a role.[33] The occurrence of no-reflow with rotational atherectomy is more frequent with longer device activation times, right coronary artery intervention, unstable angina, or recent infarction in the territory of the treated vessel, long lesions, and recent use of β-blockers.[28,29] No-reflow after rotational atherectomy is reversible in the majority of instances, unlike no-reflow seen after extraction atherectomy.[11]

4. Clinical Manifestations and Outcomes

The majority of patients with angiographic no-reflow develop clinical evidence of ischemia. The typical features include chest pain and ST-segment changes (elevation or depression). In the early series, 78%–86% of patients displayed one or more of these manifestations, the remainder being clinically silent.[10,11] With reversal of no-reflow the ischemic changes can be expected to resolve. However, in the setting of acute infarct PCI an improvement in epicardial flow may be seen although impaired microvascular perfusion may persist as demonstrated by poor myocardial blushing. In this instance symptoms and ECG changes may not resolve rapidly. Less common accompaniments of no-reflow include con-

duction system disturbances and hypotension. The lack of symptoms in some patients has been attributed to the presence of collateral flow or nonviable myocardium in the distal territory.[11] Conversely the more dramatic presentations may be related to the amount of myocardium subtended by the vessel with no-reflow, the presence and severity of coronary disease in remote vessels, or the degree of baseline ventricular dysfunction.

The short- and long-term clinical outcomes in patients with no-reflow after PCI are serious. The risk of in-hospital mortality is increased as much as 10-fold compared to patients without this complication.[11] Other studies have also found a high incidence of death associated with no-reflow.[10,22] In these studies no-reflow has been associated with mortality rates of 7.4% and 15%. The incidence of Q-wave and non–Q-wave MI is 5 to 10 times greater in patients with no-reflow.[10,11,22] Indeed, no-reflow has been found to be a strong independent predictor of death or MI after PCI with an odds ratio of 3.6.[22]

Morishima and colleagues found that myocardial rupture was more frequent in the setting of acute infarct angioplasty complicated by no-reflow, with more severe coronary flow disturbances being associated with a worse prognosis.[34] In an extension of their initial report, these investigators followed 120 patients with acute infarction treated with balloon angioplasty alone for a mean of nearly 6 years.[35] No-reflow (TIMI flow ≥2) occurred in 25% of their study group, and death was nearly four times more common in this group. Multivariate analysis showed that angiographic no-reflow was an independent predictor of cardiac death, and of other cardiac events including malignant nonfatal arrhythmias and cardiac failure over the follow-up period. No-reflow was associated with an adverse impact on left ventricular remodeling. In keeping with these findings, large multicenter trials of angioplasty and stenting in acute infarction also demonstrate worse outcomes when normal coronary flow cannot be re-established.[36,37] An interesting observation from the Stent PAMI (Primary Angioplasty in Myocardial Infarction) study was the lower rate of TIMI grade 3 flow in patients receiving stents compared to balloon angioplasty.[36] This effect has been attributed to distal embolization of thrombus extruded through the stent struts. However, in the more recent CADILLAC (Controlled Abciximab and Device Investigation to Lower Late Angioplasty Complications) trial, stenting and angioplasty were associated with similar rates of postprocedural TIMI grade 3 flow.[38]

5. Pathophysiology of Coronary No-Reflow

Although its etiology is incompletely understood, several factors have been postulated based on experimental studies and clinical observations. These are summarized

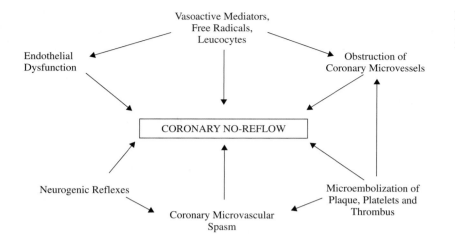

FIGURE 8-2. A schematic diagram depicting the various factors involved in the pathophysiology of coronary no-reflow.

in Figure 8-2. It is conceivable that some or all of these mechanisms may be operative in the pathophysiology of coronary no-reflow seen during PCI. Moreover, one etiologic factor may predominate depending on the particular setting such as during acute infarct PCI, high-speed rotational atherectomy, or vein graft PCI. In the seminal study by Kloner and colleagues, mechanical obstruction of the coronary microvasculature was observed.[3] Edema of the capillary endothelium and endothelial cell protrusions compromises the lumen of the microvessels within the region of no-reflow. Extrinsic microvascular compression may also occur from extracellular and intracellular edema in adjacent injured cardiomyocytes.[39] An additional cause of mechanical compression is ischemic contracture of the myocardium. These factors may be particularly relevant to coronary no-reflow seen in the setting of reperfusion in acute MI.

Physical obstruction of the microcirculation may occur as a result of luminal occlusion by platelets, fibrin thrombi, and atherosclerotic plaque components. Clinical studies indicate that these elements may embolize into the microvessels from upstream locations after plaque disruption during angioplasty.[40–42] Furthermore, disrupted plaque and activated platelets may elaborate a host of potent vasoactive factors such as endothelin-1, serotonin, thromboxane, and urotensin-II, which may alter the balance of microvascular tone in favor of constriction in a setting where vasodilator endothelial function may already be impaired.[43] It is likely that these factors are important in the etiology of no-reflow occurring during percutaneous PCI, as suggested by the salutary response to intracoronary vasodilator therapy. Activated tissue factor may also be released from disrupted plaques into the distal coronary circulation leading to microvascular thrombosis and no-reflow.[44] Microvascular spasm and reduced flow may be promoted by α-adrenergic coronary vasoconstriction during angioplasty and stenting.[45] It is thought that ischemia and arterial stretch with balloon inflation elicits a neural reflex leading to α-receptor–mediated vasoconstriction.

In experimental models of reperfusion after myocardial ischemia, neutrophils may contribute to no-reflow by plugging the microvessels,[46] and by generating oxygen-derived free radicals.[47] These reactive species cause cellular injury and endothelial vasodilator dysfunction by reducing the bioactivity of nitric oxide. Evidence for the production of free radicals has been found in humans after angioplasty.[48] Under the stimulus of inflammatory mediators and cytokines, neutrophils migrate from the vascular space into ischemic myocardium by initially interacting with endothelial cellular adhesion molecules, perhaps leading to persistence or worsening of no-reflow.

6. Management of No-Reflow

6.1. General Measures

Care should be taken to ensure the guiding catheter is not deeply seated as this may limit coronary flow. A mechanical cause for obstruction by intracoronary instrumentation must be excluded as discussed previously. Epicardial coronary spasm should be treated with boluses of intracoronary nitroglycerin, repeated as required (50–200 μg per dose). A patent airway and good oxygenation should be ensured, and hypotension aggressively treated to maintain adequate coronary perfusion pressure with intravenous fluid loading and inotropic or vasopressor drugs if required. Hemodynamically significant bradycardia should be treated with intravenous atropine or a temporary pacemaker. Titrated analgesia and sedation should be provided for the relief of chest pain and agitation, and the adequacy of procedural anticoagulation should be assessed by drawing a blood sample to determine the activated clotting time (ACT). Forceful hand injection of saline or blood drawn through the guiding catheter into the involved coronary artery has been suggested as a simple maneuver to dislodge fragments of thrombus or cellular debris that are occluding the microcirculation. Although there are anecdotal reports of success, this method has not been formally evaluated.

6.2. Specific Measures

Although several therapies have been advocated, no treatment is universally efficacious at reversing no-reflow (Table 8-2). Existing evidence to support the use of pharmacologic strategies is derived mainly from small non-randomized studies. Verapamil, adenosine, and nitroprusside can all be considered for use as first-line agents. Drugs can be delivered into the coronary artery proximally via the guiding catheter, or distally through an infusion catheter or central lumen of a balloon catheter once the guidewire has been removed. Distal delivery is strongly recommended when antegrade coronary flow is severely impaired (TIMI flow <2), or when using a guiding catheter with side holes.

6.2.1. Calcium Channel Antagonists

Calcium channel antagonists were among the first pharmacologic agents used in the treatment of coronary no-reflow.[8] They act by inhibiting L-type voltage-dependent calcium channels found on vascular smooth muscle, thereby inducing coronary vasodilatation. Most experience is with verapamil.[10,11,21,49] Dose ranging studies in angiographically normal human coronary arteries have shown that intracoronary verapamil produces a graded increase in coronary blood flow with the maximal effect reached upon administration of 1000 μg.[50] Piana and

TABLE 8-2. Vasodilator agents used to treat established no-reflow.

Drug	Intracoronary dosage
Verapamil	100–250 μg boluses to a total of 100–1250 μg, or 500 μg distal infusion over 1 min to a total dose of 1000 μg.
Adenosine	18–24 μg rapid bolus repeated 5–10 times with 2–3 rapid saline boluses after each adenosine bolus.
Sodium nitroprusside	50–200 μg per bolus to a total dose of 1400 μg.
Nicorandil	1–2 mg over 30–60 s.
Diltiazem	0.5–2.5 mg over 1 min to a total of 8.5 mg.
Papaverine	10–15 mg bolus.
Epinephrine	For use in no-reflow with hypotension: 50–200 μg bolus depending on blood pressure.
Nicardipine	200 μg bolus.

Verapamil, adenosine, and nitroprusside are considered first line agents, as there is most experience with the use of these drugs. Refer to text for details.

colleagues documented an improvement in TIMI flow grade and coronary flow in 89% of patients with no-reflow treated with intracoronary verapamil using a mean dose of 234 ± 142 μg (maximum dose 600 μg in 100-μg boluses delivered proximally or distally).[10] Systemic hypotension was not observed and bradycardia requiring temporary pacing was seen in only 2.7% of patients. Abbo and colleagues noted an improvement in no-reflow in 67% of patients treated with intracoronary verapamil.[11] Kaplan and colleagues compared intracoronary nitroglycerin (200 μg) with verapamil (total dose range 250–1250 μg per patient in boluses of 100–250 μg) to treat no-reflow in the setting of PCI on degenerated saphenous vein grafts.[21] Nitroglycerin had no effect in reversing no-reflow, but verapamil resulted in an improvement in TIMI flow by at least 1 grade in all cases, with normalization of flow in 88% of cases. In these studies, the outcomes for patients who responded to verapamil were better compared to poor responders.

The effect of intracoronary verapamil (500 μg infused into the infarct-related artery over 1 min) on microvascular function assessed by myocardial contrast echocardiography in the setting of acute infarct angioplasty has been studied in a randomized trial.[51] Compared to control, verapamil reduced no-/low-reflow zones assessed by echocardiography, and improved TIMI frame counts. Others have also found verapamil to be effective at reversing no-reflow in the setting of infarct angioplasty.[49] Improvement in TIMI flow grade was seen in 87% of patients after a mean dose of 910 ± 190 μg administered through an infusion catheter over 2 minutes into the distal coronary bed. A transient change in arteriovenous (AV) conduction was seen after verapamil in 43% of patients with no-reflow, with 13% of these patients requiring intravenous atropine for high-degree AV block. In contrast to these studies, Resnic and colleagues found that intracoronary verapamil was not more effective than nitroglycerin at improving TIMI frame counts after no-reflow.[22]

Subselective intracoronary diltiazem injections in increments of 0.5 to 2.5 mg (mean, 3.5 mg; total dose range, 0.5–8.5 mg) can also induce rapid improvement of no-reflow.[52] Nicardipine, a vasoselective dihydropyridine, may produce more potent and prolonged vasodilation than verapamil or diltiazem without significant effects on the cardiac conducting system.[53] These findings imply that it may be useful in treating no-reflow.

6.2.2. Adenosine

Adenosine is an endogenous purine nucleoside that predominantly dilates the small coronary microvessels, through adenosine A_2 receptors, leading to activation of vascular adenosine triphosphate (ATP)-sensitive potassium channels and release of nitric oxide.[54] Thus, it has both endothelium-dependent and -independent vasodilator activity. Other advantageous effects include inhibition of neutrophil-mediated injury, reduction of local tumor necrosis factor production, and diminution of cellular calcium overload.[55] Studies in humans indicate that intracoronary adenosine at doses of 12 μg in the right coronary artery and 16 μg in the left coronary artery induce comparable hyperemic response to intracoronary papaverine at a mean dose of 10 ± 2 mg.[56] The duration of hyperemic effect is about 40 seconds due to the short half-life of adenosine. Two studies have examined the effect of adenosine in treating established no-reflow, both in vein grafts.[57,58] Fischell and colleagues reported that forceful administration of multiple doses of adenosine (18–24 μg per bolus given at least 10 times) into the guiding catheter with two or three saline boluses after each adenosine bolus was successful in improving 10 of 11 no-reflow episodes (mean TIMI flow, pre 1.0 ± 0.3 to post 2.9 ± 0.3) within a short time frame (mean, 3.8 ± 1.7 min) during vein graft PCI.[57,59] Adenosine and saline injections were given with 3-mL Luer lock syringes, enabling higher pressure and velocity boluses to be delivered than larger syringes. Comparable results have been reported by others using similar doses (24 μg per bolus) and methods of administration, with the best success seen with higher total doses of adenosine (≥5 boluses of adenosine).[58] In these studies, adenosine was not associated with significant changes to systemic hemodynamics or cardiac rhythm.

6.2.3. Nitrovasodilators

Endothelium-derived nitric oxide is an important contributor to the maintenance of coronary conduit and microvascular tone. Nitric oxide induces vasodilation by relaxing vascular smooth muscle principally through a cyclic guanosine monophosphate (cGMP)-dependent mechanism. In addition to its vasodilator properties, nitric oxide has other effects including anti-inflammatory and antiplatelet actions, which may be of benefit in treating no-reflow. Nitroglycerin is primarily a dilator of the conduit coronary arteries rather than the microvessels, and requires bioconversion into nitric oxide for its vasodilator effect.[60] Several clinical studies indicate that it is not beneficial in reversing no-reflow, and this has been attributed to its primary action on large coronary vessels.[10,21,49] In contrast, nitroprusside is a direct nitric oxide donor that does not require intracellular metabolic processing and dilates both coronary conduit vessels and microvessels.[60] The efficacy of intracoronary sodium nitroprusside in treating no-reflow has been investigated by Hillegass and colleagues.[60] They reviewed 20 consecutive cases of no-reflow (TIMI flow <3) treated with nitroprusside, of which 60% occurred during native vessel

interventions and 40% in saphenous vein grafts. Patients received a mean dose of 435 ± 419 μg (50–200 μg per injection; total dose range, 50–1400 μg) delivered via the guide catheter or directly into the distal circulation. An improvement in angiographically determined coronary blood flow velocity was observed in 75% of patients. Statistically significant improvements in TIMI flow grades were also seen. Notably, no adverse hemodynamic effects of nitroprusside were documented. A prospective comparison of nitroprusside with other agents has yet to be carried out; however, one study suggests more complete resolution of no-reflow with nitroprusside compared with nitroglycerin or verapamil.[22]

6.2.4. Papaverine

Papaverine is an opiate derivative with direct smooth-muscle relaxing properties. Its precise mechanism of action is unknown, but appears involve the inhibition of phosphodiesterase. Studies in humans indicate that intracoronary papaverine is a potent microvascular dilator with minimal effect on epicardial arteries and a short duration of action of 2 to 3 minutes.[61] Maximum coronary vasodilation is observed after doses of 12 mg in the left coronary artery and 8 mg in the right coronary artery. Papaverine has been successfully used to treat no-reflow (TIMI flow <3) during acute infarct angioplasty.[62] In contrast to nitroglycerin, which had no significant effect on coronary flow, intracoronary papaverine (10 mg over 10 s given through the guiding catheter) resulted in an improvement of TIMI flow grade in 78% of cases and angiographic frame counts in this small study. Papaverine can induce QT prolongation, but ventricular arrhythmias are uncommon.[63] It is considered a safe agent with minimal effects on systemic hemodynamics at these doses.[61,62] When mixed with ionic contrast dye, opalescence may be seen due to precipitation, thus non-ionic agents should be used with papaverine.

6.2.5. Epinephrine

Epinephrine is an endogenous catecholamine with coronary vasoactive properties that produces its effects by binding to α- and β-adrenoceptors found in the coronary vasculature. Stimulation of vascular α-adrenoceptors induces vasoconstriction, whereas activation of $β_2$-adrenoceptors mediates vasodilation. Increased myocardial metabolism due to activation of myocardial $β_1$-adrenoreceptors may indirectly result in vasodilation. Intracoronary epinephrine (50–200 μg per dose) has been used to treat refractory no-reflow during PCI, defined as TIMI flow ≤2 after the use of single or combination drug therapy including nitroglycerin, verapamil, urokinase, or abciximab.[64] In this retrospective study of 29 no-reflow cases, 76% occurred in the setting of acute coronary syndromes and 48% were hypotensive before epinephrine was given. A mean total epinephrine dose of 139 ± 189 µg was administered with an improvement in TIMI flow grade from a mean of 1.0 ± 1.0 to 2.66 ± 0.55. Not surprisingly, there were associated changes in systemic hemodynamic parameters with a tolerable increase in heart rate and recovery of blood pressure. In view of the potential for adverse effects such as proarrhythmia, it has been suggested that intracoronary epinephrine not be used as a routine first-line agent, but rather to treat no-reflow in the hypotensive patient.[65]

6.2.6. Nicorandil

Nicorandil is a vasodilator that activates ATP-sensitive potassium channels on vascular smooth muscle cells and also has a nitrate moiety. These channels have been found in the human coronary circulation and play a role in the regulation of coronary blood flow.[66] Activation of these channels in cardiac tissue by nicorandil may invoke the protective mechanism of ischemic preconditioning, which may protect against no-reflow.[25] This drug is used to treat no-reflow in Japan, but at the time of writing is not available in the United States. Intracoronary bolus administration of 1.0 mg in the right coronary artery and 1.5 mg in the left coronary artery results in potent microvascular vasodilation similar to the effect induced by 10 mg and 12 mg of papaverine, respectively, but with minimal effect on systemic blood pressure.[67] Using myocardial contrast echocardiography, nicorandil has been shown to reduce no-reflow in patients having acute anterior infarct angioplasty by direct intracoronary administration (2 mg over 30–60 s into the left coronary artery),[68] or intravenously.[69]

6.2.7. Glycoprotein IIb/IIIa Antagonists

The basic mechanism of action of this class of drug is inhibition of the final common pathway of platelet aggregation by blocking the platelet surface glycoprotein (GP) IIb/IIIa receptor, thus reducing thrombus and platelet microemboli formation. These agents also improve microvascular endothelial function and myocardial perfusion, and have anti-inflammatory properties.[70–73] A number of clinical trials have demonstrated improved periprocedural outcomes with adjunctive GP IIb/IIIa receptor blockade in a range of PCI settings.[74] However, these agents do not appear to improve outcomes after vein graft PCI, perhaps due to the importance of microvascular obstruction by atheroemboli in this setting.[75] There is limited published data for GP IIb/IIIa inhibitor use in the treatment of no-reflow during PCI. There have been case reports using intravenous abciximab for this indication with complete reversal of impaired flow occurring after the initial bolus was administered.[76] Recent data suggests that high local doses

achieved with an initial intracoronary bolus followed by intravenous administration may be more efficacious in reducing adverse events than standard intravenous therapy during PCI for MI or unstable angina.[77] However, in this study the incidence of no-reflow was no different between the strategies. The timing of administration appears to be important, with better microvascular perfusion noted with early (pre–catheterization laboratory) administration of GP IIb/IIIa inhibitors in the setting of acute infarct PCI.[78]

6.2.8. Other Agents

Intracoronary thrombolytic therapy has been used to treat no-reflow, but success rates are low with resolution in only 10% of cases.[11] Inhibition of leukocyte adhesion and the complement system as an adjunct to reperfusion in acute MI have been studied in randomized trials;[79,80] however, there is not enough evidence to recommend these treatment approaches at the current time.

6.2.9. Intraaortic Balloon Counterpulsation

Intraaortic balloon counterpulsation has been advocated as an adjunct to the pharmacologic treatment of no-reflow after PCI, primarily to support the circulation. As discussed, no-reflow and subsequent ischemia have a detrimental impact on left ventricular function. Optimal use of the balloon pump will result in reduction of cardiac afterload. Moreover, intraaortic balloon pumping can result in augmentation of distal coronary blood flow and myocardial perfusion after successful treatment of the epicardial obstruction.[81] Such beneficial effects on coronary blood flow may be advantageous. Although prophylactic placement of a balloon pump may not prevent no-reflow from occurring in high-risk settings, there is evidence to suggest that this treatment is associated with a lower risk of non–Q-wave MI in the setting of no-reflow.[82]

7. Prevention of No-Reflow

In view of the serious sequelae resulting from established no-reflow and the variable efficacy of currently available therapies, recent attention has been focused on preventive measures.

7.1. Pharmacologic Strategies

Some of the previously discussed drug therapies have been administered immediately prior to PCI in an effort to prevent no-reflow. The Vasodilator Prevention of No-Reflow (VAPOR) trial was a small randomized study of intragraft verapamil pretreatment (200µg) before saphenous vein graft PCI ($n = 22$).[83] No-reflow occurred in 33% of grafts in the placebo group, but in none of the verapamil-treated patients ($P = 0.10$). There was a significant improvement in corrected TIMI frame counts and a trend to improvement in myocardial perfusion grades in the verapamil-treated group.

There is conflicting data regarding the utility of adenosine to prevent no-reflow. In a nonrandomized study of vein graft PCI, adenosine given before first balloon inflation (1 bolus, 24µg; mean dose, 1.7 ± 0.9 boluses) did not prevent the occurrence of no-reflow compared to patients not receiving adenosine.[58] However, a randomized study of adenosine (4mg administered over 1 min through an over-the-wire balloon catheter during first balloon inflation) showed that it could prevent no-reflow and result in better outcomes compared to saline placebo during acute infarct PCI.[55] Similar acute results were observed in a retrospective study using smaller doses of intracoronary adenosine (24–48µg before and after balloon inflations) during acute infarct PCI.[84] The discordant findings of these studies using adenosine may reflect the different settings involved, dose, and method of administration.

Patients undergoing rotational atherectomy represent another high-risk subset for no-reflow. The use of a drug cocktail containing verapamil, nitroglycerin, and heparin mixed with pressurized normal saline and infused through the Teflon® sheath of the rotablator system has been advocated to reduce vasospasm and no-reflow. In the observational Cocktail Attenuation of Rotational Ablation Flow Effects (CARAFE) Pilot Study, transient no-reflow was seen in only 1 of 27 patients (3.7%), which compared favorably with the incidence of no-reflow described in earlier reports.[85] There is some evidence to suggest that nicorandil in place of verapamil in the cocktail may be more efficacious at reducing no-reflow.[86] Intracoronary adenosine boluses before and after each atherectomy run (24–48µg) have been shown to reduce no-reflow.[87] In view of the ability of high-speed rotational atherectomy to activate platelets, the adjunctive use of GP IIb/IIIa antagonists may lower the risk of no-reflow and myocardial hypoperfusion.[33,88,89] Other recommendations to prevent no-reflow include using a maximum burr to artery ratio ≥ 0.70 and lower rotational speeds (140,000–150,000 rpm).[30,89,90]

7.2. Direct Stenting

In native coronary arteries of patients with acute coronary syndromes, direct stenting does not reduce the occurrence of no-reflow.[91] In contrast, direct stenting may have a particular role in vein graft PCI. In this setting, the burden of embolic debris is less when direct stenting is performed compared to balloon predilatation and stenting, perhaps because direct stenting results in entrapment of friable plaque between the stent and vessel wall.[41]

7.3. Intracoronary Thrombectomy

Catheter-based removal of thrombus from coronary arteries to minimize distal embolization and no-reflow has some intuitive appeal; however, results to date have been variable. The AngioJet rheolytic thrombectomy system (Possis Medical, Inc., Minneapolis, MN) utilizes a dual lumen catheter passed over a coronary guidewire through which high-velocity saline jets flow to create a localized low-pressure area adjacent to the catheter tip. The resulting Bernoulli effect enables the breakdown and suction of thrombus into the catheter. In the randomized Vein Graft AngioJet Study (VeGAS 2) trial, patients with thrombus-containing lesions in vein grafts or native vessels received an intracoronary urokinase infusion or AngioJet treatment, followed by angioplasty and stenting.[92] Distal embolization and no-reflow were not significantly different between the two arms. This device has also been used in the setting of acute MI and the reported incidence of transient or sustained no-reflow was 18.6%, which is similar to historical controls.[93] Another thrombectomy device, the X-Sizer catheter system (EndiCOR Medical, San Clemente, CA), consists of a high-speed rotating helical cutter connected to a vacuum source to fragment and remove thrombus. In a randomized study, patients having PCI with thrombectomy for acute coronary syndromes had lower corrected TIMI frame counts and more complete early ST-segment resolution than a conventionally treated group, although coronary flow reserve and myocardial blush grades were not different.[94] Positive results with this device have been reported in another study, where no cases of sustained no-reflow were observed in a high-risk population.[95]

7.4. Embolic Protection

The biggest recent advance in the prevention of no-reflow has been the development of the embolic protection device. Several systems are available or under evaluation, but they all serve to capture and retrieve embolic debris dislodged during intracoronary manipulations.[96] The early clinical experience was with the PercuSurge GuardWire (Medtronic, Inc., Santa Rosa, CA) distal embolic protection system. This device consists of a 0.014-inch "balloon-on-a-hypotube-wire" with an elastomeric occlusion balloon on its tip. Once the wire is across the lesion, the balloon is inflated, thus occluding blood flow into the distal vessel. Angioplasty and stenting is performed over the wire, and the static column of blood in the vessel containing the embolic debris can be removed with an aspiration catheter before balloon occlusion is released and blood flow re-established. Using this system, Webb and colleagues were able to retrieve predominantly acellular atheromatous microparticulate debris from vein grafts in 21 of 23 cases.[41] The efficacy of the PercuSurge device was demonstrated in the multi-center Saphenous vein graft Angioplasty Free of Emboli Randomized (SAFER) trial, which recruited 801 patients.[97] Compared with conventional PCI, there was a 42% relative reduction in major adverse cardiac events at 30 days ($P = 0.004$) due to fewer no-reflow events (3% vs. 9%; $P = 0.02$) and myocardial infarcts (8.6% vs. 14.7%; $P = 0.008$) in the PercuSurge arm.

Filter-based devices consisting of a guidewire with an expandable porous filter at its tip with delivery and retrieval sheaths are also available for distal embolic protection (Figure 8-3, see color plate, part E). Filter-based systems allow maintenance of antegrade blood flow and myocardial perfusion during PCI, unlike the balloon occlusion devices. The lesion can be visualized with contrast dye and the procedure completed in a more leisurely manner due to the lack of ischemia. Using the Angio-Guard Emboli Capture Guidewire (Cordis Corp., Warren, NJ), which has a filter pore size of 100 μm, capture

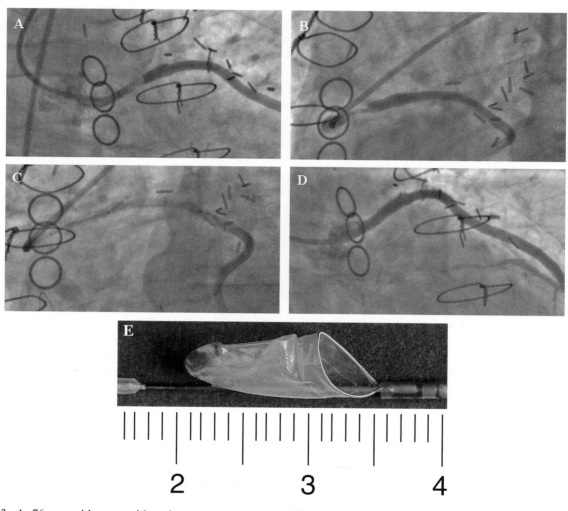

FIGURE 8-3. A 76-year-old man with prior coronary artery bypass surgery presented with unstable angina. Coronary angiography revealed a severe, ulcerated stenosis in the proximal segment of an 11-year-old saphenous vein graft to the left anterior descending artery in the right anterior oblique (A) and left anterior oblique (B) projections. A FilterWire EX distal embolic protection system was deployed in the graft body and the lesion was directly stented with a 4.0 × 23-mm Multilink Ultra bare-metal stent (C), yielding an excellent angiographic result with TIMI grade low (D). Examination of the retrieved filter showed a large quantity of embolized atherothrombotic debris (E). The pores can be clearly seen in the polyurethane filter. Postprocedural cardiac enzymes were within normal limits, and the patient was discharged home after an uneventful in-hospital course. (See color plate, part E only.)

of embolic debris was documented in all cases of vein graft and native coronary PCI ($n = 26$), and no-reflow did not occur in any procedure.[42] The FilterWire EX (Boston Scientific Corp., Natick, MA) also has a distal polyurethane filter with a pore size of 80 to 110μm mounted on a 0.014-inch guidewire. In the FilterWire EX Randomized Evaluation (FIRE) trial, this device was compared with the PercuSurge Guardwire system in 651 patients undergoing saphenous vein graft PCI.[98] In-hospital and 30-day event rates were similar, and the FilterWire EX system was found to be noninferior to the PercuSurge Guardwire. Both devices could be successfully used in over 95% of procedures. Apart from vein graft PCI, the Filterwire EX has been safely used in acute infarct PCI. Compared to a matched control group who had PCI without distal protection, the FilterWire group had lower corrected TIMI frame counts, improved myocardial blush grades, and ST-segment resolution indicative of better myocardial reperfusion.[99] Care needs to be taken when using such devices to achieve maximum efficacy.[100] Other approaches under investigation utilize proximal embolic protection, which has the theoretic advantage of protection before the lesion is instrumented. Embolic protection has now become the standard of care in vein graft PCI to prevent no-reflow and its complications. As refinements to existing devices are made and new technologies develop, the indications for their use will expand.

8. Conclusion

Coronary no-reflow during PCI is a serious albeit uncommon complication. It may turn an otherwise straightforward procedure into a difficult and prolonged affair with adverse clinical implications for the patient. The pathophysiology of no-reflow is complex and involves a variety of elements. For this reason no single treatment is consistently effective in ameliorating it. An awareness of clinical, angiographic, and procedural factors that may predispose to this complication will help the interventionalist in anticipating its occurrence. The benefit of preparedness will be in utilizing available strategies to prevent no-reflow and to treat it promptly with the best available therapies should it occur.

References

1. Majno G, Ames A III, Chiang J, Wright RL. No reflow after cerebral ischemia. Lancet. 1967;2:569–570.
2. Krug A, Du Mesnil de Rochemont W, Korb G. Blood supply of the myocardium after temporary coronary occlusion. Circ Res. 1966;19:57–62.
3. Kloner RA, Ganote CE, Jennings RB. The "no-reflow" phenomenon after temporary coronary occlusion in the dog. J Clin Invest. 1974;54:1496–1508.
4. Schofer J, Montz R, Mathey DG. Scintigraphic evidence of the "no reflow" phenomenon in human beings after coronary thrombolysis. J Am Coll Cardiol. 1985;5:593–598.
5. Bates ER, Krell MJ, Dean EN, et al. Demonstration of the "no-reflow" phenomenon by digital coronary arteriography. Am J Cardiol. 1986;57:177–178.
6. Kitazume H, Iwama T, Kubo I, et al. No-reflow phenomenon during percutaneous transluminal coronary angioplasty. Am Heart J. 1988;116:211–215.
7. Wilson RF, Laxson DD, Lesser JR, White CW. Intense microvascular constriction after angioplasty of acute thrombotic coronary arterial lesions. Lancet. 1989;1:807–811.
8. Pomerantz RM, Kuntz RE, Diver DJ, et al. Intracoronary verapamil for the treatment of distal microvascular coronary artery spasm following PTCA. Catheter Cardiovasc Diagn. 1991;24:283–285.
9. Feld H, Lichstein E, Schachter J, Shani J. Early and late angiographic findings of the "no-reflow" phenomenon following direct angioplasty as primary treatment for acute myocardial infarction. Am Heart J. 1992;123:782–784.
10. Piana RN, Paik GY, Moscucci M, et al. Incidence and treatment of 'no-reflow' after percutaneous coronary intervention. Circulation. 1994;89:2514–2518.
11. Abbo KM, Dooris M, Glazier S, et al. Features and outcome of no-reflow after percutaneous coronary intervention. Am J Cardiol. 1995;75:778–782.
12. Eeckhout E, Kern MJ. The coronary no-reflow phenomenon: a review of mechanisms and therapies. Eur Heart J. 2001;22:729–739.
13. The Thrombolysis in Myocardial Infarction (TIMI) trial. Phase I findings. TIMI Study Group. N Engl J Med. 1985;312:932–936.
14. Gibson CM, Cannon CP, Daley WL, et al. TIMI frame count: a quantitative method of assessing coronary artery flow. Circulation. 1996;93:879–888.
15. van't Hof AW, Liem A, Suryapranata H, et al. Angiographic assessment of myocardial reperfusion in patients treated with primary angioplasty for acute myocardial infarction: myocardial blush grade. Zwolle Myocardial Infarction Study Group. Circulation. 1998;97:2302–2306.
16. Gibson CM, Cannon CP, Murphy SA, et al. Relationship of TIMI myocardial perfusion grade to mortality after administration of thrombolytic drugs. Circulation. 2000;101:125–130.
17. Gibson CM, Cannon CP, Murphy SA, et al. Relationship of the TIMI myocardial perfusion grades, flow grades, frame count, and percutaneous coronary intervention to long-term outcomes after thrombolytic administration in acute myocardial infarction. Circulation. 2002;105:1909–1913.
18. Sherman JR, Anwar A, Bret JR, Schreibfeder MM. Distal vessel pullback angiography and pressure gradient measurement: an innovative diagnostic approach to evaluate the no-reflow phenomenon. Catheter Cardiovasc Diagn. 1996;39:1–6.
19. Iwakura K, Ito H, Takiuchi S, et al. Alternation in the coronary blood flow velocity pattern in patients with no reflow and reperfused acute myocardial infarction. Circulation. 1996;94:1269–1275.

20. Fearon WF, Balsam LB, Farouque HM, et al. Novel index for invasively assessing the coronary microcirculation. Circulation. 2003;107:3129–3132.

21. Kaplan BM, Benzuly KH, Kinn JW, et al. Treatment of no-reflow in degenerated saphenous vein graft interventions: comparison of intracoronary verapamil and nitroglycerin. Catheter Cardiovasc Diagn. 1996;39:113–118.

22. Resnic FS, Wainstein M, Lee MK, et al. No-reflow is an independent predictor of death and myocardial infarction after percutaneous coronary intervention. Am Heart J. 2003;145:42–46.

23. Sdringola S, Assali AR, Ghani M, et al. Risk assessment of slow or no-reflow phenomenon in aortocoronary vein graft percutaneous intervention. Catheter Cardiovasc Interv. 2001;54:318–324.

24. Yip HK, Chen MC, Chang HW, et al. Angiographic morphologic features of infarct-related arteries and timely reperfusion in acute myocardial infarction: predictors of slow-flow and no-reflow phenomenon. Chest. 2002;122:1322–1332.

25. Takahashi T, Anzai T, Yoshikawa T, et al. Absence of pre-infarction angina is associated with a risk of no-reflow phenomenon after primary coronary angioplasty for a first anterior wall acute myocardial infarction. Int J Cardiol. 2000;75:253–260.

26. Tanaka A, Kawarabayashi T, Nishibori Y, et al. No-reflow phenomenon and lesion morphology in patients with acute myocardial infarction. Circulation. 2002;105:2148–2152.

27. Iwakura K, Ito H, Kawano S, et al. Predictive factors for development of the no-reflow phenomenon in patients with reperfused anterior wall acute myocardial infarction. J Am Coll Cardiol. 2001;38:472–477.

28. Sharma SK, Dangas G, Mehran R, et al. Risk factors for the development of slow flow during rotational coronary atherectomy. Am J Cardiol. 1997;80:219–222.

29. Ellis SG, Popma JJ, Buchbinder M, et al. Relation of clinical presentation, stenosis morphology, and operator technique to the procedural results of rotational atherectomy and rotational atherectomy-facilitated angioplasty. Circulation. 1994;89:882–892.

30. Whitlow PL, Bass TA, Kipperman RM, et al. Results of the study to determine rotablator and transluminal angioplasty strategy (STRATAS). Am J Cardiol. 2001;87:699–705.

31. Safian RD, Niazi KA, Strzelecki M, et al. Detailed angiographic analysis of high-speed mechanical rotational atherectomy in human coronary arteries. Circulation. 1993;88:961–968.

32. Warth DC, Leon MB, O'Neill W, et al. Rotational atherectomy multicenter registry: acute results, complications and 6-month angiographic follow-up in 709 patients. J Am Coll Cardiol. 1994;24:641–648.

33. Koch KC, vom Dahl J, Kleinhans E, et al. Influence of a platelet GPIIb/IIIa receptor antagonist on myocardial hypoperfusion during rotational atherectomy as assessed by myocardial Tc-99m sestamibi scintigraphy. J Am Coll Cardiol. 1999;33:998–1004.

34. Morishima I, Sone T, Mokuno S, et al. Clinical significance of no-reflow phenomenon observed on angiography after successful treatment of acute myocardial infarction with

percutaneous transluminal coronary angioplasty. Am Heart J. 1995;130:239–243.

35. Morishima I, Sone T, Okumura K, et al. Angiographic no-reflow phenomenon as a predictor of adverse long-term outcome in patients treated with percutaneous transluminal coronary angioplasty for first acute myocardial infarction. J Am Coll Cardiol. 2000;36:1202–1209.

36. Grines CL, Cox DA, Stone GW, et al. Coronary angioplasty with or without stent implantation for acute myocardial infarction. Stent Primary Angioplasty in Myocardial Infarction Study Group. N Engl J Med. 1999;341:1949–1956.

37. A clinical trial comparing primary coronary angioplasty with tissue plasminogen activator for acute myocardial infarction. The Global Use of Strategies to Open Occluded Coronary Arteries in Acute Coronary Syndromes (GUSTO IIb) Angioplasty Substudy Investigators. N Engl J Med. 1997;336:1621–1628.

38. Stone GW, Grines CL, Cox DA, et al. Comparison of angioplasty with stenting, with or without abciximab, in acute myocardial infarction. N Engl J Med. 2002;346:957–966.

39. Manciet LH, Poole DC, McDonagh PF, et al. Microvascular compression during myocardial ischemia: mechanistic basis for no-reflow phenomenon. Am J Physiol. 1994;266:H1541–H1550.

40. Kotani J, Nanto S, Mintz GS, et al. Plaque gruel of atheromatous coronary lesion may contribute to the no-reflow phenomenon in patients with acute coronary syndrome. Circulation. 2002;106:1672–1677.

41. Webb JG, Carere RG, Virmani R, et al. Retrieval and analysis of particulate debris after saphenous vein graft intervention. J Am Coll Cardiol. 1999;34:468–475.

42. Grube E, Gerckens U, Yeung AC, et al. Prevention of distal embolization during coronary angioplasty in saphenous vein grafts and native vessels using porous filter protection. Circulation. 2001;104:2436–2441.

43. Taylor AJ, Bobik A, Berndt MC, et al. Experimental rupture of atherosclerotic lesions increases distal vascular resistance: a limiting factor to the success of infarct angioplasty. Arterioscler Thromb Vasc Biol. 2002;22:153–160.

44. Bonderman D, Teml A, Jakowitsch J, et al. Coronary no-reflow is caused by shedding of active tissue factor from dissected atherosclerotic plaque. Blood. 2002;99:2794–2800.

45. Gregorini L, Marco J, Farah B, et al. Effects of selective alpha1- and alpha2-adrenergic blockade on coronary flow reserve after coronary stenting. Circulation. 2002;106:2901–2907.

46. Engler RL, Schmid-Schonbein GW, Pavelec RS. Leukocyte capillary plugging in myocardial ischemia and reperfusion in the dog. Am J Pathol. 1983;111:98–111.

47. Przyklenk K, Kloner RA. "Reperfusion injury" by oxygen-derived free radicals? Effect of superoxide dismutase plus catalase, given at the time of reperfusion, on myocardial infarct size, contractile function, coronary microvasculature, and regional myocardial blood flow. Circ Res. 1989;64:86–96.

48. Roberts MJ, Young IS, Trouton TG, et al. Transient release of lipid peroxides after coronary artery balloon angioplasty. Lancet. 1990;336:143–145.

49. Werner GS, Lang K, Kuehnert H, Figulla HR. Intracoronary verapamil for reversal of no-reflow during coronary angioplasty for acute myocardial infarction. Catheter Cardiovasc Interv. 2002;57:444–451.

50. Oldenburg O, Eggebrecht H, Herrmann J, et al. Dose-dependent effects of intracoronary verapamil on systemic and coronary hemodynamics. Cardiovasc Drugs Ther. 2000;14:651–655.

51. Taniyama Y, Ito H, Iwakura K, et al. Beneficial effect of intracoronary verapamil on microvascular and myocardial salvage in patients with acute myocardial infarction. J Am Coll Cardiol. 1997;30:1193–1199.

52. Weyrens FJ, Mooney J, Lesser J, Mooney MR. Intracoronary diltiazem for microvascular spasm after interventional therapy. Am J Cardiol. 1995;75:849–850.

53. Fugit MD, Rubal BJ, Donovan DJ. Effects of intracoronary nicardipine, diltiazem and verapamil on coronary blood flow. J Invasive Cardiol. 2000;12:80–85.

54. Hein TW, Belardinelli L, Kuo L. Adenosine A(2A) receptors mediate coronary microvascular dilation to adenosine: role of nitric oxide and ATP-sensitive potassium channels. J Pharmacol Exp Ther. 1999;291:655–664.

55. Marzilli M, Orsini E, Marraccini P, Testa R. Beneficial effects of intracoronary adenosine as an adjunct to primary angioplasty in acute myocardial infarction. Circulation. 2000;101:2154–2159.

56. Wilson RF, Wyche K, Christensen BV, et al. Effects of adenosine on human coronary arterial circulation. Circulation. 1990;82:1595–1606.

57. Fischell TA, Carter AJ, Foster MT, et al. Reversal of "no reflow" during vein graft stenting using high velocity boluses of intracoronary adenosine. Catheter Cardiovasc Diagn. 1998;45:360–365.

58. Sdringola S, Assali A, Ghani M, et al. Adenosine use during aortocoronary vein graft interventions reverses but does not prevent the slow-no reflow phenomenon. Catheter Cardiovasc Interv. 2000;51:394–399.

59. Fischell TA, Foster MT 3rd. Adenosine for reversal of "no reflow." Catheter Cardiovasc Interv. 1999;46:508.

60. Hillegass WB, Dean NA, Liao L, et al. Treatment of no-reflow and impaired flow with the nitric oxide donor nitroprusside following percutaneous coronary interventions: initial human clinical experience. J Am Coll Cardiol. 2001;37:1335–1343.

61. Wilson RF, White CW. Intracoronary papaverine: an ideal coronary vasodilator for studies of the coronary circulation in conscious humans. Circulation. 1986;73:444–451.

62. Ishihara M, Sato H, Tateishi H, et al. Attenuation of the no-reflow phenomenon after coronary angioplasty for acute myocardial infarction with intracoronary papaverine. Am Heart J. 1996;132:959–963.

63. Talman CL, Winniford MD, Rossen JD, et al. Polymorphous ventricular tachycardia: a side effect of intracoronary papaverine. J Am Coll Cardiol. 1990;15:275–278.

64. Skelding KA, Goldstein JA, Mehta L, et al. Resolution of refractory no-reflow with intracoronary epinephrine. Catheter Cardiovasc Interv. 2002;57:305–309.

65. Baim DS. Epinephrine: a new pharmacologic treatment for no-reflow? Catheter Cardiovasc Interv. 2002;57:310–311.

66. Farouque HM, Worthley SG, Meredith IT, et al. Effect of ATP-sensitive potassium channel inhibition on resting coronary vascular responses in humans. Circ Res. 2002;90:231–236.

67. Hongo M, Takenaka H, Uchikawa S, et al. Coronary microvascular response to intracoronary administration of nicorandil. Am J Cardiol. 1995;75:246–250.

68. Sakata Y, Kodama K, Komamura K, et al. Salutary effect of adjunctive intracoronary nicorandil administration on restoration of myocardial blood flow and functional improvement in patients with acute myocardial infarction. Am Heart J. 1997;133:616–621.

69. Ito H, Taniyama Y, Iwakura K, et al. Intravenous nicorandil can preserve microvascular integrity and myocardial viability in patients with reperfused anterior wall myocardial infarction. J Am Coll Cardiol. 1999;33:654–660.

70. Heitzer T, Ollmann I, Koke K, et al. Platelet glycoprotein IIb/IIIa receptor blockade improves vascular nitric oxide bioavailability in patients with coronary artery disease. Circulation. 2003;108:536–541.

71. Aymong ED, Curtis MJ, Youssef M, et al. Abciximab attenuates coronary microvascular endothelial dysfunction after coronary stenting. Circulation. 2002;105:2981–2985.

72. Gibson CM, Cohen DJ, Cohen EA, et al. Effect of eptifibatide on coronary flow reserve following coronary stent implantation (an ESPRIT substudy). Enhanced Suppression of the Platelet IIb/IIIa Receptor with Integrilin Therapy. Am J Cardiol. 2001;87:1293–1295.

73. Nannizzi-Alaimo L, Alves VL, Phillips DR. Inhibitory effects of glycoprotein IIb/IIIa antagonists and aspirin on the release of soluble CD40 ligand during platelet stimulation. Circulation. 2003;107:1123–1128.

74. Lincoff AM, Califf RM, Topol EJ. Platelet glycoprotein IIb/IIIa receptor blockade in coronary artery disease. J Am Coll Cardiol. 2000;35:1103–1115.

75. Roffi M, Mukherjee D, Chew DP, et al. Lack of benefit from intravenous platelet glycoprotein IIb/IIIa receptor inhibition as adjunctive treatment for percutaneous interventions of aortocoronary bypass grafts: a pooled analysis of five randomized clinical trials. Circulation. 2002;106:3063–3067.

76. Rawitscher D, Levin TN, Cohen I, Feldman T. Rapid reversal of no-reflow using Abciximab after coronary device intervention. Catheter Cardiovasc Diagn. 1997;2:187–190.

77. Wohrle J, Grebe OC, Nusser T, et al. Reduction of major adverse cardiac events with intracoronary compared with intravenous bolus application of abciximab in patients with acute myocardial infarction or unstable angina undergoing coronary angioplasty. Circulation. 2003;107:1840–1843.

78. Lee DP, Herity NA, Hiatt BL, et al. Adjunctive platelet glycoprotein IIb/IIIa receptor inhibition with tirofiban before primary angioplasty improves angiographic outcomes: results of the TIrofiban Given in the Emergency Room before Primary Angioplasty (TIGER-PA) pilot trial. Circulation. 2003;107:1497–1501.

79. Baran KW, Nguyen M, McKendall GR, et al. Double-blind, randomized trial of an anti-CD18 antibody in conjunction with recombinant tissue plasminogen activator for acute myocardial infarction: limitation of myocardial infarction following thrombolysis in acute myocardial infarction (LIMIT AMI) study. Circulation. 2001;104:2778–2783.

80. Granger CB, Mahaffey KW, Weaver WD, et al. Pexelizumab, an anti-C5 complement antibody, as adjunctive therapy to primary percutaneous coronary intervention in acute myocardial infarction: the COMplement inhibition in Myocardial infarction treated with Angioplasty (COMMA) trial. Circulation. 2003;108:1184–1190.

81. Kern MJ, Aguirre F, Bach R, et al. Augmentation of coronary blood flow by intra-aortic balloon pumping in patients after coronary angioplasty. Circulation. 1993;87:500–511.

82. O'Murchu B, Foreman RD, Shaw RE, et al. Role of intraaortic balloon pump counterpulsation in high risk coronary rotational atherectomy. J Am Coll Cardiol. 1995;26:1270–1275.

83. Michaels AD, Appleby M, Otten MH, et al. Pretreatment with intragraft verapamil prior to percutaneous coronary intervention of saphenous vein graft lesions: results of the randomized, controlled vasodilator prevention on no-reflow (VAPOR) trial. J Invasive Cardiol. 2002;14:299–302.

84. Assali AR, Sdringola S, Ghani M, et al. Intracoronary adenosine administered during percutaneous intervention in acute myocardial infarction and reduction in the incidence of "no reflow" phenomenon. Catheter Cardiovasc Interv. 2000;51:27–31, discussion 32.

85. Cohen BM, Weber VJ, Blum RR, et al. Cocktail attenuation of rotational ablation flow effects (CARAFE) study: pilot. Catheter Cardiovasc Diagn. 1996;(suppl 3):69–72.

86. Tsubokawa A, Ueda K, Sakamoto H, et al. Effect of intracoronary nicorandil administration on preventing no-reflow/slow flow phenomenon during rotational atherectomy. Circ J. 2002;66:1119–1123.

87. Hanna GP, Yhip P, Fujise K, et al. Intracoronary adenosine administered during rotational atherectomy of complex lesions in native coronary arteries reduces the incidence of no-reflow phenomenon. Catheter Cardiovasc Interv. 1999;48:275–278.

88. Kini A, Reich D, Marmur JD, et al. Reduction in periprocedural enzyme elevation by abciximab after rotational atherectomy of type B2 lesions: results of the Rota ReoPro randomized trial. Am Heart J. 2001;142:965–969.

89. Williams MS, Coller BS, Vaananen HJ, et al. Activation of platelets in platelet-rich plasma by rotablation is speed-dependent and can be inhibited by abciximab (c7E3 Fab; ReoPro). Circulation. 1998;98:742–748.

90. Reisman M, Shuman BJ, Dillard D, et al. Analysis of low-speed rotational atherectomy for the reduction of platelet aggregation. Catheter Cardiovasc Diagn. 1998;45:208–214.

91. Sabatier R, Hamon M, Zhao QM, et al. Could direct stenting reduce no-reflow in acute coronary syndromes? A randomized pilot study. Am Heart J. 2002;143:1027–1032.

92. Kuntz RE, Baim DS, Cohen DJ, et al. A trial comparing rheolytic thrombectomy with intracoronary urokinase for coronary and vein graft thrombus (the Vein Graft AngioJet Study [VeGAS 2]). Am J Cardiol. 2002;89:326–330.

93. Silva JA, Ramee SR, Cohen DJ, et al. Rheolytic thrombectomy during percutaneous revascularization for acute myocardial infarction: experience with the AngioJet catheter. Am Heart J. 2001;141:353–359.

94. Beran G, Lang I, Schreiber W, et al. Intracoronary thrombectomy with the X-sizer catheter system improves epicardial flow and accelerates ST-segment resolution in patients with acute coronary syndrome: a prospective, randomized, controlled study. Circulation. 2002;105:2355–2360.

95. Stone GW, Cox DA, Low R, et al. Safety and efficacy of a novel device for treatment of thrombotic and atherosclerotic lesions in native coronary arteries and saphenous vein grafts: results from the multicenter X-Sizer for treatment of thrombus and atherosclerosis in coronary applications trial (X-TRACT) study. Catheter Cardiovasc Interv. 2003;58:419–427.

96. Sangiorgi G, Colombo A. Embolic protection devices. Heart. 2003;89:990–992.

97. Baim DS, Wahr D, George B, et al. Randomized trial of a distal embolic protection device during percutaneous intervention of saphenous vein aorto-coronary bypass grafts. Circulation. 2002;105:1285–1290.

98. Stone GW, Rogers C, Hermiller J, et al. Randomized comparison of distal protection with a filter-based catheter and a balloon occlusion and aspiration system during percutaneous intervention of diseased saphenous vein aorto-coronary bypass grafts. Circulation. 2003;108:548–553.

99. Limbruno U, Micheli A, De Carlo M, et al. Mechanical prevention of distal embolization during primary angioplasty: safety, feasibility, and impact on myocardial reperfusion. Circulation. 2003;108:171–176.

100. Stone GW, Rogers C, Ramee S, et al. Distal filter protection during saphenous vein graft stenting: technical and clinical correlates of efficacy. J Am Coll Cardiol. 2002;40:1882–1888.

9
Early versus Late Complications

Albert W. Chan and Christopher J. White

One stitch in time saves nine.

1. Case

A 70-year-old woman had acute onset of groin pain and hypotension about 3 hours after removal of an arterial sheath. The patient was brought to the catheterization laboratory and antegrade contrast injection via the contralateral access identified the location of the bleeding (Figure 9-1A, arrow). After the advancement of the stiff-angled guidewire and the insertion of a crossover sheath, balloon inflation was performed across the extravasation site (Figure 9-1B). A total of 3000 U of diluted 1:10,000 thrombin was injected percutaneously while the balloon was inflated within the artery (Figure 9-1C, blocked arrow). Repeat angiography revealed minimal residual leak (Figure 9-1D, arrow), but an intra-arterial thrombus was identified in the common femoral artery and part of it migrated distally to the superficial femoral artery (Figure 9-1E, arrowhead) and to the tibioperoneal trunk (Figure 9-1F, arrowhead). Angiojet, Percusurge Guardwire, and Filterwire were used sequentially in both the anterior and posterior tibial artery to reduce the thrombus burden (Figures 9-1G,H). Tissue plasminogen activator and papaverine were given through a Transit catheter. Because of residual thrombotic occlusion in the infrapopliteal arteries (Figure 9-1I), intra-arterial thrombolysis was administered overnight. To avoid bleeding in the common femoral artery, a Wallgraft was placed to seal the original extravasation site in the common femoral artery. The patient was discharged on the next day after an uneventful recovery.

2. Introduction

Patients who have undergone a successful percutaneous coronary intervention (PCI) are conventionally observed in the hospital overnight. However, procedure-related complications do happen beyond the hospitalization period (Table 9-1). Appropriate selections of arterial access, antithrombotic regimen, guide catheters, guidewires, and balloon and stent catheters, combined with meticulous techniques, contribute to the lowering of the periprocedural risk and late complications. Indeed, with a routine stent strategy and improved antiplatelet and anticoagulation regimens, complications associated with PCI are much less common in recent years; and when combined with the use of vascular closure devices, same-day discharge has become possible, and even advocated by some for low-risk patients.[1-7] The objective of this chapter is to discuss and contrast several major early and late complications of PCI, and include possible preventive measures as well as management strategies for their resolution.

3. Complications with Arterial Access

Arterial access-site complications are the most common complications of PCI, occurring in ~3%–5% of all cases.[8] Dissection, hematoma, pseudoaneurysm, and retroperitoneal hemorrhage represent examples of the early arterial access complications, while pseudoaneurysm and infection may sometimes be noted only days after the index procedure. Arterial access complications may cause major morbidity, prolongation of hospital stay, increased cost, and even mortality. Hence, operators should pay as much attention to the arterial access as to the coronary anatomy, and meticulous technique and advanced planning are the keys to prevent these complications.

While diagnostic and interventional coronary procedures can be performed via radial or brachial access, the femoral artery is the most common choice of vascular access. When arterial access is established too close to, or above, the inguinal ligament, it may become difficult to achieve hemostasis with manual pressure at the end of

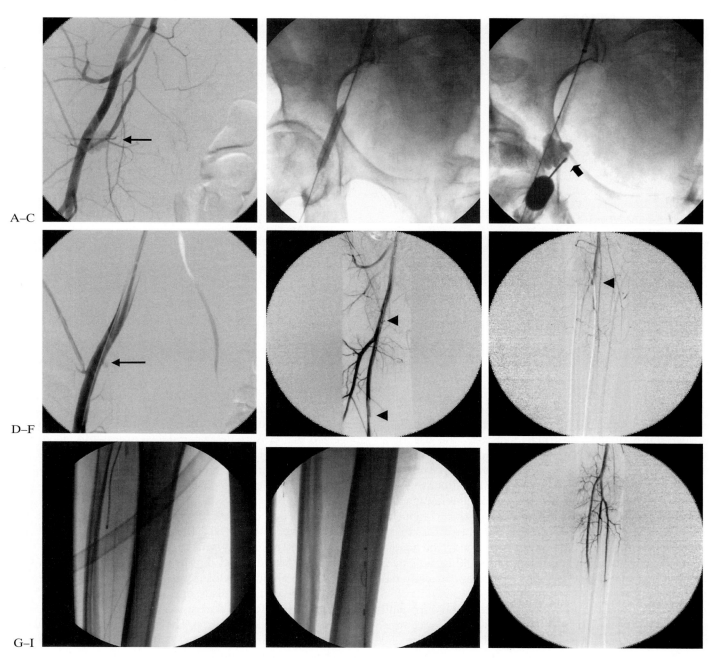

A–C

D–F

G–I

FIGURE 9-1. Catheterization laboratory management of severe access-site bleeding. Refer to the text for details of the case.

TABLE 9-1. Early versus late complications associated with percutaneous coronary interventions.

Early complications with	Late complications with
Arterial access	**Arterial access**
• Hematoma	• Pseudoaneurysm
• Retroperitoneal bleeding	• Arteriovenous fistula
• Arterial dissection	• Ischemic limb or arterial closure
• Acute limb ischemia	• Complications specific for vascular closure devices
	• Infection
Catheterization	
• Atheroembolization (stroke, lower extremity embolization)	**Catheterization**
	• Atheroembolization (lower extremity, renal)
Coronary intervention	
• Dissections of aorta, coronary arteries, and abrupt vessel closure	**Coronary intervention**
• Coronary perforation and cardiac tamponade	• Subacute or late (stent) thrombosis
• Distal embolization, acute thrombosis, and no reflow	• Late coronary perforation
• Periprocedural myocardial infarction	• Antiplatelet drugs
• Side-branch occlusion	• Thrombocytopenia (abciximab)
	• Neutropenia (ticlopidine)
Anticoagulation	• Thrombotic thrombocytopenic purpura (thienopyridines)
• Coronary thrombosis	
• Heparin-induced thrombocytopenia	**Contrast**
	• Contrast-associated nephropathy
Contrast	
• Anaphylatoid reactions	

the procedure and the risk of hemorrhage into the retroperitoneum or into the rectus sheath is increased. In the presence of iliac obstructive disease, the use of a steerable floppy tip wire (e.g., Wholey wire) may increase the chance of successful arterial canalization and may reduce the risk of dissection. Under no circumstances should a wire be advanced retrogradely unless pulsatile blood flow returns through the needle. If resistance is encountered while passing the wire, the wire should be pulled back into the needle or out of the body, the needle should be repositioned and its angle should be adjusted, so that pulsatile blood is seen returning through the needle before re-advancing the wire.

When a glycoprotein (GP) IIb/IIIa antagonist and unfractionated heparin are used during the procedure, the target activated clotting time (ACT) should be 250 to 300 seconds.[9] Postprocedural heparin should be avoided unless there is a clear need, such as in a patient requiring an intra-aortic balloon pump. At the end of the procedure, a closure device could be placed, or the arterial sheath can be removed as soon as the ACT is normalized (e.g., <180s). Bivalirudin has a relatively short half-life (~25min), but manual removal of the sheath is still delayed at least 1 to 2 hours (or more in case of the presence of renal insufficiency), unless a closure device can be implanted immediately postprocedure. If intravenous enoxaparin is used for anticoagulation, a longer waiting period (~4h) is needed before sheath removal.

The use of a closure device after arterial access allows early ambulation after procedure. Although some reports suggested that closure devices reduced access-site bleeding and were cost effective,[10–12] others reported no difference, or worsening, in bleeding rates among various devices or when compared with manual pressure, irrespective of the types of anticoagulation given.[13–17] Regardless, each of these devices is associated with a learning curve, and the rates of successful deployment of these devices are closely related to the operators' experience with the particular device. Other factors that play a role in the choice of closure devices include presence of peripheral vascular disease, calcification, location of entry site, prior closure device use in the same location, and need for early ambulation. The management decision of access-site complications is also affected by whether a closure device has been used or not.

Before implantation of any closure device, a limited angiogram of the arterial access site should be performed. In our opinion, the presence of calcification is a relative contraindication for suture-mediated devices (e.g., Perclose) and for collagen-based closure devices (e.g., Angioseal). Deployment of a closure device below the common femoral artery (at the bifurcation, superficial femoral artery, or profundus femoris), or at the origin of a side branch, is not recommended. If there is any doubt about whether a closure device can be deployed successfully, manual pressure remains the standard for hemostasis after sheath removal.

3.1. Specific Complications Involving the Access Site

3.1.1. Hematoma, Retroperitoneal Bleeding, and Pseudoaneurysm

Access bleeding accounts for more than 50% of all bleeding complications associated with PCI procedures.[18] Almost always an early complication, late pseudoaneurysm pain or bleeding are possible, more so in this era of more aggressive anticoagulation regimens. Risk factors of developing hematomas include obesity, low body weight, female gender, old age, large sheath size, patient movement, prolonged procedure, anticoagulation after the procedure, severe hypertension or high pulse pressure, access site above or below the common femoral artery, or multiple or posterior wall punctures. Hematomas in the groin, lower abdomen, or thigh are related to bleeding from the front wall of the artery, while retroperitoneal hematoma is often due to extravasation in the posterior wall of the artery that is created with the needle during initial arterial access.

Use of relatively low dose unfractionated heparin (60–70 U/kg) when combined with a GP IIb/IIIa antagonist, avoidance of postprocedural heparin administration, and early sheath removal have markedly reduced the incidence of hematoma formation.[19] Immediate management of hematoma or retroperitoneal bleeding includes manual pressure applied directly over the arterial entrance site, which provides pressure to the anterior and the posterior wall of the artery against the femoral head. The maneuver also helps to dissipate the blood collection over the bleeding site and allows more direct pressure onto the extravasation site. The amount of pressure should be strong enough to stop any bleeding but not to compromise the perfusion of the distal extremity. Rapid volume replacement (e.g., pressurized normal saline infusion), vasopressors, or atropine may be used to stabilize the patient's hemodynamics. When a moderate to large-sized hematoma occurs, or retroperitoneal bleeding is suspected, protamine should be given to reverse the effect of unfractionated heparin and any GP IIb/IIIa inhibitor infusion should be stopped. Platelet transfusion may be considered if abciximab was given. The clinical effectiveness of protamine in reversing low-molecular-weight heparin is undetermined because it is effective in reversing the anti-IIa activity but not the anti-Xa activity of low-molecular-weight heparin. There is currently no antidote for bivalirudin.

Track oozing is not uncommon after an apparently successful closure device deployment. When this happens, manual pressure is usually all that is required, but if bleeding persists, local injection of approximately 10 mL of 2% lidocaine with 1:100,000 epinephrine around the track can facilitate hemostasis.

Pseudoaneurysms represent communication between the arterial lumen and the adventitial or subcutaneous tissue, and are characterized by a narrow neck at the exit site on the Duplex ultrasound. A pseudoaneurysm may cause no symptom, but could be painful if it enlarges. For small pseudoaneurysms (e.g., <2 cm in diameter), observation, compression manually or with ultrasound probe for 15 to 30 minutes may be all that is needed to completely seal the entry site. If this enlarges or is associated with hemodynamic compromise, ultrasound-guided thrombus injection may be attempted.[20,21] To do this, an ultrasound probe is placed directly over the suspected bleeding site and the location of the pseudoaneurysm and its neck are identified. A 21-gauge spinal needle is introduced parallel to the beam of the ultrasound probe. The location of the needle tip within the pseudoaneurysm is confirmed by (1) direct visualization on the ultrasound, (2) ability to aspirate blood, and (3) identifying a small amount of saline contrast injected through the needle. Attention should be paid so as not to allow the needle to inadvertently advance into the main artery during thrombin injection as this can result in an acute ischemic leg. Using a 1-mL tuberculin syringe, about 1000 U of thrombin is then injected into the pseudoaneurysm through the spinal needle. Flow into the pseudoaneurysm will disappear instantaneously if the thrombin is injected correctly. When this is done, the ultrasound should be used to confirm patency of the arterial and venous systems, and should confirm the absence of any other pseudoaneurysms. An ultrasound may be repeated at 24 hours after thrombin injection to exclude recurrent pseudoaneurysm formation.

When bleeding continues despite manual pressure (e.g., location of bleeding is above the inguinal ligament), the patient may be brought back to the catheterization laboratory and the bleeding site can be directly visualized under fluoroscopy. Antegrade injection of contrast can be performed with a 5F internal mammary artery (IMA) diagnostic catheter advanced across the aortic bifurcation. Once a pseudoaneurysm is confirmed, a 6F crossover sheath can replace the IMA catheter via a 0.035-inch wire, and a low-pressure balloon inflation (e.g., with 5–6 mm diameter balloon catheter) can be used to seal the extravasation. Usually, hemostasis can be achieved after 5 to 10 minutes of balloon inflation. In addition, while the balloon is inflated, percutaneous thrombin injection into the pseudoaneurysm can be done safely. If bleeding continues despite these measures, placement of a stent graft (e.g., Wallgraft) may be considered as surgical consultation is obtained.

3.1.2. Arterial Dissection

Atherosclerosis occurs systemically in both coronary and noncoronary circulations. The presence of peripheral vascular disease increases the risk of access site complications. A tortuous femoral or iliac artery with or without atherosclerotic plaque may also increase the risk of dissection when advancing guidewires. When an arterial sheath is placed subintimally and a dissection flap is raised (Figure 9-2), antegrade blood flow can be reestablished with sheath removal alone. In other occasions, when a spiral dissection occurs and antegrade blood flow is compromised (such as in the case when the guidewire enters and exits an atheroma as in Figure 9-3), it would be prudent to perform angioplasty via retrograde access in the contralateral extremity as described in the last section.

3.1.3. Infections

The risk of access-site infection with manual compression after sheath removal is uncommon, but this occurs in about 0.5% of all cases when arterial closure devices are employed.[11,22] Patients with access-site infection may present with localized pain, tenderness, erythema, drainage, fever, and rigor that begin within a few days after the procedure. Female gender has been suggested as a risk factor for access-site infection.[11] Most of these infections are related to *Staphylococcal* species.

In many institutions, surgical scrub prior to the procedure is mandated but this practice does not eliminate the risk of infections. Other centers have been routinely giving one dose of a systemic antibiotic at the end of the procedure, but the effectiveness of this practice has not been reported. Although there is no evidence suggesting one closure device is associated with more infections than the others, any infection associated with closure device is considered serious. The treatment of an access-site infection depends on whether a closure device has been used. Surgical debridement and reconstruction may be required if a closure device has been utilized.[23]

4. Coronary Perforation

Coronary perforation is one of the most devastating complications associated with PCI. While usually manifest during the procedure it may occasionally become apparent after the patient's departure from the catheterization laboratory (Figures 9-4 and 9-5). Coronary perforation is defined as any extravasation of blood beyond the boundary of the vessel. Based on the angiographic morphology and the extent of extravasation, Ellis and colleagues

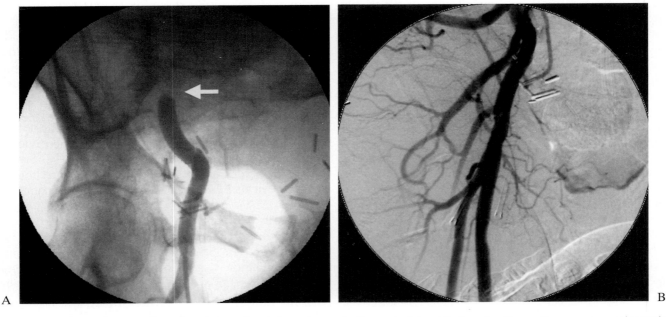

A   B

FIGURE 9-2. Femoral artery dissection during sheath insertion. Resistance was encountered during advancement of a 0.035-inch J-tipped guidewire after placement of the 6F sheath in the right common femoral artery. Digital angiography confirmed entry of the arterial sheath within a false lumen, as suggested by the blunt cut-off of the contrast during the limited common femoral angiography (arrow, A). Arterial access was established in the contralateral limb and a diagnostic coronary angiography was accomplished via the new access. Using an IMA diagnostic catheter engaged in the proximal right common iliac artery, antegrade flow was present in the common femoral artery, superficial femoral artery, as well as in the profundus femoris, assuring that the arterial sheath can be safely removed without intervention and adverse sequelae (B).

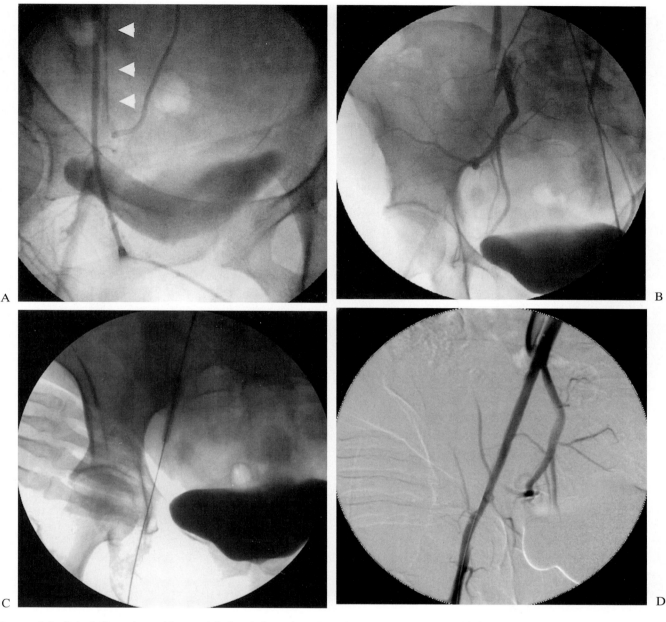

FIGURE 9-3. Spiral dissection with arterial sheath insertion. A 6F arterial sheath was inserted into the right common femoral artery via a J-tipped guidewire, which was initially advanced with mild resistance. After the completion of the apparently unremarkable diagnostic coronary procedure, a limited common femoral artery angiogram prior to anticipated closure device placement showed spiral dissection of the common femoral artery that extended to the external iliac artery (arrowhead) and compromises distal flow to the right lower extremity (A). This was confirmed with antegrade contrast injection via the contralateral access (B). Through the IMA catheter, a stiff-angled guidewire was advanced carefully across the common femoral artery and the IMA catheter was advanced forward over the guidewire. After confirming that the catheter was in the true lumen, the original arterial sheath was removed and manual pressure was applied. Balloon angioplasty was performed via the crossover sheath in the contralateral access and the dissection was successful sealed off (C). Normal flow was achieved with no residual stenosis (D).

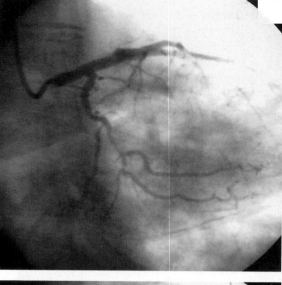

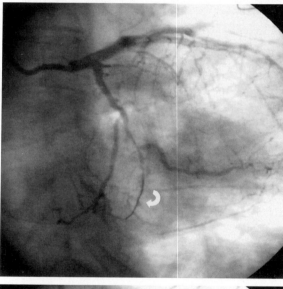

FIGURE 9-4. Guidewire perforation. This 84-year-old female patient had Canadian Cardiovascular Society (CCS) class IV angina associated with severe and diffuse stenosis in the mid and distal circumflex artery (A). Initial intention was to wire into the third obtuse marginal branch and was unsuccessful. Angioplasty was performed with a 1.5-mm balloon catheter while the BMW guidewire was inadvertently put across the arterial wall (B). Free extravasation was noted around the tip of the guidewire during angiography (C). Anticoagulation with heparin was reversed with protamine, and integrilin was stopped. The guidewire was redirected into the second obtuse marginal branch and balloon inflation was performed across the mid circumflex artery into the second obtuse marginal branch for 2 minutes (D), followed by a 2.25 × 18-mm stent catheter inflation for 90 seconds. Final angiogram revealed no further extravasation and an occluded distal circumflex artery (E). The patient remained hemodynamically stable throughout the case. The peak CKMB level was measured at 33 IU at 12 hours after the procedure, and the patient was discharged on aspirin and clopidogrel the next day.

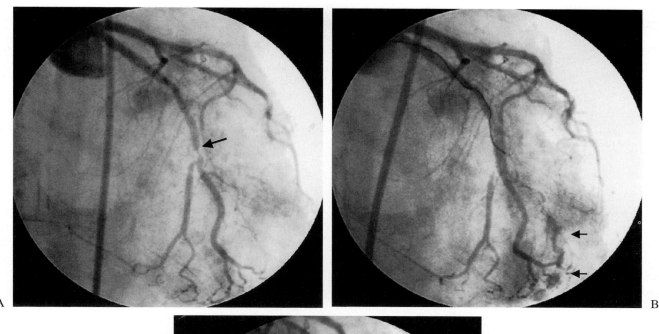

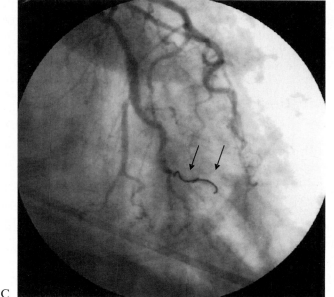

FIGURE 9-5. Guidewire perforation. An 80-year-old woman underwent ad-hoc PCI of the circumflex artery after a successful right coronary artery (RCA) stent placement (A). She received chronic warfarin therapy and her international normalized ratio (INR) was 1.9 on the day of the procedure. Because of the heavy calcification in the proximal coronary artery, the operator elected to exchange the 6F JL4 guide catheter to a 6F XB3.5 guide catheter through a 300-cm Platinum-Plus wire placed within the circumflex artery. The stent was successfully placed in the target lesion, though guidewire perforation was noted (B). The intergrilin infusion was stopped and protamine was given to reverse the effect of heparin. The patient was observed in the catheterization laboratory for 15 minutes and blood pressure was maintained within normal range. About half an hour later, the patient was noted hypotensive in the intensive care unit, and the patient responded to intravenous bolus of saline solution. Echocardiogram confirmed moderate-sized pericardial effusion. The patient was transferred to the catheterization laboratory where a pericardiocentesis drainage was placed and 200 mL of blood was removed. Free extravasation was noted in the distal circumflex artery. A Transit catheter was advanced over a Choice PT wire to the distal circumflex artery and the wire was then removed. Two detachable microembolization coils were deployed to the distal circumflex artery and the patient remained hemodynamically stable over the next 24 hours and no further pericardial drainage was observed (C). The pericardial drain was then removed.

TABLE 9-2. Classification of coronary perforation proposed by Ellis.

Perforation type	Angiographic definitions	Complications (%)		
		Death	Tamponade	Emergency surgery
I	A crater extending outside of the lumen only and in the absence of linear staining angiographically suggestive of a dissection	0	0	15
II	Pericardial or myocardial blush without a ≥1-mm exit hole	0	10	6
IIIa	Frank streaming of contrast through a >1-mm exit hole	20	53	57
IIIb	Perforation with cavity spilling (e.g., coronary sinus)	0	0	0

Source: Adapted from Ellis et al.[24] and Dippel et al.[26]

proposed a classification scheme for coronary perforation that assists interventionalists in predicting the likelihood of acute decompensation in the catheterization laboratory (Table 9-2).[24] Patients with type I coronary perforations typically require temporary balloon tamponade across or proximal to the extravasation site, without the need for reversal of anticoagulation. Type III perforations demonstrate continuous streaming of blood through a large (>1 mm) exit hole into the pericardium (Figure 9-6). This usually requires reversal of anticoagulation, balloon tamponade, and sometimes a covered stent to seal the exit site; urgent pericardiocentesis is similarly required for the accompanying cardiac tamponade.

4.1. Predictors of Coronary Perforation

4.1.1. Patient Factors

Interventionalists aware of the risk factors for coronary perforation can alter case and equipment selections to minimize the risk (Table 9-3). Old age and female gender have been associated with a higher incidence of perforation. Heavy calcification, eccentricity, proximal tortuosity, and angulated lesions, as well as chronic total occlusions, are anatomic characteristics associated with higher risk of perforation.[24–26]

4.1.2. Device Selection

The use of guidewires with hydrophilic coatings or increased stiffness may facilitate recanalization of high-risk lesions such as heavily calcified, chronically occluded lesions, but these also pose an increased risk of perforation and therefore care needs to be taken while using these wires. Although guidewire perforation is often benign and usually responds to guidewire withdrawal alone or with brief balloon occlusion proximally, inadvertent passage of a balloon catheter across the exit site may create a hemodynamically important extravasation. Delayed tamponade has been reported with guidewire perforation, and close observation is recommended within the first 24 hours or more after the incident.[24]

When crossing a chronically occluded lesion, a soft-tipped guidewire should be used first; an over-the-wire balloon placed across the guidewire transition often helps to improve support. The over-the-wire balloon catheter is preferable because of the ease of exchanging guidewires, superior pushability, and ability to perform contrast injection through the balloon catheter to confirm passage into the true lumen once it passes the occlusion. Although an 8F guide catheter may provide extra support, a 6F catheter allows deep seating of the guide. Guide catheters with specific shapes (XB, EBU, Amplatz, or Voda) may also provide extra support and further enhance the pushability of the guidewires. Once the lesion is successfully crossed and the true lumen position is confirmed, a less stiff, nonhydrophilic wire should replace the hydrophilic wire through the balloon catheter in order to avoid inadvertent guidewire perforation during subsequent device manipulation. The Frontrunner™ coronary catheter (LuMend Inc., Redwood City, CA), a device that is approved for recanalization of occluded coronary arteries that fail conventional techniques, has also been linked to coronary perforation.[27]

Potent antithrombotic therapies using GP IIb/IIIa inhibitors or clopidogrel pretreatment did not appear to increase the risk of perforation in several large series to date,[28–32] although there was no information in these series about the morbidity of the patients when a type III perforation did occur.

Atheroablative devices, such as rotational or directional atherectomy, and cutting balloons have consistently been associated with a higher incidence of perforation.[24–26,33–41] New technologies that are intended to overcome the limitations of balloon angioplasty through ablation, cutting, or thromboaspiration are associated with a higher risk of perforation,[24–26,33–39,41–54] especially when these devices are intended for more high-risk lesions.

Regardless of the type of device, device sizing is one of the main determining factors for perforation risk. When stent placement is intended, an undersized balloon is usually sufficient for predilatation in order to ensure the lesion is compliant with balloon inflation, and a stent with size not greater than 1.1 times the reference diameter of the vessel should be used. For rotational atherectomy, the burr size should be less than 0.7 times the reference

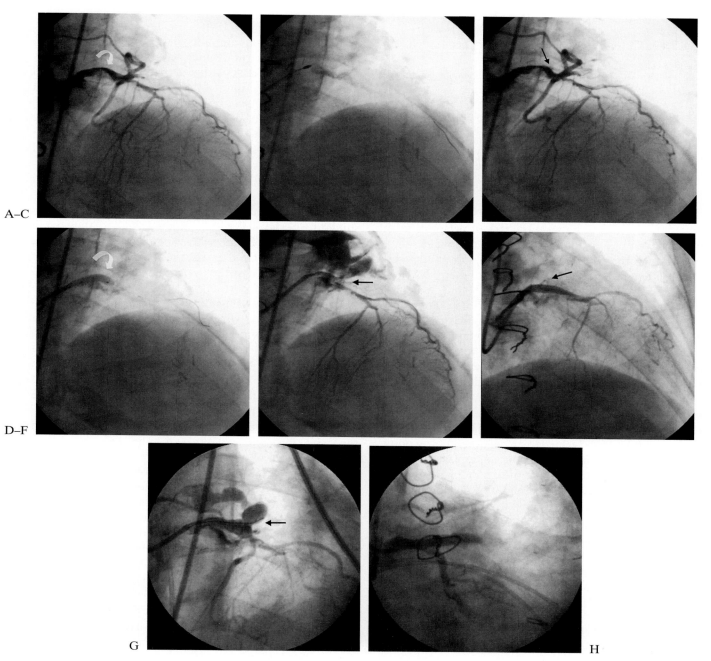

A–C

D–F

G　　　　　　　　　　　　　　　　　　　H

FIGURE 9-6. Coronary perforation and pseudoaneurysm formation. The 81-year-old man had CCS class III angina. He had a patent bypass internal mammary arterial bypass graft to the left anterior descending artery. After the administration of unfractionated heparin and initial bolus and infusion of abciximab, an attempt of revascularization of the left main coronary artery that supplied the diagonal branch was begun with rotational atherectomy using 1.5-mm burr (A, curved arrow; B). Mild stream of extravasation was present after the first pass of the burr but it was not noticed by the operator (C, arrow). Balloon angioplasty followed by stent deployment (4.0 × 16 mm) was performed and a type III perforation was noted along the stent (D, E). Cardiac tamponade ensued despite immediate balloon tamponade within the vessel. A pericardial drain was inserted and protamine and platelets were given. A JOMED stent (16 mm) was deployed across the extravasation site with a 4.0 mm noncompliant balloon. Mild extravasation persisted but responded to prolonged balloon inflation (F). Although the patient remained hemodynamically stable and there was no pericardial drainage over the subsequent hours, a repeat angiogram on the next day demonstrated a large pseudoaneurysm coming off the left main coronary artery (G). Another JOMED stent was placed distal to the first one but still failed to completely seal the exit site. Although thrombosis of the pseudoaneursym was finally achieved by prolonged balloon inflation within the left main coronary artery, this also resulted in thrombosis in the septal perforators and the diagonal artery (H). The patient, who had left bundle branch block on his electrocardiogram prior to the procedure, developed complete heart block, necessitating implantation of permanent pacemaker prior to discharge.

TABLE 9-3. Factors associated with coronary perforation.

Patient's factors	Female
	Elderly
Lesion morphology	Heavy calcification
	Eccentric lesion
	Angulated lesion
	Chronic total occlusion
	Small vessel diameter
Procedural factors	Atheroablative devices
	Hydrophilic wire
	Over-sized balloon or stent diameter

diameter in order to balance the risk of perforation and yet achieve optimal amount of plaque removal.

Although the Cutting Balloon™ angioplasty catheter (Boston Scientific Scimed Inc., Maple Grove, NM) was proposed to be advantageous for in-stent restenosis, ostial lesions, and calcified stenosis,[55–59] its utility for in-stent restenosis has been disputed in two randomized controlled trials.[60,61] Coronary perforation, inability to retrieve balloon catheter when used in dilatating heavily calcified lesions, and late aneurysm formation have also been reported.[25,41,62,63] Indeed, the incidence of coronary perforation reported in cutting balloon series (0.3%) was slightly higher than conventional balloon angioplasty (0.1%) but not as high as stents (0.7%) or atheroablative devices (~1.5%).[25,41] Delayed perforation after an apparently uneventful cutting balloon angioplasty has also been reported,[40] and therefore a high index of suspicion is required when dealing with high-risk lesions.

4.2. Management of Coronary Perforation

Immediate management is determined by the extent of extravasation. Low-pressure balloon inflation across or proximal to the lesion usually is all that is required for a type I perforation, with or without reversal of anticoagulation. Irrespective of the perforation type, the GP IIb/IIIa antagonist infusion should be stopped. Type III perforation necessitates reversal of anticoagulation, and immediate balloon tamponade across the lesion with a balloon catheter (using low pressure, e.g., 4 atm for 5–20 min depending on the patient's tolerence to ischemia). The size of the balloon should be the same or slightly smaller than the reference diameter of the vessel. A perfusion balloon can be used if the patient is not tolerant of the ischemia due to prolonged balloon inflation. Protamine sulfate (10–50 mg) should be given to reverse the heparin effect, but, as mentioned in the section on Access Bleeding, the effect of protamine on reversing the effect of low-molecular-weight heparin is undetermined.[64,65] Platelet transfusion (~6 units) should be provided to reverse abciximab. Platelet transfusion would not be effective if small molecule GP IIb/IIIa antagonists are given because they are less tightly bound to the

platelets and copious amounts of these free molecules are available in the serum, which would bind to the newly transfused platelets. A cardiac surgeon should be notified immediately at the onset of type III perforation so that an operating room can be ready for emergency surgery.

The diagnosis of cardiac tamponade is prompted by hypotension immediately following angiographic evidence of perforation, and the absence of synchronized movement of the cardiac silouette on fluoroscopy. Tachycardia is almost always the rule, but electromechanical dissociation may ensue if pericardiocentesis is not performed immediately. Emergency pericardiocentesis should be performed with equipment immediately available on the field. Echocardiographic confirmation is not required. The needle that was used to gain arterial access may be used to access the pericardial space through subxiphoid, apical, or parasternal approach. When nonpulsatile blood flow is returning from the needle, a 0.035-inch J-tipped wire is then advanced through the needle and its position within the pericardial space can be confirmed on fluoroscopy. If the wire is within a cardiac chamber, the wire should be withdrawn, and a new access into the pericardial space should be attempted. Once the wire is successfully passed into the pericardial space, the small skin incision is made and a 6F dilator (one for the arterial sheath) is introduced through the wire into the pericardium. The dilator is then removed and a 6F pigtail catheter is advanced into the pericardial space. Manual aspiration of the blood through the pigtail catheter should be immediately performed after the removal of the wire, and should be continued until no re-accumulation of blood is demonstrated in the laboratory and the patient's hemodynamics returns to baseline. At this time, the pigtail catheter should be attached to a suction drainage.

When repeat angiography demonstrates reduction of the extent of leakage causing balloon tamponade, additional balloon inflation may be all that is needed for successful closure. If there is no sign of decreasing extravasation despite prolonged balloon inflation, the use of a covered stent [e.g., polytetrafluorethylene (PTFE)-covered stent] may be considered. A covered stent may also be useful if a local hematoma is compressing the coronary artery, causing myocardial ischemia. The size of the covered stent is based on the length of the vessel segment that needs to be covered. The stent is mounted on a noncompliant balloon catheter that matches the reference diameter of the target vessel. The use of this type of stent requires minimal resistance in the proximal coronary segment for successful stent delievery because of its relatively large profile. After the stent is mounted onto the balloon catheter, the balloon should be inflated and deflated at 1 atm outside of the body in order to increase the balloon profile and decrease the risk of stent dislodgement during delivery. After the covered stent is hand crimped onto the balloon, it is then centered across the extravasation site and should be deployed at high pressure (12–18 atm). The patient should be observed for 10 to 15 minutes in the laboratory after successful sealing of the extravasation site and no blood can be aspirated through the pericardial drain. The drain should be left for 24 hours during the observation period. A prolonged course of aspirin and thienopyridine therapy should be given because a stent graft may take a longer time than conventional stents for complete endothelialization. If type III extravasation occurs at the distal end of a vessel, coil embolization may be performed (Figure 9-5). Any further elective coronary intervention should be aborted once perforation occurs.

Surgery is the last resort for treatment if the extravasation is not amendable to a percutaneous approach. The balloon catheter should remain inflated across the extravasation site en route to the operation suite. Another situation when surgical treatment should be considered is when the leakage is located at a coronary bifurcation, where the placement of a covered stent would compromise the flow of a major side branch (e.g., ≥2.5-mm diameter). Surgical treatment can offer definitive sealing of the extravasation site and also provide bypasses to all the diseased coronary arteries.

5. Acute, Subacute, and Late Stent Thrombosis

5.1. Incidence and Risk Factors

Stent implantation lowers the rate of target vessel revascularization and is now employed in more than 85% of all PCI procedures, except for very small coronary arteries (i.e., reference diameter <2.5 mm) in which the efficacy of routine stent use is still debatable. Along with coronary perforation and stroke, stent thrombosis is one of the most devastating complications encountered by interventional cardiologists and their patients. When stent thrombosis occurs, two-thirds of these events are fatal or associated with myocardial infarction, and up to 10% of patients may die within 6 months.[66]

In a large consecutive series of patients who had received bare-metal stents, stent thrombosis occurred in 0.5%–1.5% of all patients within the first month of the procedure.[66–71] Most of these events occur within 48 hours after the index procedure (Figure 9-7).[66] While suboptimal anticoagulation may be related to periprocedural stent thrombosis, mechanical factors such as incomplete stent expansion, residual dissection, and tissue prolapse could cause stent thrombosis periprocedurally or up to the first week (Figures 9-8 and 9-9).[70] A small final minimal lumen diameter, long stents, multiple stents, poor left ventricular ejection fraction, old age, and low blood

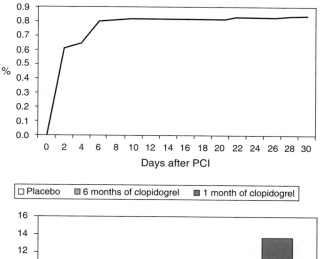

FIGURE 9-7. Early and late stent thrombosis. (A) After coronary stent implantation, acute stent thrombosis occurs mostly within 48 hours, and further event beyond 1 week is rare (data adapted from Cutlip et al.[66]). (B) After gamma brachytherapy for in-stent restenosis, subacute thrombosis is associated with early thienopyridine withdrawal. As such, a long course of dual antiplatelet regimen has been recommended (data adapted from Waksman et al.[84]).

pressure are additional predictors for stent thrombosis.[66,67,72,73]

5.2. Prevention and Management

Optimal antiplatelet and anticoagulation therapies for PCI are still evolving. When a GP IIb/IIIa inhibitor is used together with unfractionated heparin, stent thrombosis is rare during the procedure. Dual antiplatelet therapy using aspirin and a thienopyridine improves the safety and efficacy of stent implantation by effectively preventing stent thrombosis.[74–77] A minimum of a 2- to 4-week course of aspirin and clopidogrel has been recommended after bare-metal stent placement.[78] A loading dose of 300 mg clopidogrel prior to PCI may offer additional myocardial protection even with planned administration of GP IIb/IIIa antagonist.[30] The Intracoronary Stenting and Antithrombotic Regimen-Rapid Early

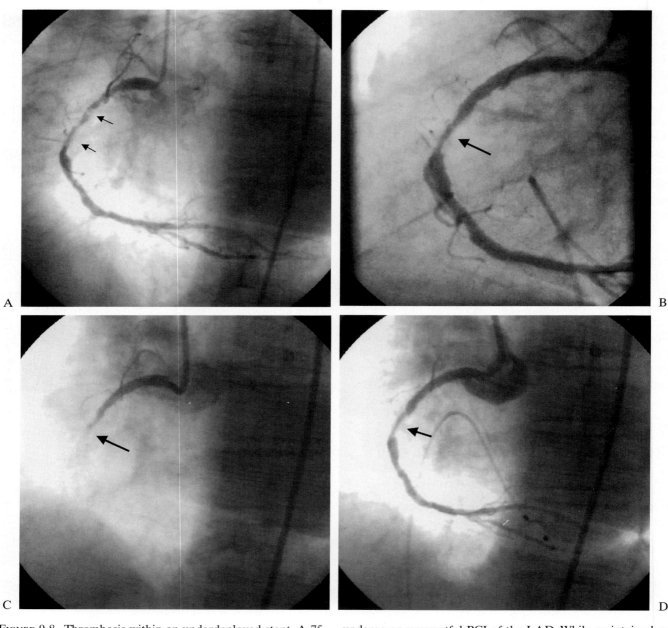

FIGURE 9-8. Thrombosis within an underdeployed stent. A 75-year-old woman with chronic hypertension was admitted for unstable angina. She had heavily calcified coronary arteries with severe lesions in the mid dominant RCA (A) and left anterior descending coronary artery (LAD). Rotational atherectomy using 1.5-mm burr was used via a 6F guide-catheter. Subsequent balloon dilatation across the lesion showed inadequate expansion but the operator elected to deploy a 3.0-mm stent across the lesion. The stent was inadequately expanded despite rupture of several noncompliant balloon catheters with high-pressure inflation (B). The patient received abciximab during the procedure, and was brought back 2 days later to undergo an uneventful PCI of the LAD. While maintained on aspirin and clopidogrel, the patient presented 5 days later with acute transmural inferior myocardial infarction (C). Reperfusion therapy using emergency balloon angioplasty alone was successful across the stent in the RCA (D). While the patient was awaiting surgical revascularization in the hospital together with discontinuation of clopidogrel, the patient suffered from re-occlusion of the stent in the RCA associated with ST-elevation myocardial infarction. The patient was brought to the operating suite and underwent successful single-vessel coronary bypass surgery.

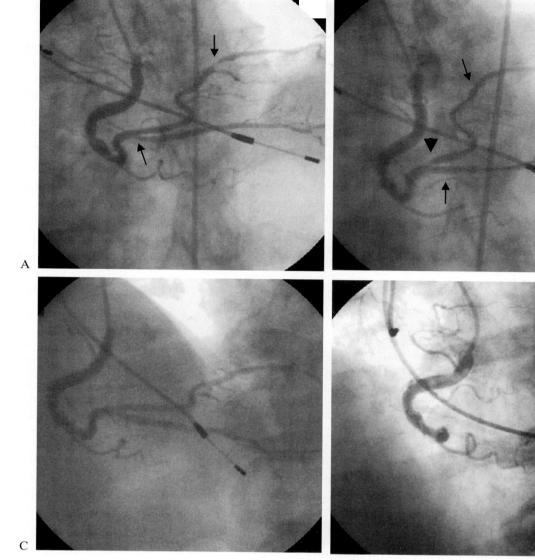

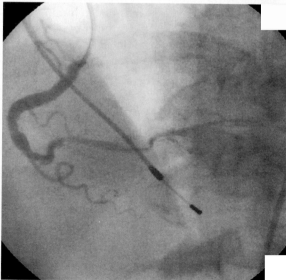

FIGURE 9-9. Stent thrombosis with suboptimal antiplatelet therapy. This 80-year-old man underwent an ad hoc PCI of the lesions at the ostial posterior descending artery and the mid segment of the posterolateral branch for stable angina associated with inferior ischemia on the myocardial stress test (A, arrows). The procedure involved placement of a sirolimus-eluting stent in each of the mid posterolateral branch and in the ostial posterior descending artery (B, arrows). Stent-jail of the ostial posterolateral branch associated with plaque shift (B, arrowhead) necessitated an additional sirolimus-eluting stent placed in the ostial posterolateral branch using T-stenting technique (C). Clopidogrel 300 mg loading dose was given to the patient immediately postprocedure but the patient failed to continue the medication after discharge. Six days later, he presented with acute transmural inferior myocardial infarction (D). Attempt of recanalization revealed partial flow return to the posterolateral branch associated with thrombus, and unsuccessful reperfusion to the posterior descending artery (E). The patient was discharged 3 days later after uneventful recovery.

Action for Coronary Treatment (ISAR-REACT) trial,[79] which demonstrated similar efficacies obtained by 600 mg clopidogrel loading and by abciximab administration in PCI among low-risk patients, further highlights the importance of clopidogrel pretreatment prior to the procedure.

Since the introduction of brachytherapy and drug-eluting stents (DES), physicians have become aware of the phenomenon of subacute (within 30 days) and late (>30 days) stent thrombosis. Following brachytherapy and angioplasty for treatment of in-stent restenosis, the process of re-endothelialization may take more than 6 months, and late stent thrombosis could occur if antiplatelet therapy is withdrawn within this period.[80,81] Placement of new stents at the time of brachytherapy markedly increases the risk of subacute or late stent thrombosis, and therefore should be avoided unless flow-limiting dissection or significant residual stenosis is present.[82] Aspirin and clopidogrel are now recommended for 9 to 12 months after brachytherapy in order to minimize the risk of late stent thrombosis.[83,84]

The salutary clinical benefits of DES lie in their predictable ability to lower clinical restenosis rates by more than 75% by inhibiting cell migration and proliferation.[85,86] Similar to brachytherapy, DES cause delay in complete endothelialization and hence a prolonged course of dual antiplatelet therapy (e.g., 3–6 months) has been used within both clinical trials and clinical practice settings. Summarizing the results of four clinical trials involving Cypher™ stent (Cordis Inc, Miami Lakes, FL),[85–88] the incidence of stent thrombosis was similar to those of bare-metal stents (0.6% vs. 0.6%). In the post-marketing surveillance of the Cypher stent for off-labelled stent use, the event rates of subacute and late stent thrombosis were comparable to those of bare metal stents.[89]

Regardless of the type of stent used, it is important to optimize the deployment in order to minimize the risk of stent thrombosis,[90] although an intravascular ultrasound study suggested that incomplete stent apposition was not a critical predictor for adverse clinical outcome with DES.[91] The reference diameter of the vessel should be determined as accurately as possible (e.g., assisted by the predilatation balloon), such that the diameter of the stent at nominal pressure should match the reference diameter of the vessel. Optimal stent deployment can be achieved by routine high-pressure inflation (12–18 atm) and complete lesion coverage, and intravascular ultrasound can be used in selected cases, particularly for vessel sizing or when it is uncertain if a dissection is present at the edges of the stent.[92,93] While the length of the bare-metal stents is chosen in order to match the lesion length, it is prudent to extend the stent coverage by 3 to 5 mm with the DES because, in the early clinical trial, resteno-

sis appears to be more prevalent when residual plaque exists at the edges.[86]

When stent thrombosis occurs, it is imperative to identify the etiology of stent thrombosis in the catheterization laboratory. Rheolytic thrombectomy (e.g., Angiojet) appears to be a useful adjunct for reducing thrombus burden and optimizing distal coronary flow.[94–97] Dissections should be treated with additional stents, and malapposed stents should be re-inflated, typically at higher pressures, if possible.

6. Renal Function Deterioration after Catheterization

Renal function deterioration, while uncommon after angiography, is associated with increased mortality, morbidity, and hospitalization costs, and a prolonged hospital stay. Contrast-induced nephropathy (CIN) and atheroembolism are important considerations for renal deterioration after catheterization.

6.1. Contrast-Induced Nephropathy

Depending on the definition used, the incidence of CIN varies between 2% and 15% of all patients undergoing angiography, with dialysis required in less than 1% of patients.[98–100] Among various definitions of CIN, a greater than 25% increase in baseline serum creatinine has been more commonly used in clinical trials. While many clinicians may debate whether such an arbitrary selection of a level of serum creatinine should be used to reflect CIN, serum creatinine does provide a convenient means for clinicians to monitor renal function and its response to treatment of CIN. When CIN occurs, the mortality rate varies between 5% and 34%, depending on the comorbidities of the patient.[101–104] Therefore, every effort should be made to avoid this complication.

Contrast-induced nephropathy is typically noted at 48 hours after the procedure, with renal function typically returning to baseline by days 4 to 10. Urinalysis is often benign, with nonspecific findings such as proteinuria, granular casts, or epithelial cells present. The pathogenesis of CIN is still not clearly understood. Direct contrast toxicity, vasoconstriction leading to renal medullary ischemia, and oxygen free radical production in the glomerular basement membrane and the mesangium are now considered the mechanism of CIN.[105–107]

Baseline renal insufficiency is the most important predictor for the development of CIN.[100] Other risk factors include diabetes mellitus, congestive heart failure, dehydration, concomitant renal toxic medications (e.g., nonsteroidal anti-inflammatory drugs), contrast volume, and repeat contrast administration within 72 hours.[100,108] In a randomized trial that included 1196 patients with preexisting renal insufficiency, those who received low osmolality nonionic contrast (iohexol) had less incidence of CIN (>1.0 mg/dL in serum creatinine) as compared to those who received high osmolality ionic contrast (diatrizoate) (3% vs. 7%, $P < 0.002$).[99] Among 126 patients with diabetes and renal insufficiency (serum creatinine, 1.5–3.5 mg/dL) undergoing angiography, patients who were randomized to iso-osmolar nonionic contrast (iodixanol) had significantly less incidence of CIN (>0.5 mg/dL rise in serum creatinine) than those who received low osmolar nonionic contrast (iohexol) (3% vs. 26%, $P = 0.002$).[109] The results of these studies suggest that patients who have baseline abnormal renal function should receive iso-osmolar nonionic contrast in order to minimize the risk of CIN.

There are two methods that can lower the risk of CIN. Infusion of normal saline has been the most effective regimen in lowering the risk of CIN and it remains the benchmark against which other methods are compared. Isotonic saline infusion reduces the incidence of CIN by 65% when compared to half normal saline administration among patients with renal insufficiency undergoing cardiac catheterization.[98]

The second method is administration of acetylcysteine. The use of this medication has been gaining increased popularity in prophylaxis against CIN. Apart from its antioxidant property, acetylcysteine promotes vasodilatation through the reduction of angiotensin-converting enzyme activity and the enhancement of the production of nitric oxide by increasing nitric oxide synthase.[110–112] There have been nine published randomized controlled trials that examined the utility of this medication among contrast recipients. In seven trials, which enrolled more than 600 high-risk patients, 600 mg acetylcysteine twice a day started at least 24 hours prior to angiography resulted in a significant (70%–90%) reduction in the incidence of CIN.[113–119] Another study that enrolled 183 patients with lower risk of renal insufficiency demonstrated a 50% reduction in the incidence of CIN but this did not reach the prespecified statistical significance.[120] In a randomized controlled trial that tested the efficacy of 1200 mg acetylcysteine given at 1 hour before and 3 hours after the index procedure, there was no significant benefit demonstrated.[121] We can conclude that among high-risk patients who are already receiving intravenous hydration, acetylcysteine administration may further minimize the risk of CIN; however, this medication has to be given at least 24 hours prior to the procedure in order to achieve such an effect.

Several other modalities have been considered as a primary prophylaxis for CIN in patients with renal insufficiency. Among these include furosemide, mannitol, calcium channel blockers, dopamine, and endothelin antagonists, but they all failed to produce significant benefits, or even harm, in clinical studies.[122–130] Though several small observational studies had suggested that dopaminergic agonist fenoldopam mesylate was effective in preventing CIN,[131–134] a large randomized control trial, the Evaluation of Corlopam in Patients at Risk for Renal Failure—A Safety and Efficacy Trial (CONTRAST),[135] confirmed that no such benefit was present in fenoldopam when given to patients with renal insufficiency and who were already receiving intravenous hydration prior to catheterization. Recently, hemofiltration was shown to be effective in eliminating CIN.[136] However, there are logistic issues associated with offering this therapy to all renal dysfunction patients as a prophylactic treatment including the associated high cost; further investigation is required to examine whether this is cost-effective.

6.2. Atheroembolism

Renal atheroembolism is manifested by continuous worsening of renal function, which plateaus at approximately 4 weeks postcatheterization. While atheromatous debris has been reported in up to 50% of guide catheters,[137,138] clinically detectable systemic atheroembolism associated with catheterization occurs in only 1%–2% of overall cases, but 60% may be associated with renal function deterioration.[139] Severe peripheral vascular disease, presence of an aortic aneurysm, large guide catheters (e.g., 8F), and specific guide-catheter shapes (e.g., XB, Voda, Amplatz), but not the femoral approach, are associated with increased risk of dislodgement of atheromatous debris.[137–139] Patients may have associated evidence of distal embolization in the lower extremities (livedo reticularis, blue-toe syndrome, and digital gangrene), and eosinophilia may be present.

To reduce the risk of atheroembolism, the guide catheters should be advanced and removed through guidewires in order to straighten the catheters and to prevent them from scrapping along the aortic wall. Once atheroembolism occurs, management is usually supportive. Hydration and blood pressure control are essential. Analgesics may be required for painful ulceration due to digital embolization, and amputation may be required in severe instances.

7. Future Perspectives

Complications related to PCI may occur within the first 24 hours and also extend beyond the hospitalization period. We have described the presentation and management of several major complications associated with

PCI. With the continuous refinement of interventional technologies, the number of PCI procedures will continue to grow, and physicians are going to operate on more challenging lesions; however, the incidence of these complications are not expected to decrease. Prevention remains the best way to avoid these events.

References

1. Dalby M, Davies J, Rakhit R, et al. Feasibility and safety of day-case transfemoral coronary stenting. Catheter Cardiovasc Interv. 2003;60:18–24.

2. Khatri S, Webb JG, Carere RG, et al. Safety and cost benefit of same-day discharge after percutaneous coronary intervention. Am J Cardiol. 2002;90:425–427.

3. Carere RG, Webb JG, Buller CE, et al. Suture closure of femoral arterial puncture sites after coronary angioplasty followed by same-day discharge. Am Heart J. 2000; 139:52–58.

4. Ziakas AA, Klinke BP, Mildenberger CR, et al. Safety of same-day-discharge radial percutaneous coronary intervention: a retrospective study. Am Heart J. 2003; 146:699–704.

5. Banning AP, Ormerod OJ, Channon K, et al. Same day discharge following elective percutaneous coronary intervention in patients with stable angina. Heart. 2003;89:665.

6. Slagboom T, Kiemeneij F, Laarman GJ, et al. Actual outpatient PTCA: results of the OUTCLAS pilot study. Catheter Cardiovasc Interv. 2001;53:204–208.

7. Ormiston JA, Shaw BL, Panther MJ, et al. Percutaneous coronary intervention with bivalirudin anticoagulation, immediate sheath removal, and early ambulation: a feasibility study with implications for day-stay procedures. Catheter Cardiovasc Interv. 2002;55:289–293.

8. Piper WD, Malenka DJ, Ryan TJ Jr, et al. Predicting vascular complications in percutaneous coronary interventions. Am Heart J. 2003;145:1022–1029.

9. Chew DP, Bhatt DL, Lincoff AM, et al. Defining the optimal activated clotting time during percutaneous coronary intervention: aggregate results from 6 randomized, controlled trials. Circulation. 2001;103:961–966.

10. Chevalier B, Lancelin B, Koning R, et al. Effect of a closure device on complication rates in high-local-risk patients: results of a randomized multicenter trial. Catheter Cardiovasc Interv. 2003;58:285–291.

11. Eggebrecht H, Haude M, Woertgen U, et al. Systematic use of a collagen-based vascular closure device immediately after cardiac catheterization procedures in 1,317 consecutive patients. Catheter Cardiovasc Interv. 2002;57:486–495.

12. Rickli H, Unterweger M, Sutsch G, et al. Comparison of costs and safety of a suture-mediated closure device with conventional manual compression after coronary artery interventions. Catheter Cardiovasc Interv. 2002;57:297–302.

13. Eggebrecht H, Haude M, von Birgelen C, et al. Early clinical experience with the 6 French Angio-Seal device: immediate closure of femoral puncture sites after diagnostic and interventional coronary procedures. Catheter Cardiovasc Interv. 2001;53:437–442.

14. Shammas NW, Rajendran VR, Alldredge SG, et al. Randomized comparison of Vasoseal and Angioseal closure devices in patients undergoing coronary angiography and angioplasty. Catheter Cardiovasc Interv. 2002;55:421–425.

15. Kahn ZM, Kumar M, Hollander G, Frankel R. Safety and efficacy of the Perclose suture-mediated closure device after diagnostic and interventional catheterizations in a large consecutive population. Catheter Cardiovasc Interv. 2002;55:8–13.

16. Rinder MR, Tamirisa PK, Taniuchi M, et al. Safety and efficacy of suture-mediated closure after percutaneous coronary interventions. Catheter Cardiovasc Interv. 2001;54: 146–151.

17. Dangas G, Mehran R, Kokolis S, et al. Vascular complications after percutaneous coronary interventions following hemostasis with manual compression versus arteriotomy closure devices. J Am Coll Cardiol. 2001;38:638–641.

18. Juran NB. Minimizing bleeding complications of percutaneous coronary intervention and glycoprotein IIb-IIIa antiplatelet therapy. Am Heart J. 1999;138:297–306.

19. Platelet glycoprotein IIb/IIIa receptor blockade and low-dose heparin during percutaneous coronary revascularization. The EPILOG Investigators. N Engl J Med. 1997;336:1689–1696.

20. Olsen DM, Rodriguez JA, Vranic M, et al. A prospective study of ultrasound scan-guided thrombin injection of femoral pseudoaneurysm: a trend toward minimal medication. J Vasc Surg. 2002;36:779–782.

21. Edgerton JR, Moore DO, Nichols D, et al. Obliteration of femoral artery pseudoaneurysm by thrombin injection. Ann Thorac Surg. 2002;74:S1413–S1415.

22. Cherr GS, Travis JA, Ligush J Jr, et al. Infection is an unusual but serious complication of a femoral artery catheterization site closure device. Ann Vasc Surg. 2001;15: 567–570.

23. Johanning JM, Franklin DP, Elmore JR, Han DC. Femoral artery infections associated with percutaneous arterial closure devices. J Vasc Surg. 2001;34:983–985.

24. Ellis SG, Ajluni S, Arnold AZ, et al. Increased coronary perforation in the new device era. Incidence, classification, management, and outcome. Circulation. 1994;90:2725–2530.

25. Stankovic G, Ferraro M, Kostov J, et al. Coronary artery perforations: incidence, predictors and clinical outcomes. Circulation. 2002;106:II-444.

26. Dippel EJ, Kereiakes DJ, Tramuta DA, et al. Coronary perforation during percutaneous coronary intervention in the era of abciximab platelet glycoprotein IIb/IIIa blockade: an algorithm for percutaneous management. Catheter Cardiovasc Interv. 2001;52:279–286.

27. Orlic D, Stankovic G, Sangiorgi G, et al. Preliminary experience with the frontrunner coronary catheter: novel device dedicated to mechanical revascularization of chronic total occlusions. Catheter Cardiovasc Interv. 2005;64:146–152.

28. Bajzer CT, Whitlow PL, Lincoff AM, et al. Coronary perforation and pericardial tamponade risk in the abciximab era. J Am Coll Cardiol. 1999;34:72A.

29. Topol EJ, Moliterno DJ, Herrmann HC, et al. Comparison of two platelet glycoprotein IIb/IIIa inhibitors, tirofiban and abciximab, for the prevention of ischemic events with percutaneous coronary revascularization. N Engl J Med. 2001;344:1888–1894.

30. Chan AW, Moliterno DJ, Berger PB, et al. Triple antiplatelet therapy during percutaneous coronary intervention is associated with improved outcomes including one-year survival: results from the Do Tirofiban and Reo-ProGive Similar Efficacy Outcome Trial (TARGET). J Am Coll Cardiol. 2003;42:1188–1195.

31. Mehta SR, Yusuf S, Peters RJ, et al. Effects of pretreatment with clopidogrel and aspirin followed by long-term therapy in patients undergoing percutaneous coronary intervention: the PCI-CURE study. Lancet. 2001;358: 527–533.

32. Steinhubl SR, Berger PB, Mann JT, et al. Early and sustained dual oral antiplatelet therapy following percutaneous coronary intervention. JAMA. 2002;288:2411–2420.

33. Ajluni SC, Glazier S, Blankenship L, et al. Perforations after percutaneous coronary interventions: clinical, angiographic, and therapeutic observations. Catheter Cardiovasc Diagn. 1994;32:206–212.

34. Vlietstra RE, Abbotsmith CW, Douglas JS Jr, et al. Complications with directional atherectomy. Experience at eight centers. Circulation. 1989;80:II–582.

35. Vetter JW, Robertson G, Selmon M, et al. Perforation with directional coronary atherectomy. J Am Coll Cardiol. 1992;19:76A.

36. Johnson D, Hinohara T, Reberson G, et al. Acute complications of directional coronary atherectomy are related to the morphology of excised stenosis. J Am Coll Cardiol. 1992;19:76A.

37. Reifart N, Vandormael M, Krajcar M, et al. Randomized comparison of angioplasty of complex coronary lesions at a single center. Excimer Laser, Rotational Atherectomy, and Balloon Angioplasty Comparison (ERBAC) Study. Circulation. 1997;96:91–98.

38. Takagi T, Toutouzas K, Stankovic G, et al. Initial experience with a new 8 French compatible directional coronary atherectomy catheter: a comparison with GTO device. J Am Coll Cardiol. 2002;39:7A.

39. Cox DA, Stuckey T, Babb J, et al. The endicor X-Sizer AMI registry: improvement in myocardial blush scores with adjunctive thrombectomy combined with stenting for AMI. Circulation. 2001;104:II–504.

40. Maruo T, Yasuda S, Miyazaki S. Delayed appearance of coronary artery perforation following cutting balloon angioplasty. Catheter Cardiovasc Interv. 2002;57:529–531.

41. Takano Y, Bastani S, Guttman OT, et al. Intravascular ultrasound guidance optimizes cutting balloon angioplasty. J Am Coll Cardiol. 2002;39:55A.

42. Gruberg L, Pinnow E, Flood R, et al. Incidence, management, and outcome of coronary artery perforation during percutaneous coronary intervention. Am J Cardiol. 2000;86:680–682.

43. Holmes DR Jr, Reeder GS, Ghazzal ZM, et al. Coronary perforation after excimer laser coronary angioplasty: the Excimer Laser Coronary Angioplasty Registry experience. J Am Coll Cardiol. 1994;23:330–335.

44. Bittl JA, Ryan TJ Jr, Keaney JF Jr, et al. Coronary artery perforation during excimer laser coronary angioplasty. The percutaneous Excimer Laser Coronary Angioplasty Registry. J Am Coll Cardiol. 1993;21:1158–1165.

45. Flood RD, Popma JJ, Chuang YC, et al. Incidence, angiographic predictors, and clinical significance of coronary perforation occurring after new device angioplasty. J Am Coll Cardiol. 1994;23:301A.

46. Cowley MJ, Dorros G, Kelsey SF, et al. Acute coronary events associated with percutaneous transluminal coronary angioplasty. Am J Cardiol. 1984;53:12C–16C.

47. Haase KK, Baumbach A, et al. Success rate and incidence of restenosis following coronary excimer laser angioplasty: results of a single center experience. J Interv Cardiol. 1992;5:15–23.

48. Colombo A, Hall P, Nakamura S, et al. Intracoronary stenting without anticoagulation accomplished with intravascular ultrasound guidance. Circulation. 1995;91:1676–1688.

49. Fukutomi I, Suzuki I, Hosokawa H, et al. Incidence and management of coronary perforation occurring during various coronary interventions. Jpn J Interrent Cardiol. 1996;II:189–193.

50. Baim DS, Cutlip DE, Sharma SK, et al. Final results of the Balloon vs Optimal Atherectomy Trial (BOAT). Circulation. 1998;97:322–331.

51. Bonnier H, Grube E, Koolen J. Crossing total occlusions with a forward-looking guidance system. Circulation. 2000;102:II–508.

52. Heuser RR, Underwood PL, Schroeder W, et al. Experience with OCR guidance in the treatment of chronic total occlusion. Circulation. 2001;104:II–416.

53. Condado JA, Lansky AJ, Saucedo J, et al. Five year clinical and angiographic follow-up after intracoronary 192-Iridium radiation therapy. Circulation. 2000;102:II–750.

54. Sanmartin M, Goicolea J, Ruiz-Salmeron R, et al. Coronary perforation as a potential complication derived from coronary thrombectomy with the X-Sizer device. Catheter Cardiovasc Interv. 2002;56:378–382.

55. Adamian M, Colombo A, Briguori C, et al. Cutting balloon angioplasty for the treatment of in-stent restenosis: a matched comparison with rotational atherectomy, additional stent implantation and balloon angioplasty. J Am Coll Cardiol. 2001;38:672–679.

56. Izumi M, Tsuchikane E, Funamoto M, et al. Final results of the CAPAS trial. Am Heart J. 2001;142:782–789.

57. Karvouni E, Stankovic G, Albiero R, et al. Cutting balloon angioplasty for treatment of calcified coronary lesions. Catheter Cardiovasc Interv. 2001;54:473–481.

58. Kondo T, Kawaguchi K, Awaji Y, Mochizuki M. Immediate and chronic results of cutting balloon angioplasty: a matched comparison with conventional angioplasty. Clin Cardiol. 1997;20:459–463.

59. Muramatsu T, Tsukahara R, Ho M, et al. Effectiveness of cutting balloon angioplasty for small vessels less than 3.0 mm in diameter. J Interv Cardiol. 2002;15:281–286.

60. Albiero R, Silber S, Di Mario C, et al. Cutting balloon versus conventional balloon angioplasty for the treatment of instent restenosis: results of the restenosis cutting

balloon evaluation trial (RESCUT). J Am Coll Cardiol. 2004;43:943–949.

61. Suzuki T. Restenosis reduction by cutting balloon evaluation (REDUCE II). Available at: http://www.theheart.org.

62. Bertrand OF, Mongrain R, Soualmi L, et al. Development of coronary aneurysm after cutting balloon angioplasty: assessment by intracoronary ultrasound. Catheter Cardiovasc Diagn. 1998;44:449–452.

63. Kawamura A, Asakura Y, Ishikawa S, et al. Extraction of previously deployed stent by an entrapped cutting balloon due to the blade fracture. Catheter Cardiovasc Interv. 2002;57:239–243.

64. Massonnet-Castel S, Pelissier E, Bara L, et al. Partial reversal of low molecular weight heparin (PK 10169) anti-Xa activity by protamine sulfate: in vitro and in vivo study during cardiac surgery with extracorporeal circulation. Haemostasis. 1986;16:139–146.

65. Crowther MA, Berry LR, Monagle PT, Chan AK. Mechanisms responsible for the failure of protamine to inactivate low-molecular-weight heparin. Br J Haematol. 2002;116: 178–186.

66. Cutlip DE, Baim DS, Ho KK, et al. Stent thrombosis in the modern era: a pooled analysis of multicenter coronary stent clinical trials. Circulation. 2001;103:1967–1671.

67. Orford JL, Lennon R, Melby S, et al. Frequency and correlates of coronary stent thrombosis in the modern era: analysis of a single center registry. J Am Coll Cardiol. 2002;40:1567–1572.

68. Schuhlen H, Kastrati A, Pache J, et al. Incidence of thrombotic occlusion and major adverse cardiac events between two and four weeks after coronary stent placement: analysis of 5,678 patients with a four-week ticlopidine regimen. J Am Coll Cardiol. 2001;37:2066–2073.

69. Moussa I, Oetgen M, Roubin G, et al. Effectiveness of clopidogrel and aspirin versus ticlopidine and aspirin in preventing stent thrombosis after coronary stent implantation. Circulation. 1999;99:2364–2366.

70. Cheneau E, Leborgne L, Mintz GS, et al. Predictors of subacute stent thrombosis: results of a systematic intravascular ultrasound study. Circulation. 2003;108:43–47.

71. Lotan C, Bakst A, Rozenman Y, et al. Initial and long-term results with the CrossFlex stent—data from a national registry. Int J Cardiovasc Intervent. 1999;2:237–240.

72. Hausleiter J, Kastrati A, Mehilli J, et al. Predictive factors for early cardiac events and angiographic restenosis after coronary stent placement in small coronary arteries. J Am Coll Cardiol. 2002;40:882–889.

73. Wang F, Stouffer GA, Waxman S, Uretsky BF. Late coronary stent thrombosis: early vs. late stent thrombosis in the stent era. Catheter Cardiovasc Interv. 2002;55:142–147.

74. Schomig A, Neumann FJ, Kastrati A, et al. A randomized comparison of antiplatelet and anticoagulant therapy after the placement of coronary-artery stents. N Engl J Med. 1996;334:1084–1089.

75. Bertrand ME, Legrand V, Boland J, et al. Randomized multicenter comparison of conventional anticoagulation versus antiplatelet therapy in unplanned and elective coronary stenting. The full anticoagulation versus aspirin and ticlopidine (fantastic) study. Circulation. 1998;98:1597–1603.

76. Leon MB, Baim DS, Popma JJ, et al. A clinical trial comparing three antithrombotic-drug regimens after coronary-artery stenting. Stent Anticoagulation Restenosis Study Investigators. N Engl J Med. 1998;339:1665–1671.

77. Urban P, Macaya C, Rupprecht HJ, et al. Randomized evaluation of anticoagulation versus antiplatelet therapy after coronary stent implantation in high-risk patients: the multicenter aspirin and ticlopidine trial after intracoronary stenting (MATTIS). Circulation. 1998;98:2126–2132.

78. Berger PB, Mahaffey KW, Meier SJ, et al. Safety and efficacy of only 2 weeks of ticlopidine therapy in patients at increased risk of coronary stent thrombosis: results from the Antiplatelet Therapy alone versus Lovenox plus Antiplatelet therapy in patients at increased risk of Stent Thrombosis (ATLAST) trial. Am Heart J. 2002;143: 841–846.

79. Kastrati A, Mehilli J, Schuhlen HA, et al. Clinical trial of abciximab in elective percutaneous coronary intervention after pretreatment with clopidogrel. N Engl J Med. 2004; 350:232–238.

80. Farb A, Burke AP, Kolodgie FD, Virmani R. Pathological mechanisms of fatal late coronary stent thrombosis in humans. Circulation. 2003;108:1701–1706.

81. Cheneau E, John MC, Fournadjiev J, et al. Time course of stent endothelialization after intravascular radiation therapy in rabbit iliac arteries. Circulation. 2003;107: 2153–2158.

82. Waksman R, Bhargava B, Mintz GS, et al. Late total occlusion after intracoronary brachytherapy for patients with in-stent restenosis. J Am Coll Cardiol. 2000;36: 65–68.

83. Waksman R, Ajani AE, Pinnow E, et al. Twelve versus six months of clopidogrel to reduce major cardiac events in patients undergoing gamma-radiation therapy for in-stent restenosis: Washington Radiation for In-Stent restenosis Trial (WRIST) 12 versus WRIST PLUS. Circulation. 2002;106:776–778.

84. Waksman R, Ajani AE, White RL, et al. Prolonged antiplatelet therapy to prevent late thrombosis after intracoronary gamma-radiation in patients with in-stent restenosis: Washington Radiation for In-Stent Restenosis Trial Plus 6 Months of Clopidogrel (WRIST PLUS). Circulation. 2001;103:2332–2335.

85. Morice MC, Serruys PW, Sousa JE, et al. A randomized comparison of a sirolimus-eluting stent with a standard stent for coronary revascularization. N Engl J Med. 2002;346:1773–1780.

86. Moses JW, Leon MB, Popma JJ, et al. Sirolimus-eluting stents versus standard stents in patients with stenosis in a native coronary artery. N Engl J Med. 2003;349:1315–1323.

87. Schofer J, Schluter M, Gershlick AH, et al. Sirolimus-eluting stents for treatment of patients with long atherosclerotic lesions in small coronary arteries: double-blind, randomised controlled trial (E-SIRIUS). Lancet. 2003; 362:1093–1099.

88. Schluter M, et al. The Canadian study of the sirolimus-eluting stent in the treatment of patients with long de novo lesions in small native coronary arteries (C-SIRIUS). J Am Coll Cardiol. 2004;43:1110–1115.

89. Lemos PA, Serruys PW, Van Domburg RT, et al. Unrestricted utilization of sirolimus-eluting stents compared with conventional bare stent implantation in the "Real world". The rapamycin-eluting stent evaluated at Rotterdam Cardiology Hospital (RESEARCH) Registry. Circulation 2004;109:190–195.

90. Takebayashi H, Kobayashi Y, Dangas G, et al. Restenosis due to underexpansion of sirolimus-eluting stent in a bifurcation lesion. Catheter Cardiovasc Interv. 2003;60: 496–499.

91. Degertekin M, Serruys PW, Tanabe K, et al. Long-term follow-up of incomplete stent apposition in patients who received sirolimus-eluting stent for de novo coronary lesions: an intravascular ultrasound analysis. Circulation. 2003;108:2747–2750.

92. De Servi S, Repetto S, Klugmann S, et al. Stent thrombosis: incidence and related factors in the R.I.S.E. Registry (Registro Impianto Stent Endocoronarico). Catheter Cardiovasc Interv. 1999;46:13–18.

93. Nakamura S, Hall P, Gaglione A, et al. High pressure assisted coronary stent implantation accomplished without intravascular ultrasound guidance and subsequent anticoagulation. J Am Coll Cardiol. 1997;29:21–27.

94. Silva JA, White CJ, Ramee SR, et al. Treatment of coronary stent thrombosis with rheolytic thrombectomy: results from a multicenter experience. Catheter Cardiovasc Interv. 2003;58:11–17.

95. Waksman R, Bhargava B, Leon MB. Late thrombosis following intracoronary brachytherapy. Catheter Cardiovasc Interv. 2000;49:344–347.

96. Rinfret S, Cutlip DE, Katsiyiannis PT, et al. Rheolytic thrombectomy and platelet glycoprotein IIb/IIIa blockade for stent thrombosis. Catheter Cardiovasc Interv. 2002;57:24–30.

97. Adams MR, Blake GJ, Kinlay S, Rogers C. Rheolytic thrombectomy for in-stent thrombosis: creating a diagnostic window. J Interv Cardiol. 2001;14:27–31.

98. Mueller C, Buerkle G, Buettner HJ, et al. Prevention of contrast media-associated nephropathy: randomized comparison of 2 hydration regimens in 1620 patients undergoing coronary angioplasty. Arch Intern Med. 2002;162: 329–336.

99. Rudnick MR, Goldfarb S, Wexler L, et al. Nephrotoxicity of ionic and nonionic contrast media in 1196 patients: a randomized trial. The Iohexol Cooperative Study. Kidney Int. 1995;47:254–261.

100. McCullough PA, Wolyn R, Rocher LL, et al. Acute renal failure after coronary intervention: incidence, risk factors, and relationship to mortality. Am J Med. 1997;103: 368–375.

101. Berns AS. Nephrotoxicity of contrast media. Kidney Int. 1989;36:730–740.

102. Levy EM, Viscoli CM, Horwitz RI. The effect of acute renal failure on mortality. A cohort analysis. JAMA. 1996;275:1489–1494.

103. Gruberg L, Mintz GS, Mehran R, et al. The prognostic implications of further renal function deterioration within 48 h of interventional coronary procedures in patients with pre-existent chronic renal insufficiency. J Am Coll Cardiol. 2000;36:1542–1548.

104. Gruberg L, Mehran R, Dangas G, et al. Acute renal failure requiring dialysis after percutaneous coronary interventions. Catheter Cardiovasc Interv. 2001;52:409–416.

105. Bakris GL, Lass N, Gaber AO, et al. Radiocontrast medium-induced declines in renal function: a role for oxygen free radicals. Am J Physiol. 1990;258:F115–F120.

106. Baliga R, Ueda N, Walker PD, Shah SV. Oxidant mechanisms in toxic acute renal failure. Drug Metab Rev. 1999; 31:971–997.

107. Deray G. Festschrift for Professor Claude Jacobs. Nephrotoxicity of contrast media. Nephrol Dial Transplant. 1999;14:2602–2606.

108. Rihal CS, Textor SC, Grill DE, et al. Incidence and prognostic importance of acute renal failure after percutaneous coronary intervention. Circulation. 2002;105:2259–2264.

109. Aspelin P, Aubry P, Fransson SG, et al. Nephrotoxic effects in high-risk patients undergoing angiography. N Engl J Med. 2003;348:491–499.

110. Boesgaard S, Aldershvile J, Poulsen HE, et al. N-acetylcysteine inhibits angiotensin converting enzyme in vivo. J Pharmacol Exp Ther. 1993;265:1239–1244.

111. Muller B, Kleschyov AL, Stoclet JC. Evidence for N-acetylcysteine-sensitive nitric oxide storage as dinitrosyl-iron complexes in lipopolysaccharide-treated rat aorta. Br J Pharmacol. 1996;119:1281–1285.

112. Brunet J, Boily MJ, Cordeau S, Des Rosiers C. Effects of N-acetylcysteine in the rat heart reperfused after low-flow ischemia: evidence for a direct scavenging of hydroxyl radicals and a nitric oxide-dependent increase in coronary flow. Free Radic Biol Med. 1995;19:627–638.

113. Tepel M, van der Giet M, Schwarzfeld C, et al. Prevention of radiographic-contrast-agent-induced reductions in renal function by acetylcysteine. N Engl J Med. 2000;343: 180–184.

114. Diaz-Sandoval LJ, Kosowsky BD, Losordo DW. Acetylcysteine to prevent angiography-related renal tissue injury (the APART trial). Am J Cardiol. 2002;89:356–358.

115. Adamian MG, Moussa I, Mehran R, et al. The role of mucomyst administration prior to percutaneous interventions on renal function in patients with chronic renal failure. J Am Coll Cardiol. 2002;39:1A.

116. Mouhayar EN, Tadros G, Akin AO, et al. Prevention of contrast-induced renal dysfunction with acetylcysteine in patients undergoing coronary angiography. J Am Coll Cardiol. 2002;39:1A.

117. Kay J, Chow WH, Chan TM, et al. Acetylcysteine for prevention of acute deterioration of renal function following elective coronary angiography and intervention: a randomized controlled trial. JAMA. 2003;289:553–558.

118. Shyu KG, Cheng JJ, Kuan P. Acetylcysteine protects against acute renal damage in patients with abnormal renal function undergoing a coronary procedure. J Am Coll Cardiol. 2002;40:1383–1388.

119. MacNeill BD, Harding SA, Bazari H, et al. Prophylaxis of contrast-induced nephropathy in patients undergoing coronary angiography. Catheter Cardiovasc Interv. 2003; 60:458–461.

120. Briguori C, Manganelli F, Scarpato P, et al. Acetylcysteine and contrast agent-associated nephrotoxicity. J Am Coll Cardiol. 2002;40:298–303.

121. Durham JD, Caputo C, Dokko J, et al. A randomized controlled trial of N-acetylcysteine to prevent contrast nephropathy in cardiac angiography. Kidney Int. 2002; 62:2202–2207.

122. Weinstein JM, Heyman S, Brezis M. Potential deleterious effect of furosemide in radiocontrast nephropathy. Nephron. 1992;62:413–415.

123. Solomon R, Werner C, Mann D, et al. Effects of saline, mannitol, and furosemide to prevent acute decreases in renal function induced by radiocontrast agents. N Engl J Med. 1994;331:1416–1420.

124. Stevens MA, McCullough PA, Tobin KJ, et al. A prospective randomized trial of prevention measures in patients at high risk for contrast nephropathy: results of the P.R.I.N.C.E. Study. Prevention of Radiocontrast Induced Nephropathy Clinical Evaluation. J Am Coll Cardiol. 1999;33:403–411.

125. Russo D, Testa A, Della Volpe L, Sansone G. Randomised prospective study on renal effects of two different contrast media in humans: protective role of a calcium channel blocker. Nephron. 1990;55:254–257.

126. Neumayer HH, Junge W, Kufner A, Wenning A. Prevention of radiocontrast-media-induced nephrotoxicity by the calcium channel blocker nitrendipine: a prospective randomised clinical trial. Nephrol Dial Transplant. 1989;4: 1030–1036.

127. Weisberg LS, Kurnik PB, Kurnik BR. Dopamine and renal blood flow in radiocontrast-induced nephropathy in humans. Ren Fail. 1993;15:61–68.

128. Abizaid AS, Clark CE, Mintz GS, et al. Effects of dopamine and aminophylline on contrast-induced acute renal failure after coronary angioplasty in patients with preexisting renal insufficiency. Am J Cardiol. 1999;83: 260–263, A5.

129. Gare M, Haviv YS, Ben-Yehuda A, et al. The renal effect of low-dose dopamine in high-risk patients undergoing coronary angiography. J Am Coll Cardiol. 1999;34:1682–1688.

130. Margulies KB, Hildebrand FL, Heublein DM, Burnett JC Jr. Radiocontrast increases plasma and urinary endothelin. J Am Soc Nephrol. 1991;2:1041–1045.

131. Kini AA, Sharma SK. Managing the high-risk patient: experience with fenoldopam, a selective dopamine receptor agonist, in prevention of radiocontrast nephropathy during percutaneous coronary intervention. Rev Cardiovasc Med. 2001;2(suppl 1):S19–S25.

132. Madyoon H, Croushore L, Weaver D, Mathur V. Use of fenoldopam to prevent radiocontrast nephropathy in high-risk patients. Catheter Cardiovasc Interv. 2001;53: 341–345.

133. Madyoon H, Croushore L. Use of fenoldopam for prevention of radiocontrast nephropathy in the cardiac catheterization laboratory: a case series. J Interv Cardiol. 2001;14:179–185.

134. Tumlin JA, Wang A, Murray PT, Mathur VS. Fenoldopam mesylate blocks reductions in renal plasma flow after radiocontrast dye infusion: a pilot trial in the prevention of contrast nephropathy. Am Heart J. 2002;143:894–903.

135. Stone GW, McCullough PA, Tumlin JA, et al. Fenoldopam mesylate for the prevention of contrast-induced nephropathy: a randomized controlled trial. JAMA. 2003;290:2284–2291.

136. Marenzi G, Marana I, Lauri G, et al. The prevention of radiocontrast-agent-induced nephropathy by hemofiltration. N Engl J Med. 2003;349:1333–1340.

137. Keeley EC, Grines CL. Scraping of aortic debris by coronary guiding catheters: a prospective evaluation of 1,000 cases. J Am Coll Cardiol. 1998;32:1861–1865.

138. Eggebrecht H, Oldenburg O, Dirsch O, et al. Potential embolization by atherosclerotic debris dislodged from aortic wall during cardiac catheterization: histological and clinical findings in 7,621 patients. Catheter Cardiovasc Interv. 2000;49:389–394.

139. Fukumoto Y, Tsutsui H, Tsuchihashi M, et al. The incidence and risk factors of cholesterol embolization syndrome, a complication of cardiac catheterization: a prospective study. J Am Coll Cardiol. 2003;42:211–216.

10
Complications of Radiation Exposure and Therapy

William L. Ballard

A 64-year-old man with a past medical history of hypertension, hyperlipidemia, and strong family history of heart disease presented with angina in June 2000. A cardiac catheterization revealed single vessel disease in the dominant right coronary artery (RCA) with normal left ventricular (LV) function. Balloon angioplasty was performed successfully on the mid RCA.

In January 2001, recurrent angina developed and restenosis of the mid RCA was found with repeat angioplasty performed. In April 2001 recurrent angina developed and the recurrent restenosis of the mid RCA was treated with a 3.0 × 15-mm Quantum balloon followed by Novoste β-cath radiation for 190-second dwell time, using a 40-mm source train. A S770 3.0 × 15-mm stent was placed after the radiation therapy.

In February 2003, after withholding aspirin for a planned colonoscopy, the patient developed an acute inferior infarct immediately postprocedure (removal of 3 polyps). An emergent angiogram revealed an occluded mid RCA due to thrombus at the proximal end of the stent (Figure 10-1). The ejection fraction was 55% with inferior hypokinesis. Initially a 2.5 × 15-mm Maverick balloon followed by Angiojet thrombectomy were used after a 4Fr transvenous pacing wire was placed. The patient fibrillated and was successfully defibrillated, and the procedure was concluded with a 3.0 × 8-mm EXPRESS stent at the distal end of the prior stent. The patient has done well since, remaining on aspirin and clopidogrel indefinitely.

This case demonstrates a relatively rare phenomenon before brachytherapy, that of delayed or subacute thrombosis of a stent, occurring more than 30 days after the coronary intervention. As discussed under the heading of Intravascular Brachytherapy, this problem may best be avoided with more prolonged clopidogrel treatment.[1]

1. Introduction

The topic of complications as it pertains to radiation exposure and therapy is an interesting blend of recent and distant history.[2–5] As the use of X-ray as a diagnostic tool is fundamental to cardiology, an understanding of its safe use is critical. The use of therapeutic radiation is an important topic as well. Whether this involves the cardiovascular effects of external radiation treatment, or the direct effects of intravascular brachytherapy, the potential for complications is still significant.

2. Therapeutic Use of Radiation

External beam radiation as a therapeutic tool is commonly used in cancer treatments. The bulk of knowledge of the adverse effects on the cardiovascular system comes from the treatment of Hodgkin's disease. Possible cardiac complications include pericarditis, constriction, myocardial fibrosis, coronary artery disease, and myocardial infarction.[6,7] Other vascular effects include fibrosis and aneurysm formation as well as rare reports of vessel rupture. Intravascular brachytherapy is a newer treatment modality and has evolved into the treatment of choice for in-stent restenosis.[8,9] We will review the complications that may take place with this treatment and the strategies used to avoid their occurrence.

3. Diagnostic Use of Radiation

The use of X-rays to image the coronary arteries is a vital diagnostic technique in cardiology. Both fluoroscopy and cineangiography impart a significant amount of radiation

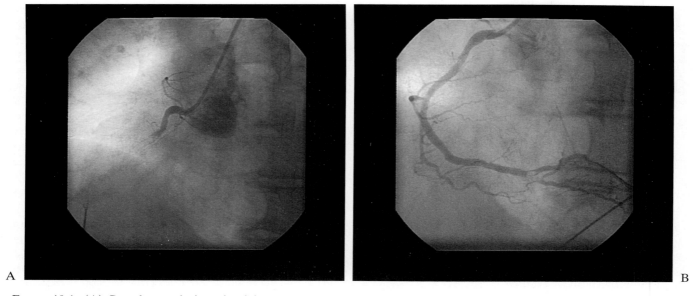

FIGURE 10-1. (A) Complete occlusion of a right coronary artery more than 6 months following successful IVBT. (B) Thrombus embolized distally in the same right coronary artery after flow was re-established.

to patients and staff, particularly in long procedures. Though uncommon, radiation complications such as dermatitis, ulceration, and infections can be avoided by changing camera angles, reducing imaging time, and weighing the risks of extreme exposure with alternative methods of revascularization in selected patients.[10–12] This will be discussed in more detail later in the chapter.

4. External Beam Radiation

Before we review the topic of intravascular brachytherapy (IVBT), a few words on external beam radiation therapy (XRT) are warranted. The clinical lessons learned from therapeutic XRT also provided some of the basis for IVBT. Much of the knowledge of the cardiovascular effects of radiation treatments has been learned from treatment of Hodgkin's lymphoma. This tumor typically occurs in the chest, and therapy thus involves chest and mediastinal radiation. The cardiac effects include inflammation and fibrosis of the pericardium, myocardium, and vessel walls. There have been case reports of vascular aneurysms, as well as rare vessel rupture.[13,14] These vascular effects have been shown to be dose dependent, and thus can be avoided by dose reduction and shielding. Case reports and historical registries of Hodgkin's survivors have shown an increased incidence of myocardial infarction and coronary disease, more often at younger ages than the general population.[15,16] The coronary lesions are often aorta–ostial fibrosis and coronary aneurysm formation. Avoidance of these complications in XRT patients includes dose adjustment,

interrupted therapies (temporal spacing of several, shorter radiation treatments), and shielding of sensitive tissues.[17]

5. Intravascular Brachytherapy

Complications occurring with IVBT, some common to all forms of percutaneous intervention and others particularly unique to IVBT, are discussed in this section. The initial preclinical work on IVBT, begun in the early 1990s, evaluated the safety of this technique in animal models.[18–20] The balance between the intended therapeutic effect on the monocytes, macrophages, and endothelial cells and the potential deleterious effects on vessel wall integrity is achieved by careful dosing of the radiotherapy. The optimal dose has been determined, and careful centering of the radiation in the vessel lumen achieves uniform application of the β or γ rays.[21,22] There have been anecdotal reports of coronary aneurysms after brachytherapy, and their relation to the brachytherapy in a cause-and-effect role is debatable.[23–25]

The use of radiation treatments in the coronary vascular tree dates to the early to mid 1990s. Experimentation and success in the preclinical arena led to application of this technique in human subjects. Successful clinical trials resulted in the approval of both the β- and γ-emitting brachytherapy systems by the Food and Drug Administration in November 2000.[9]

One of the first problems with these devices relates to their delivery in the coronary artery. The devices currently approved consist of an irradiated wire segment or radiation seeds delivered via a centering balloon or hydraulic catheter system, respectively. Complications related to device delivery include, from most to least common, coronary spasm, impaired distal blood flow, dissection, and perforation, as well as potential delayed healing of balloon-induced dissections after radiation treatment (Table 10-1).[20,26,27]

5.1. Coronary Spasm

This is the case of a 75-year-old man with a history of known coronary disease, a previous stroke, and long-standing hypertension who continued to smoke. In April 2003, a cardiac catheterization to further evaluate his angina revealed normal LV function, minor disease of a dominant right coronary artery, moderate disease in the left circumflex artery, and serial 80% lesions in the proximal-through-mid left anterior descending coronary artery (LAD). The patient had a 4.0×18-mm Zeta stent placed in the proximal LAD, and a 2.75×8-mm Zeta stent in the mid LAD. Intravascular ultrasound (IVUS) was used for stent placement, and the procedure was successful and uneventful.

In August 2003, after recurrent anginal symptoms developed, cardiac catheterization revealed long in-stent restenosis in the mid LAD. A 2.75×10-mm cutting balloon was used over a 300 cm Luge wire. This was followed by β-radiation (Galileo, Guidant, Inc., Indianapolis, IN) using a 3.0×32-mm delivery catheter. At the end of the 190-second dwell time, the patient developed severe chest pain and hypotension. The angiogram revealed severe spasm of the entire left coronary vessel (Figure 10-2). Despite placement of a perfusion balloon, intracoronary nitroglycerin, and advanced cardiac life support (ACLS) protocol, the patient did not suvive the procedure. This is the only case to date in our laboratory of such intense vasospasm, and the only brachytherapy-related in-hospital death.

Pretreatment and intraprocedural intracoronary nitroglycerin and an adequate level of anticoagulation are important strategies employed to avoid complications with IVBT.

TABLE 10-1. Complications specific to intracoronary brachytherapy.

Device-related
  Coronary spasm
  Impaired distal flow with or without myocardial ischemia
  Coronary thrombosis
  Loss of radiation seeds
Radiation-injury related
  Restenosis edge effect
  Late coronary thrombosis
  Late aneurysm development

The case cited above occurred despite these measures, but fortunately has been the only occurrence of such profound spasm seen in our laboratory. There is a case report of a similar experience in treating a right coronary restenosis reported in 2001.[28]

Procedural differences between β- and γ-radiation therapy principally involve different dwell times. β IVBT requires 2 to 5 minutes, while γ IVBT generally is in the range of 20 minutes. The other advantage of β over γ treatment is the lower degree of radiation exposure to patient and staff, related to the diminished depth of penetration of β emitters. We performed our initial β-radiation case in October 1997 and our first γ-radiation case in 2000. There have been a total of 954 β- and γ-radiation cases at the Fuqua Heart Center through December 2003, predominantly β-radiation cases. The number of IVBT cases in our laboratory in 2003 represented 8.8% of our total interventions, giving some idea of the clinical occurrence rate of in-stent restenosis. Whether this number remains the same in the era of drug-eluting stents awaits the results of forthcoming prospective clinical trials.

5.2. Coronary Thrombosis

The immediate or acute problem of intracoronary thrombosis (*acute thrombosis*), defined as stent thrombosis within the first 24 hours after implantation, is now uncommon given standard pharmacology measures discussed elsewhere. This complication does not appear to be any more prevalent with the use of brachytherapy and is a topic well covered elsewhere in this book. There have been some reports, however, of creatine kinase–MB (CPK-MB) elevations after intracoronary radiation of potential but unproven clinical significance.[29]

The next complication in this timeline is *subacute thrombosis*, defined as stent thrombosis occurring between 24 hours and 30 days after the interventional procedure. It should be noted that both acute and subacute thrombosis, though infrequent, are much more likely when the initial procedure is performed during an acute coronary syndrome (ACS), particularly with visible thrombus.[30–32] Clinical trials of vascular brachytherapy for in-stent restenosis excluded patients with ACS. Therefore, it may be prudent to avoid the use of brachytherapy during the acute intervention in patients who present with true in-stent restenosis combined with thrombosis or with visible thrombus but incomplete thrombosis. Our practice is to stage the procedure, first treating the stenosis and thrombosis, and then electively performing brachytherapy at a later date.

The new phenomenon of *late stent thrombosis*, defined as stent thrombosis more than 30 days after the procedure, was initially reported and recognized in the era of vascular brachytherapy.[33–36] There is also a defined cate-

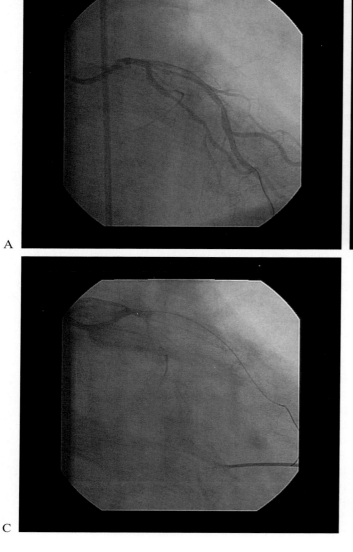

FIGURE 10-2. (A) Angiogram at beginning of β-catheter intervention, with mild wire-induced spasm only. (B) Angiogram of the Galileo system in position in the mid LAD. (C) Angiogram at the end of the β-radiation dwell time, with intense spasm which now involves the entire left coronary tree.

gory of *late–late thrombosis* occurring more than 6 months after treatment, first described by Ron Waksman in 1999.[37] Delayed re-endothelialization with any treatment modality appears to increase the risk of either problem, both of which are simply referred to collectively as late thrombosis in this chapter. A pathologic study found the unifying morphologic finding in 12 of 13 cases of fatal late stent thrombosis (at autopsy) to be impaired neointimal healing.[38] Placement of a new stent at the time of brachytherapy adds significantly to this risk because there is bare or exposed metal present in the setting of delayed healing.[39] A goal in the treatment of in-stent restenosis should thus be to obtain an excellent result with debulking or balloon therapies, and avoid placement of new stents.

There is an increased incidence of late stent thrombosis with brachytherapy even without the placement of a new stent.[39,40] The case that opens this chapter is an example of this dangerous problem that occurred at our institution, a late thrombosis resulting in an acute myocardial infarction (Figure 10-1). This patient had successful IVBT for in-stent restenosis months before the acute thrombotic occlusion and had appropriately discontinued the clopidogrel just before the event.

This experience, as well as clopidogrel trial results in other patient subsets, has resulted in prolonged therapy, now recommended for at least 6 months after brachytherapy or drug-eluting stent implantation.[41] Our current practice is at least 6 months of combined aspirin and clopidogrel, more often 9 months, and typically extended for 12 months after IVBT. This practice is supported by a recent report of the WRIST 12 study (Washington Radiation for In-Stent restenosis trial).[1] In this study, clopidogrel treatment was carried out for 12 months, and major adverse cardiac events were compared to a historical WRIST registry, a group treated with 6 months of clopidogrel. Although there were similar late stent thrombosis rates in both groups, there was a significant reduction in major adverse coronary events (MACE) and target lesion revascularization (TLR) in the 12-month therapy arm, from approximately 35% to 20%.

5.3. The "Edge" Effect

Another common problem associated with intravascular radiation is the "edge" effect, first described with the use of irradiated stents and subsequently noted with catheter-based brachytherapy.[42,43] This is defined as recurrent stenosis seen at the edges of stents, noted in follow-up angiograms after intravascular brachytherapy.[8] The edge effect is related to two factors: geographic miss with the radiation source at the stent ends, and balloon injury outside of the stent struts.[44] Thus, restenosis created by the new overstretch injury is left untreated with brachytherapy at adequate dose levels. By using longer source trains or treatment lengths, and using balloon lengths confined to the stent segments, this problem is much less prevalent.[45–47] Animal studies have thus far shown no negative effects of intravascular brachytherapy on normal, untouched endothelium. Thus, there appears to be no danger in extending the margins of radiation treatment to avoid the edge effect. The following is another case from our institution illustrating the edge effect of brachytherapy.

A 58-year-old man with hyperlipidemia and a family history of heart disease developed crescendo anginal symptoms in February 2002. A cardiac catheterization revealed normal LV function with minor disease in the dominant RCA and left circumflex artery. The LAD had complex proximal disease. As a participant in the Deliver trial, a 2.5 × 15-mm PENTA stent (Guidant, Inc.), paclitaxel versus bare metal, was delivered after balloon predilatation (trial mandated) with a 2.25 × 15-mm Raptor balloon. In July 2002, a stress imaging study revealed anterior ischema associated with anginal chest pain. In-stent restenosis was confirmed and treated with 3.0 × 15-mm cutting balloon, 3.5 × 15-mm NC Ranger, followed by Novoste β-catheter delivery (40-mm source train for 3 min, without pull-back). There was minimal edge intimal disruption noted after radiation, for which a 3.5 × 13-mm Velocity stent was placed proximally and a 3.5 × 28-mm Velocity stent was placed at the distal end. The procedure was otherwise uneventful.

In May 2003, crescendo angina developed over 2 to 3 weeks prompting an invasive evaluation. The catheterization revealed the typical edge effect restenosis pattern (Figure 10-3). The patient was presented with the option of single-vessel coronary artery bypass graft (CABG), left internal mammary artery (LIMA) to LAD by off-pump coronary bypass versus repeat percutaneous approach and repeat β-radiation. He opted for a "final try" at radiation. A 3.5 × 10-mm cutting balloon, guided by IVUS, was used followed by placement of a 30-mm Novoste β-catheter source train at the proximal edge. No additional stents were placed. The patient has remained asymptomatic.

A theoretical and real concern of intracoronary radiation relates to known vascular effects of external radiation therapy. With high doses of XRT, such as in the treatment of Hodgkin's disease, there have been reports of vascular aneurysms and, rarely, large vessel rupture.[14,48,49] Both complications result from weakening of the vessel wall from radiation exposure. Appropriately, this was a concern early in the preclinical experimentation with therapeutic intravascular radiation, particularly in dose-finding studies.[50] This has not yet been seen to any significant degree, once the appropriate therapeutic window for radiation doses was determined, but is a reason for prudence in strategies for repeat brachytherapy after recurrent restenosis. As noted and referenced earlier in this chapter, there have been only one or two anecdotal case examples of coronary aneurysm after brachytherapy, and it is unclear if these cases represent true cause and effect or simply are coincident events.[25,51] In animal models, there is a dose–response relationship, with no vessel wall weakening seen with total doses below 25 to 30 Gy.[52] Usual γ- or β-radiation treatment doses for IVBT are in the range of 12 to 15 Gy.

6. Diagnostic and Interventional Complications of X-Rays

The final topic in this chapter will be the use of diagnostic X-Rays in the cardiac catheterization laboratory. There are several good reviews of this subject, including the American College of Cardiology/Society for Cardiac Angiography and Interventions (ACC/SCA&I) guidelines for cardiac catheterization.[53]

Radiation effects are characterized as stochastic risks (DNA injury, carcinogenesis) or nonstochastic risks (cellular injury). There is little to no evidence that the level of radiation exposure in the catheterization laboratory carries a stochastic, genetic risk to the patient. There is evidence that such exposure carries a nonstochastic risk, though small.[2,54]

6.1. Patient Issues

Radiation exposure to the patient in any single diagnostic or interventional cardiac procedure in the catheterization laboratory is minimal. However, radiation exposure for multiple procedures in the same

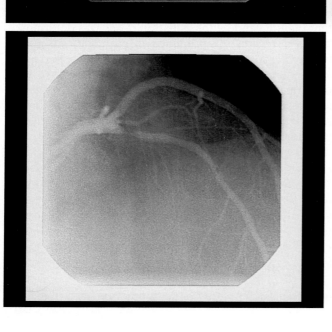

FIGURE 10-3. (A) Angiogram from the July 2002 restenotic LAD stent treatment. This shows the β-catheter in position. Note the geographic miss of the proximal radiation seeds at the site of the subsequent proximal edge stenosis. (B) Angiogram from the May 2003 re-restenosis, isolated to proximal edge effect stenosis. This angiogram is zoomed to better show the site. (C) The same view as (B), only in inverse video mode to better demonstrate the relationship of the previously radiated stent site to the edge stenosis.

patient or a single prolonged procedure may be more significant.[55] It is likely that there is an underreporting of skin lesions due to radiation injury given the presumption of excellent radiation control, safety standards, and general lack of connection between an interventional cardiac procedure and a skin lesion appearing later, however unusual in location.

There is now a significant body of case reports of radiation dermatitis and other skin effects caused by prolonged catheterization laboratory procedures[12,56–60] (Figures 10-4–10-7, see color plates.) Some of the skin injuries have been debilitating, necessitating chronic wound care, skin grafts, and a protracted recovery that may last years. Risk factors include long procedure duration and prolonged fluoroscopy without changing the camera position. Though this is an infrequent complica-

tion, awareness of the potential problem is important, and avoidance is relatively simple. If a procedure becomes lengthy and may be safely staged, then such a strategy may attenuate the potential for damage. Just as temporal spacing of XRT for cancer therapy minimizes side effects, the same applies to diagnostic X-ray exposure. However, cumulative dose is still of paramount importance.[11,61–63]

There are legal concerns with the possibility of significant damage caused by the diagnostic use of radiation as part of an interventional therapeutic procedure. Current consenting tools do not include the possibility of injury from radiation, making a defense more difficult.[56] In fact, this is not simply theory, as even having had two percutaneous coronary intervention (PCI) procedures 5 months apart led to a jury award of $1 million, as

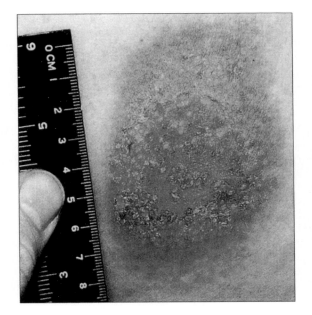

FIGURE 10-4. This 48-year-old woman underwent two stent placements within a month. Photograph of left mid back 2 months after last procedure shows well-marginated focal erythema and desquamation. (Reprinted with permission from Stone et al. J Am Acad Derm. 1998;38:333–336.) (See color plate.)

reported in *USA Today*.[57] While invisible to the naked eye, unchecked, unnecessary, or cavalier use of radiation as a diagnostic tool may lead to adverse outcomes for both physician and patient.

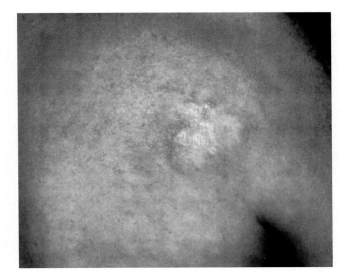

FIGURE 10-6. This 54-year-old man with stenosis of left circumflex artery. Photograph of right shoulder at 5.5 months after percutaneous transluminal coronary angioplasty shows area of depigmentation and atrophy. Injury progressed to deep ulceration, requiring skin grafting. (Reprinted with permission from Am J Roentgen. 2001:177:3–11.) (See color plate.)

6.2. Staff Issues

Radiation exposure levels in all fields are expected to be kept under ALARA standards (as low as reasonably achievable). The standard unit of measure of radiation is rem, or roentgen equivalents in man. As discussed in

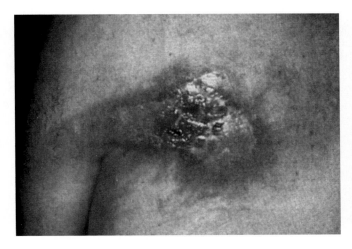

FIGURE 10-5. This 69-year-old man with history of angina underwent two angioplasties of left coronary artery within 30 hours. Photograph taken 1 to 2 months after last procedure shows secondary ulceration over left scapula. (Reprinted with permission from Granel et al. Ann Dermat Venereol. 1998;125:405–407.) (See color plate.)

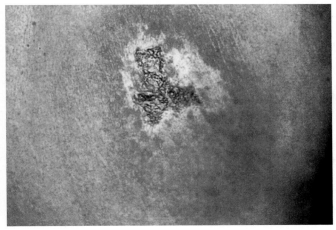

FIGURE 10-7. This 69-year-old man with history of angina underwent three coronary angiograms followed by three angioplasties within 8 months. Photograph 3 years after last procedure shows skin necrosis with surrounding erythema and hyperpigmentation in right subscapular region. (Reprinted with permission from Dandurand et al. Ann Dermat Venereol. 1999;126:413–417.) (See color plate.)

the ACC/SCA&I 2001 Cath Lab Standards, the total maximum safe exposure level per year is 5 rem.[53] It is important to limit staff exposure by using appropriate precautions, with particular attention during prolonged and/or complex cases. Simple techniques that greatly reduce the radiation exposure levels include appropriate shielding, reduction of fluoroscopy and cineangiography times, and reducing scatter whenever possible. Keeping the image intensifier as close to the patient as possible is most important in achieving this goal. Lead shielding, particularly a clear, moveable screen between the operator and the patient, dramatically reduces the amount of radiation striking the interventional cardiologist and other staff members.[12,64,65]

Collimation and equipment maintenance reduce the amount of scatter and the energy needed to produce the images, reducing the radiation emitted. Though the amount of radiation is not directly reduced by conversion from film to digital imaging and archiving, there are significant benefits. One can use reduced fluoroscopy times as well as potentially replacing some cine runs with fluoroscopy as image quality improves. There is also a benefit in interventional procedures of using pulsed fluoroscopy, intermittent fluoroscopy timed to the cardiac cycle, much as cine.[10,66,67]

All staff members should be monitored with radiation badges, both to track their individual exposure, as well as to determine any equipment that may be generating excess radiation scatter.[68,69]

7. Conclusions

In this chapter, we discussed issues and complications of radiation, in both diagnostic and therapeutic applications. The cardiac effects of therapeutic XRT for cancer therapy are currently uncommon due to changes in doses and shielding, but are still important to remember in late follow-up of patients treated before such precautions were taken.

Diagnostic X-ray exposure has some inherent risks. The use of shielding, reduction of scatter, and avoidance of repeated or prolonged procedures in a single camera position minimizes these risks to reasonable levels. As discussed, there have been significant clinical benefits as well as infrequent but significant complications related to IVBT in this era of increasingly complex percutaneous coronary interventions. With careful attention to technique, anticoagulation, and follow up, the majority of these complications are readily avoided.

References

1. Waksman R, Ajani AE, Pinnow E, et al. Twelve versus six months of clopidogrel to reduce major cardiac events in patients undergoing gamma-radiation therapy for in-stent restenosis: Washington Radiation for In-Stent restenosis Trial (WRIST) 12 versus WRIST PLUS. Circulation. 2002;106:776–778.
2. Bashore T. Fundamentals of X-ray imaging and radiation safety. Catheter Cardiovasc Interv. 2001;54:126–135.
3. Fajardo L, Lee A. Rupture of major vessels after radiation. Cancer. 1975;36:904–913.
4. Hull MC, Morris CG, Pepine CJ, et al. Valvular dysfunction and carotid, subclavian, and coronary artery disease in survivors of Hodgkin lymphoma treated with radiation therapy. JAMA. 2003;290:2831–2837.
5. Donaldson SS, Hancock SL, Hoppe RT. Hodgkin's disease—finding the balance between cure and late effects. Cancer J. 1999;5:625–634.
6. Basavaraju SR, Easterly CE. Pathophysiological effects of radiation on atherosclerosis development and progression, and the incidence of cardiovascular complications. Med Phys. 2002;29:2391–2403.
7. Adams MJ, Hadenbergh PH, Constine LS, et al. Radiation-associated cardiovascular disease. Crit Rev Oncol Hematol. 2003;45:55–75.
8. Ajani AE, Kim HS, Waksman R. Clinical trials of vascular brachytherapy for in-stent restenosis: update. Cardiovasc Radiat Med. 2001;2:107–113.
9. Del Negro A. Bringing vascular brachytherapy to the US forefront: FDA approves two radiation systems for in-stent restenosis. Cardiovasc Radiat Med. 2001;2:119–123.
10. Balter S. Radiation safety in the cardiac catheterization laboratory: basic principles. Catheter Cardiovasc Interv. 1999;47:229–236.
11. Clark AL, Brennan AG, Robertson LJ, et al. Factors affecting patient radiation exposure during routine coronary angiography in a tertiary referral centre. Br J Radiol. 2000;73:184–189.
12. Kawakami T, Saito R, Miyazaki S. Chronic radiodermatitis following repeated percutaneous transluminal coronary angioplasty. Br J Dermatol. 1999;141:150–153.
13. Gupta S. Radiation-induced carotid artery blow-out: a case report. Acta Chir Belg. 1994;94:299–300.
14. Fajardo LF, Berthrong M. Vascular lesions following radiation. Pathol Ann. 1988;23:297–330.
15. Stewart HR, Fajardo LF, Gillette SM, Constine LS. Radiation injury to the heart. Int J Radiat Oncol Biol Phys. 1995;31:1205–1211.
16. Boivin JF, Hutchinson GB, Lubin JH, Mauch P. Coronary artery disease mortality in patients treated for Hodgkin's disease. Cancer. 1992;69:1241–1247.
17. Adams MJ, Lipshultz SE, Schwartz C, et al. Radiation-associated cardiovascular disease: manifestations and management. Semin Radiat Oncol. 2003;13:346–356.
18. Waksman R, Robinson KA, Crocker IR, et al. Endovascular low dose irradiation inhibits neointima formation after coronary artery balloon injury in swine: a possible role for radiation therapy in restenosis prevention. Circulation. 1995;91:1553–1559.
19. Mazur W, Ali M, Khan M, et al. High dose rate intracoronary radiation for inhibition of neointimal formation in the stented and balloon-injured porcine models of restenosis:

angiographic, morphometric, and histopathological analyses. Int J Radiat Oncol Biol Phys. 1997;36:777–778.

20. Chapter 18, Monique MH, et al. Comparison of endovascular and external beam radiation in the prevention of restenosis. pp. 221–230, Chapter 22, Waksman R, Endovascular Beta Radiation in the Swine Model, pp. 273–286. In: Waksman R, editor. Vascular brachytherapy. 2nd ed. Mount Kisco, NY: Futura; 1999:273–286.

21. Campos L, Stabin M. Intravascular brachytherapy to prevent restenosis: dosimetric considerations. Cell Mol Biol. 2002;48:429–439.

22. Arbab-Zadeh A, Bhargava V, Russo RJ, et al. Centered versus noncentered source for intracoronary artery radiation therapy: a model based on the Scripps Trial. Am Heart J. 2002;143:342–348.

23. Vandergoten P, Brosens M, Benit E. Coronary aneurysm five months after intracoronary beta-irradiation. Acta Cardiol. 2000;55:313–315.

24. Dixon SR, Grines CL, Safian RD. Coronary artery pseudo-aneurysm after balloon angioplasty and intracoronary beta-radiation for in-stent restenosis. Catheter Cardiovasc Interv. 2004;61:214–216.

25. Bertrand OF, Meerkin D, Bonan R. Coronary aneurysm after endovascular brachytherapy: true or false? Circulation. 2000;102:E121.

26. Meerkin D, Tardif JC, Bertrand OF, et al. The effects of intracoronary brachytherapy on the natural history of postangioplasty dissections. J Am Coll Cardiol. 2000;36: 59–64.

27. Scheinert D, Strnad V, Muller R, et al. High-dose intravascular beta-radiation after de novo stent implantation induces coronary artery spasm. Circulation. 2002;105: 1420–1423.

28. Gruberg L. Severe acute coronary spasm following intracoronary radiation for in-stent restenosis: a case report. Cardiovasc Radiat Med. 2001;2:138–142.

29. Ajani AE, Waksman R, Sharma AK, et al. Usefulness of periprocedural creatinine phosphokinase-MB release to predict adverse outcomes after intracoronary radiation therapy for in-stent restenosis. Am J Cardiol. 2004;93: 313–317.

30. Harjai KJ. Frequency, determinants, and clinical implications of residual intracoronary thrombus following primary angioplasty for acute myocardial infarction. Am J Cardiol. 2003;92:377–382.

31. La Vecchia L. Subacute thrombosis after stenting in acute myocardial infarction: four-year experience in a low-volume center. Coron Artery Dis. 1999;10:521–524.

32. Silva JA. Predictors of stent thrombosis after primary stenting for acute myocardial infarction. Catheter Cardiovasc Interv. 1999;47:415–422.

33. Waksman R, Bhargava B, Mintz GS, et al. Late total occlusion after intracoronary brachytherapy for patients with in-stent restenosis. J Am Coll Cardiol. 2000;36:65–68.

34. Sianos G, Mollet N, Hofma S, et al. Images in cardiovascular medicine. Late-late occlusion after intracoronary brachytherapy. Circulation. 2003;108:69–70.

35. Krotz F, Schiele TM, Zahler S, et al. Sustained platelet activation following intracoronary beta irradiation. Am J Cardiol. 2002;90:1381–1384.

36. Ajani AE, Cheneau E, Leborgne L, et al. Have we solved the problem of late thrombosis? Minerva Cardioangiol. 2002;50:463–468.

37. Waksman R. Late thrombosis after radiation. Sitting on a time bomb. Circulation. 1999;100:780–782.

38. Farb A, Burke AP, Kolodgie FD, Virmani R. Pathological mechanisms of fatal late coronary stent thrombosis in humans. Circulation. 2003;108:1701–1712.

39. Cha DH, Malik IA, Cheneau E, et al. Use of restenting should be minimized with intracoronary radiation therapy for in-stent restenosis. Catheter Cardiovasc Interv. 2003;59:1–5.

40. Maehara A, Mintz GS, Weissman NJ, et al. Late thrombosis after gamma-brachytherapy. Catheter Cardiovasc Interv. 2003;58:455–458.

41. Tierstein P, Reilly JP. Late stent thrombosis in brachytherapy: the role of long-term antiplatelet therapy. J Invasive Cardiol. 2002;14:109–114.

42. Albiero R. Short- and intermediate-term results of (32)P radioactive beta-emitting stent implantation in patients with coronary artery disease: the Milan Dose-Response Study. Circulation. 2000;101:18–26.

43. Latchem DR. Beta-radiation for coronary in-stent restenosis. Catheter Cardiovasc Interv. 2000;51:422–429.

44. Morino Y, Bonneau HN, Fitzgerald PJ. Vascular brachytherapy: what have we learned from intravascular ultrasound? J Invasive Cardiol. 2001;13:409–416.

45. Cheneau E. Understanding and preventing the edge effect. J Interv Cardiol. 2003;16:1–7.

46. Kuchulakanti P, Novoste Corporation. Mechanisms and methods to resolve edge effect. J Invasive Cardiol. 2003;15: 363–366.

47. Giap H. Required treatment margin for coronary endovascular brachytherapy with iridium-192 seed ribbon. Cardiovasc Radiat Med. 2002;3:49–55.

48. Fajardo LF, Lee A. Rupture of major vessels after radiation. Cancer. 1975;36:904–913.

49. Donaldson SS, Hancock SL, Hoppe RT. Hodgkin's disease-finding the balance between cure and late effects. Cancer J. 1999;5:625–634.

50. Condado JA, Waksman R, Gurdiel O, et al. Long-term angiographic and clinical outcome after percutaneous transluminal coronary angioplasty and intracoronary radiation therapy in humans. Circulation. 1997;96:727–732.

51. Vandergoten P, Brosens M, Benit E. Coronary aneurysm five months after intracoronary beta-irradiation. Acta Cardiol. 2000;55:313–315.

52. Chapter 23, Raizner AE, et al. Endovascular radiation with beta and gamma sources in the porcine model, pp. 287–296. Chapter 29, Virmani R, et al. Pathology of radioactive stents, pp. 353–363. In: Waksman R, editor. Vascular brachytherapy. 2nd ed. Mount Kisco, NY: Futura; 1999:295–301, 353–363.

53. Bashore TM, O'Rourke RA, et al. ACC/SCA&I Expert Consensus Document on Cath Lab Standards. J Am Coll Cardiol. 2001;37:2170–2214.

54. Balter S. Stray radiation in the cardiac catheterisation laboratory. Radiat Prot Dosimetry. 2001;94:183–188.

55. Koenig, TR, Wolff D, Mettler FA, Wagner LK. Skin injuries from fluoroscopically guided procedures: part I, char-

acteristics of radiation injury. Am J Roentgen. 2001;177: 3–11.

56. Berlin L. Malpractice issues in radiology: radiation-induced skin injuries and fluoroscopy. Am J Roentgen. 2001;177:21–25.

57. Sternberg S. The down side of angioplasty: radiation exposure cancer risk has experts, heart patients, rethinking procedure. USA Today. November 20,2000: 9D.

58. Dehen L, Vilmer C, Humiliere C, et al. Chronic radiodermatitis following cardiac catheterisation: a report of two cases and a brief review of the literature. Heart. 1999;81:308–312.

59. Aerts A, Decraene T, van den Oord JJ, et al. Chronic radiodermatitis following percutaneous coronary interventions: a report of two cases. J Eur Acad Dermatol Venereol. 2003;17:340–343.

60. Schecter AK, Lewis MD, Robinson-Bostom L, et al. Cardiac catheterization-induced acute radiation dermatitis presenting as a fixed drug eruption. J Drugs Dermatol. 2003;2:425–427.

61. Kuon E, Glaser C, Dahm JB. Effective techniques for reduction of radiation dosage to patients undergoing invasive cardiac procedures. Br J Radiol. 2003;76:406–413.

62. Kadish AH, Mayuga KA, Yablon Z, et al. Effectiveness of shielding for patients during cardiac catheterization or electrophysiologic testing. Am J Cardiol. 2001;88:1320–1323.

63. Cusma JT, Bell MR, Wondrow MA, et al. Real-time measurement of radiation exposure to patients during diagnostic coronary angiography and percutaneous interventional procedures. J Am Coll Cardiol. 1999;33:427–435.

64. Kuon E, Schmitt M, Dahm JB. Significant reduction of radiation exposure to operator and staff during cardiac interventions by analysis of radiation leakage and improved lead shielding. Am J Cardiol. 2002;89:44–49.

65. Balter S. Radiation safety in the cardiac catheterization laboratory: operational radiation safety. Catheter Cardiovasc Interv. 1999;47:347–353.

66. McCormick VA, Schultz CC, Hollingsworth-Schuler V, et al. Reducing radiation dose in the cardiac catheterization laboratory by design alterations and staff education. Am J Cardiol. 2002;90:903–905.

67. Kuon E, Dorn C, Schmitt M, et al. Radiation dose reduction in invasive cardiology by restriction to adequate instead of optimized picture quality. Health Phys. 2003;84:626–631.

68. Giles ER, Murphy PH. Measuring skin dose with radiochromic dosimetry film in the cardiac catheterization laboratory. Health Phys. 2002;82;875–880.

69. Chong NS, Yin WS, Chan P, et al. Evaluation of absorbed radiation dose to working staff during cardiac catheterization procedures. Zhonghua Yi Xue Za Zhi (Taipei). 2000;63;816–821.

11
Complications of Closure Devices

Raghunandan Kamineni and Samuel M. Butman

1. Introduction

Obtaining adequate hemostasis following cardiac catheterization is vital in preventing subsequent complications associated with vascular access. Traditionally hemostasis has been performed with manual compression or with the use of clamplike compression devices.[1,2] Manual compression is usually associated with increased patient discomfort and prolonged immobilization, leading to a significant utilization of hospital personnel time and resources. Large-scale trials using manual compression have found the incidence of major vascular complications following cardiac catheterization to be between 0.3% and 1.0%.[3–5] More recent studies have confirmed similar rates for cardiac catheterizations (1.0%) and have also reported higher incidence rates for patients undergoing complex interventional procedures (3.0%).[6,7] Vascular closure devices (VCDs) were introduced in the 1990s, anticipating two important benefits: first, increased patient comfort and convenience with early mobilization and discharge from the hospital, and second, decreased complication rates. Although the first benefit has been achieved,[8–11] the beneficial effect of such devices on the risk of vascular complications has not been demonstrated.[12,13] In fact, the earliest randomized trials of closure devices reported a relatively higher vascular complication rate in device-treated patients compared with manual compression.[14–17] This chapter describes the various VCDs that are currently available and the associated complications with the use of these devices.

Reported complications related to these devices include:

Hematoma
Retroperitoneal bleeding
Pseudoaneurysm
Late bleeding
Groin infection
Acute femoral artery thrombosis
Distal embolization
Death related to any of the above

1.2. Case

A 74-year-old female with history of diabetes mellitus, hypertension, hyperlipidemia, coronary artery disease, and prior coronary artery bypass surgery underwent coronary angiography through a 5F sheath in the right femoral artery following a non–ST-segment elevation myocardial infarction. No coronary intervention was performed, as the disease was too extensive. The femoral puncture site was closed using the Perclose™ suture-mediated device following femoral angiography to confirm that the entry site was well above the bifurcation. The next day, the patient developed cold and white right foot with absent femoral and distal pulses. Bilateral lower extremity angiography was performed from the left femoral artery showing a normal common iliac artery bilaterally; however, the right external iliac artery was completely occluded (Figure 11-1). A selective right lower extremity angiogram was then performed showing extensive thrombus in the right external iliac artery extending to the right common femoral artery (Figure 11-2). The profunda femoris artery was patent. The right superficial femoral artery reconstituted at the level of profunda femoris and remained patent throughout its course into the lower leg. After failed attempts at crossing the occluded area with a guidewire, the patient was referred for surgical thromboembolectomy. Thrombus was confirmed intraoperatively in the distal common iliac artery extending to common femoral artery. The Perclose™ sutures were noted in the distal external iliac artery traversing through the posteromedial wall. A long segment of the common femoral artery was severely damaged requiring excision of the damaged segment and placement of an interposition polytetrafluoroethylene (PTFE) bypass graft. After re-establishing the blood flow

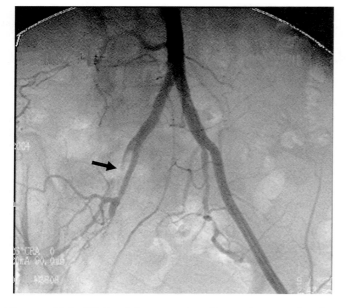

FIGURE 11-1. Bilateral lower extremity angiogram showing complete occlusion of right external iliac artery (arrow).

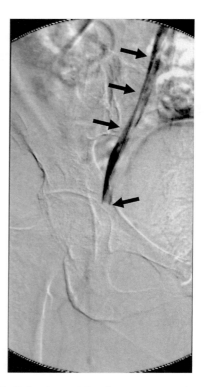

FIGURE 11-2. Selective right lower extremity angiogram showing extensive thrombus in the right external iliac artery extending to the right common femoral artery (arrows).

the patient regained the femoral pulse and recovered successfully.

VCDs can be broadly classified into the following categories (Table 11-1):

1. Suture-mediated closure devices (SCMD) (Prostar™, Techstar™, Perclose™, Perclose A-T™, Perclose Proglide™, Abbot Vascular, Inc., Redwood City, CA)
2. Collagen plugs (VasoSeal™, Datascope, Inc., Mahwah, NJ)
3. Polymer anchor and collagen (AngioSeal™, St. Jude Medical, St. Paul, MN)
4. Biosealants (Duett Pro™, Vascular Solutions, Inc., Minneapolis, MN)
5. Nonthrombogenic sealing gel (Matrix VSG™, Access Closure, Inc., Palo Alto, CA)
6. Compression girdles (Femostop™, RADI Medical Systems, Inc.)
7. Staple-mediated closure (Vascular Closure System™, Angiolink, Inc., Taunton, MA)

TABLE 11-1. Overview of the currently available vascular closure devices.

Device	Material	Mechanism of action
Perclose™	Braided polyester suture, polypropylene monofilament suture (newer generation)	Percutaneous closure of the arteriotomy site by suture
AngioSeal™	Biodegradable polymer anchor and collagen plug	Sandwich the arteriotomy site with anchor (inside the vessel) and collagen plug (outside the vessel)
VasoSeal™	Biodegradable bovine collagen plug	Extravascular closure via collagen-mediated thrombosis at the puncture site
Duett™	Procoagulant mixture containing bovine microfibrillar collagen and thrombin	Procoagulant stimulated platelet- and thrombin-based clotting mechanism sealing the arteriotomy site and tissue tract
Bioseal™	Thrombin-containing biosealant gel	Extravascular closure via thrombosis at the puncture site
Matrix VSG™	Mixture of two synthetic nonthrombogenic liquids	Two nonthrombogenic liquids when mixed together form biodegradable gel, a tissue adherent sealing the arteriotomy site
Femostop™	Compression girdle	Pneumatic compression of the arteriotomy site
Vascular Closure System™	Titanium staple	Titanium staple deployed 1 mm above the vessel adventitia achieving an anatomic purse-string closure of the arteriotomy site

2. Suture-Mediated Closure Device

Suture-mediated closure devices (SMCD) have demonstrated high efficacy rates in studies performed in non-consecutive and relatively selected populations.[11,17–21] However, the earlier-generation Perclose™ SMCD was associated with a 13% bleeding rate.[22] This was attributed to learning curve issues, use of large sheaths, and multidrug anticoagulation regimens used at the time. More recent studies have shown a decrease in complication rates in both the control- and device-treated patients.[8,12] With the newest generation Perclose™ system, one that automatically ties the knot (Perclose A-T™), a report in 72 patients found no complications except for one deployment failure.[23] With the earlier Prostar™/Techstar™ devices, a 2% complication rate was reported.[9] In a larger study of 1200 consecutive patients in whom femoral artery suture closure was performed following invasive cardiac procedures, the success rate was 91.2% and complication rate was 3.4%.[24] Several causes for failure were reported: broken suture, failure to advance the knot, failure to capture the arterial tissue with the needles, needle miss (referring to the needles not entering the receiving barrel upon deployment), persistent ooze, and iliac artery tortuosity. Complications included the development of hematoma (2.1%), retroperitoneal hemorrhage (0.3%), need for blood transfusion (0.7%), need for vascular surgery (0.6%), local infection (0.5%), and pseudoaneurysm formation (0.1%). In one patient the needles pierced and became lodged in the inguinal ligament, trapping the device and necessitating surgical removal.[24]

In a retrospective review of patients referred to vascular surgery due to peripheral vascular complications following percutaneous femoral arteriotomy, SMCD were associated with more blood loss and increased need for transfusion, and were more likely to require extensive operative procedures.[25] The pseudoaneurysms after the use of SMCD were larger and did not respond to ultrasound compression. Also, arterial infections after the use of SMCD were more common and required aggressive surgical management.

3. Collagen-Assisted Sealing Devices

Collagen-assisted sealing devices facilitate hemostasis employing bovine collagen. Earlier studies reported excessive bleeding complications (20%–33%) with the use of collagen plug devices, especially after the use of larger than 8F sheaths.[26,27] More recent studies showed no differences in bleeding or vascular complications compared to manual compression.[21,28] A prospective, single-center study of 1317 consecutive patients undergoing coronary diagnostic and interventional procedures showed similar deployment success rates but complete hemostasis after deployment was significantly lower in the interventional group (93.7% vs. 90.6%; $P = 0.05$).[29] Major complications including vascular surgery, major bleeding requiring transfusion, retroperitoneal hematoma, thrombosis, groin infections, significant groin hematoma, and death were observed in 0.53% of all patients, with no differences between diagnostic and interventional patients (0.62% vs. 0.45%; $P = NS$).

Anchor embolization or intraarterial deposition of collagen is a unique problem that is associated with the use of the Angioseal™ device.[30,31] The Manufacturer and User Facility Device Experience (MAUDE) database review reveals several anecdotal reports of distal embolization of the anchor of the AngioSeal™ device with thrombosis of femoral artery leading to acute leg ischemia[32] (Figure 11-3A,B). In the following example reported by Shaw and colleagues, the patient presented with leg ischemia 3 months following AngioSeal™ device deployment.[33]

3.1. Case

A 50-year-old female smoker underwent diagnostic coronary angiography through a 6F sheath in the right femoral artery. Coronary arteries were normal. The puncture site was closed with a 6F AngioSeal™ (St. Jude Medical). Three months later she presented with right leg claudication. Physical examination revealed a reduced right femoral pulse with an audible bruit. Popliteal and pedal pulses on the right side were also diminished. Non-invasive lower limb arterial studies showed evidence of reduced arterial blood flow with a lesion at the iliac/common femoral artery level. An abdominal aortogram with distal run off showed normal external and internal iliacs bilaterally, and a severe eccentric lesion in the right common femoral artery at the level of the femoral head (the site of previous vascular access). Debulking and balloon angioplasty of the lesion resulted in improvement of the lesion in the common femoral artery but led to sluggish flow in the superficial femoral artery. After failed initial attempts of thrombectomy in the superficial femoral artery, the object causing the angiographic filling defect was snared using a 4-mm microsnare (Microvena™, White Bear Lake, MN; Figure 11-4). As the ensnared material was too large to be removed through the indwelling 6F sheath, it had to be removed surgically, and was later confirmed to be the anchor of the AngioSeal™ device (Figure 11-5, see color plate). Fortunately, the patient had an uncomplicated recovery with no recurrent symptoms.

Inadvertent complete intraarterial deployment of the AngioSeal™ device with leg ischemia requiring surgical

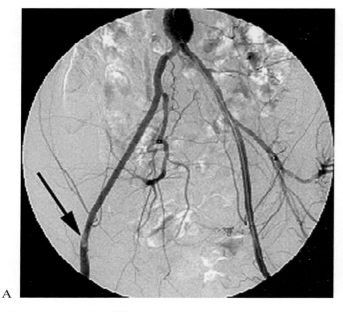

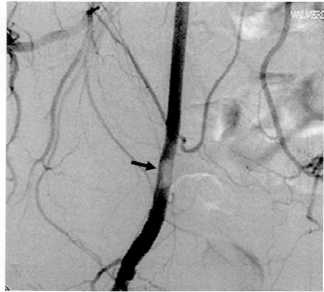

A   B

FIGURE 11-3. (A) Filling defect in the right femoral artery resulting from embolization of the anchor of the Angioseal™ device. (B) Magnified oblique view of the right femoral artery showing significant luminal compromise from the embolized anchor of the Angioseal™ device.

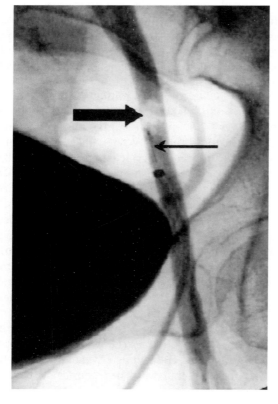

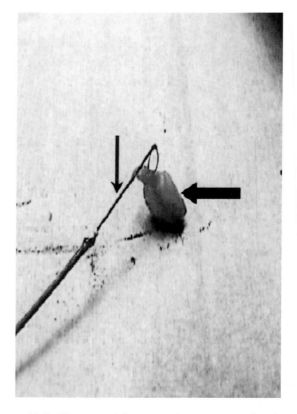

FIGURE 11-4. Angiography showing the snared object (thick black arrow) attached to the snare (thin black arrow) retracted just proximal to the sheath in the left common femoral artery.

FIGURE 11-5. The material removed at surgery showing the snare (thin black arrow) and the large object attached to it, which was the anchor of the AngioSeal™ (thick black arrow). (See color plate.)

removal of the entire system has also been reported.[34] Severe leg claudication a few days after closure with an AngioSeal™ device ultimately revealed that the plug had been placed either completely or partially through the posterior wall of the common femoral artery. This patient was successfully treated surgically.

3.2. Case

A 76-year-old woman underwent cardiac catheterization for evaluation of angina. A collagen plug device (VasoSeal™) had been used to achieve hemostasis after an uncomplicated procedure. Two weeks later she presented with a large, painful, pulsatile mass in her groin. Doppler ultrasound examination revealed a pseudoaneurysm arising from a branch of the right profunda femoris artery. Ultrasound-guided compression of the pseudoaneurysm was initially attempted but was unsuccessful. The pseudoaneurysm was eventually successfully treated with transcatheter coil embolization. The patient recovered uneventfully.

Although VasoSeal™ is an exclusively extravascular closure device, intra-arterial insertions with consecutive leg ischemia have been reported in 0.3%–2% (15/2229) of the patients.[35] One patient experienced groin discomfort for several months after the use of VasoSeal™ to achieve hemostasis due to retention of the sheath in the groin.[36]

With the Duett™ device, minor complications have been reported in 2.1% and major complications in 1% in a large single-center study, as well as in the multicenter European registry with a total of 1587 patients enrolled.[34,37] An inadvertent intra-arterial injection of the procoagulant occurred in 4 patients (0.3%) and was successfully treated by intra-arterial infusion of urokinase in three cases and surgical repair in one.[29,32]

4. Vacular Closure Devices versus Manual Compression

In a prospective analysis to evaluate the incidence of major complication rates (defined as need for transfusion, pseudoaneurysm or arteriovenous fistula requiring vascular repair, acute femoral occlusion, groin infection, or readmission for a groin complication) associated with each of the newer methods of hemostasis compared to manual compression following coronary diagnostic and interventional procedures, the incidence of complications did vary with the device selected[32] (Table 11-2). The AngioSeal™ device had the highest incidence of major complications (2.6%) followed by the VasoSeal™ device (1.5%). The Perclose™ device and manual compression had similar total complication rates (0.8% with

TABLE 11-2. Complications for each of the three closure devices compared to manual compression[32]

Complication	Manual compression	Vasoseal™	Angioseal™	Perclose™
Number	1019	937	742	1001
Surgical repair	3	6	7	2
Acute occlusion	0	0	5	1
Transfusions	2	0	3	1
Readmission	0	5	2	0
Infections	0	3	2	4
Total	5 (0.5%)	14 (1.5%)	19 (2.6%)	8 (0.8%)
P value		0.02*	0.0002*	NS*

* As compared to manual compression.

Perclose™ and 0.5% with manual compression; P = NS). In contrast, a similar randomized study failed to show differences in the major complication rates between the AngioSeal™ device and the VasoSeal™ device.[38]

In the STAND-II-trial comparing suture-mediated closure devices with manual compression, major complications occurred in 2.4% in the suture-mediated group but only 1.1% in the conventional compression group (P = NS). The complications reported included surgical repair of the femoral artery (1.2% vs. 0.4%), transfusion (1.2% vs. 0.4%), infection requiring intravenous antibiotics (0.8% vs. 0.4%), and ultrasound-guided compression for pseudoaneurysm (0.8% vs. 1.1%).[8] A larger, retrospective study comparing manual compression with the Perclose™ device involving 8906 diagnostic and 1095 interventional catheterization patients showed a dramatically higher complication rates with SMCD for diagnostic angiography (2.6% and 4.6% rates for Perclose™ major and minor complications, respectively, compared to 0.2% and 1.8% for manual compression major and minor complications, respectively; P ≥ 0.01).[9] Surprisingly, complication rates for interventional patients were similar between the Perclose™ and manual compression groups (3.4% vs. 3.3% for major complications and 7.1% vs. 6.6% for minor complications; P = NS).

In a meta-analysis of 30 randomized trials comparing any VCDs with standard manual compression, the relative risk (RR) of groin hematoma was 1.14 (P = NS); bleeding, 1.48 (P = NS); developing an arteriovenous fistula, 0.83 (P = NS); and developing a pseudoaneurysm at the puncture site, 1.19 (P = NS).[39] However, when the analysis was limited to only trials that used explicit intention-to-treat approaches, VCDs were associated with a higher risk of hematoma [RR, 1.89; 95% confidence interval (CI), 1.13–3.15] and a higher risk of pseudoaneurysm (RR, 5.40; 95% CI, 1.21–24.5). This meta-analysis indicated that there might only be marginal evidence that VCDs are effective, and these devices might increase the risk of hematoma and pseudoaneurysm formation.

3. Babu SC, Piccorelli GO, Shah PM, et al. Incidence and results of arterial complications among 16,350 patients undergoing cardiac catheterization. J Vasc Surg. 1989;10: 113–116.

4. Johnson LW, Lozner EC, Johnson S, et al. Coronary arteriography 1984–1987: a report of the Registry of the Society for Cardiac Angiography and Interventions. I. Results and complications. Catheter Cardiovasc Diagn. 1989;17: 5–10.

5. Miller GA. Local arterial complications of left heart catheterisation. J R Coll Physicians Lond. 1986;20:288–289.

6. Khoury M, Batra S, Berg R, et al. Influence of arterial access sites and interventional procedures on vascular complications after cardiac catheterizations. Am J Surg. 1992;164: 205–209.

7. Muller DW, Shamir KJ, Ellis SG, Topol EJ. Peripheral vascular complications after conventional and complex percutaneous coronary interventional procedures. Am J Cardiol. 1992;69:63–68.

8. Baim DS, Knopf WD, Hinohara T, et al. Suture-mediated closure of the femoral access site after cardiac catheterization: results of the suture to ambulate and discharge (STAND I and STAND II) trials. Am J Cardiol. 2000;85:864–869.

9. Kahn ZM, Kumar M, Hollander G, Frankel R. Safety and efficacy of the Perclose suture-mediated closure device after diagnostic and interventional catheterizations in a large consecutive population. Catheter Cardiovasc Interv. 2002;55:8–13.

10. Vetter JW, Hinohara T, Ribeiro EE, et al. Percutaneous vascular surgery: suture mediated percutaneous closure of femoral artery access site following coronary intervention. J Am Coll Cardiol. 1995;25(Supp 1):10A.

11. Gerckens U, Cattelaens N, Muller R, Lampe EG, Grube E. [Percutaneous suture of femoral artery access sites after diagnostic heart catheterization and or coronary intervention. Safety and effectiveness of a new arterial suture technic]. Herz. 1998;23:27–34.

12. Sesana M, Vaghetti M, Albiero R, et al. Effectiveness and complications of vascular access closure devices after interventional procedures. J Invasive Cardiol. 2000;12:395–399.

13. Silber S, Bjorvik A, Muhling H, Rosch A. Usefulness of collagen plugging with VasoSeal after PTCA as compared to manual compression with identical sheath dwell times. J Invasive Cardiol. 1999;11(suppl B):19B–24B.

14. Ward SR, Casale P, Raymond R, et al. Efficacy and safety of a hemostatic puncture closure device with early ambulation after coronary angiography. Angio-Seal Investigators. Am J Cardiol. 1998;81:569–572.

15. Kussmaul WG, Buchbinder M, Whitlow PL, et al. Femoral artery hemostasis using an implantable device (Angio-Seal) after coronary angioplasty. Catheter Cardiovasc Diagn. 1996;37:362–365.

16. von Hoch F, Neumann FJ, Theiss W, et al. Efficacy and safety of collagen implants for haemostasis of the vascular access site after coronary balloon angioplasty and coronary stent implantation. A randomized study. Eur Heart J. 1995;16:640–646.

17. Sanborn TA, Gibbs HH, Brinker JA, et al. A multicenter randomized trial comparing a percutaneous collagen hemostasis device with conventional manual compression after diagnostic angiography and angioplasty. J Am Coll Cardiol. 1993;22:1273–1279.

18. Shrake KL. Comparison of major complication rates associated with four methods of arterial closure. Am J Cardiol. 2000;85:1024–1025.

19. Cura FA, Kapadia SR, L'Allier PL, et al. Safety of femoral closure devices after percutaneous coronary interventions in the era of glycoprotein IIb/IIIa platelet blockade. Am J Cardiol. 2000;86:780–782, A9.

20. Chamberlin JR, Lardi AB, McKeever LS, et al. Use of vascular sealing devices (VasoSeal and Perclose) versus assisted manual compression (Femostop) in transcatheter coronary interventions requiring abciximab (ReoPro). Catheter Cardiovasc Interv. 1999;47:143–147, discussion 148.

21. Carere RG, Webb JG, Miyagishima R, et al. Groin complications associated with collagen plug closure of femoral arterial puncture sites in anticoagulated patients. Catheter Cardiovasc Diagn. 1998;43:124–129.

22. Duffin DC, Muhlestein JB, Allisson SB, et al. Femoral arterial puncture management after percutaneous coronary procedures: a comparison of clinical outcomes and patient satisfaction between manual compression and two different vascular closure devices. J Invasive Cardiol. 2001;13: 354–362.

23. Shimshak T. Vascular access site management in high-risk patients. Endovascular Today. 2003;2:48–50.

24. Fram DB, Giri S, Jamil G, et al. Suture closure of the femoral arteriotomy following invasive cardiac procedures: a detailed analysis of efficacy, complications, and the impact of early ambulation in 1,200 consecutive, unselected cases. Catheter Cardiovasc Interv. 2001;53:163–173.

25. Sprouse LR 2nd, Botta DM Jr, Hamilton IN Jr. The management of peripheral vascular complications associated with the use of percutaneous suture-mediated closure devices. J Vasc Surg. 2001;33:688–693.

26. Carere RG, Webb JG, Dodek A. Collagen plug closure of femoral arterial punctures. Are complications excessive? Circulation. 1994;90:621.

27. Webb JG, Carere RA, Dodek AA. Collagen plug hemostatic closure of femoral arterial puncture sites following implantation of intracoronary stents. Catheter Cardiovasc Diagn. 1993;30:314–316.

28. Brachmann J, Ansah M, Kosinski EJ, Schuler GC. Improved clinical effectiveness with a collagen vascular hemostasis device for shortened immobilization time following diagnostic angiography and percutaneous transluminal coronary angioplasty. Am J Cardiol. 1998;81:1502–1505.

29. Eggebrecht H, Haude M, Woertgen U, et al. Systematic use of a collagen-based vascular closure device immediately after cardiac catheterization procedures in 1317 consecutive patients. Catheter Cardiovasc Interv. 2002;57:486–495.

30. Goyen M, Manz S, Kroger K, et al. Interventional therapy of vascular complications caused by the hemostatic puncture closure device angio-seal. Catheter Cardiovasc Interv. 2000;49:142–147.

31. Stein BC, Teirstein PS. Nonsurgical removal of angio-seal device after intra-arterial deposition of collagen plug. Catheter Cardiovasc Interv. 2000;50:340–342.

32. Carey D, Martin JR, Moore CA, et al. Complications of femoral artery closure devices. Catheter Cardiovasc Interv. 2001;52:3–7, discussion 8.

33. Shaw JA, Gravereaux EC, Winters GL, Eisenhauer AC. An unusual cause of claudication. Catheter Cardiovasc Interv. 2003;60:562–565.

34. Silber S, Schon N, Seidel N, Heiss-Bogner J. [Accidental occlusion of the common femoral artery after Angio-Seal-application]. Z Kardiol. 1998;87:51–55.

35. Silber S. Rapid hemostasis of arterial puncture sites with collagen in patients undergoing diagnostic and interventional cardiac catheterization. Clin Cardiol. 1997;20: 981–992.

36. Tuli A, Lim SS, Zafari AM. An unusual case of groin discomfort. Catheter Cardiovasc Interv. 2001;52:484–485.

37. Mooney MR, Ellis SG, Gershony G, et al. Immediate sealing of arterial puncture sites after cardiac catheterization and coronary interventions: initial U.S. feasibility trial using the Duett vascular closure device. Catheter Cardiovasc Interv. 2000;50:96–102.

38. Shammas NW, Rajendran VR, Alldredge SG, et al. Randomized comparison of Vasoseal and Angioseal closure devices in patients undergoing coronary angiography and angioplasty. Catheter Cardiovasc Interv. 2002;55:421–425.

39. Koreny M, Riedmuller E, Nikfardjam M, et al. Arterial puncture closing devices compared with standard manual compression after cardiac catheterization: systematic review and meta-analysis. JAMA. 2004;291:350–357.

40. Smith TP, Cruz CP, Moursi MM, Eidt JF. Infectious complications resulting from use of hemostatic puncture closure devices. Am J Surg. 2001;182:658–662.

41. Aguirre FV, Topol EJ, Ferguson JJ, et al. Bleeding complications with the chimeric antibody to platelet glycoprotein IIb/IIIa integrin in patients undergoing percutaneous coronary intervention. EPIC Investigators. Circulation. 1995;91:2882–2890.

42. Kereiakes DJ, Lincoff AM, Miller DP, et al. Abciximab therapy and unplanned coronary stent deployment: favorable effects on stent use, clinical outcomes, and bleeding complications. EPILOG Trial Investigators. Circulation. 1998;97:857–864.

43. Applegate RJ, Grabarczyk MA, Little WC, et al. Vascular closure devices in patients treated with anticoagulation and IIb/IIIa receptor inhibitors during percutaneous revascularization. J Am Coll Cardiol. 2002;40:78–83.

44. Lunney L, Karim K, Little T. Vasoseal hemostasis following coronary interventions with abciximab. J Invasive Cardiol. 1999;11(suppl B):2B–3B.

45. Resnic FS, Blake GJ, Ohno-Machado L, et al. Vascular closure devices and the risk of vascular complications after percutaneous coronary intervention in patients receiving glycoprotein IIb-IIIa inhibitors. Am J Cardiol. 2001;88: 493–496.

46. Morice MC LT. Immediate post PTCA percutaneous suture of femoral arteries with the Perclose device: results of high volume users. J Am Coll Cardiol. 1998;31(suppl A): 1033–1104.

47. Walker SB, Cleary S, Higgins M. Comparison of the Femostop device and manual pressure in reducing groin puncture site complications following coronary angioplasty and coronary stent placement. Int J Nurs Pract. 2001;7: 366–375.

12
Legal Complications of Percutaneous Coronary Procedures

Peter Akmajian

1. Introduction

A patient arrives in the emergency department. She has classic complaints of chest pain radiating to the left arm. An electrocardiogram (ECG) is positive for an acute myocardial infarction. In consultation with a cardiologist, the emergency physician promptly refers the patient to the cardiac catheterization laboratory.

There, the cardiologist catheterizes the patient in a timely manner, finding a total occlusion of the left anterior descending coronary artery (LAD). Then the cardiologist performs an angioplasty, with reduction in the occlusion from 100% to 0%, with normal flow and perfusion. So far, so good.

The patient is transferred to the intensive care unit (ICU) for recovery. Almost immediately, the nurse records alarmingly low blood pressure. She starts dopamine and contacts the cardiologist. He orders the patient back to the catheterization laboratory for placement of an intra-aortic balloon pump. The patient continues to do poorly and is given additional vasopressors. The emergency physician arrives and intubates the patient. She continues to deteriorate and is pronounced dead almost 2 hours after arriving in the ICU.

What happened? How did this seemingly simple and efficient procedure result in death? Did the patient suffer a rupture of the artery? If so, did the healthcare providers commit malpractice? Rupture is a known complication. The patient consented to the procedure and knew of the risk of death. Yes, but did anyone recognize that complication? What if they had? What then? Perhaps coronary bypass surgery could or should have been done on an emergent basis. But what if this was a small-town hospital with no ability to have a surgical team as backup for the catheterization laboratory? Would that excuse any alleged failure to recognize the complication? After all, there would have been no time to transfer the patient to a bigger city. But should a small hospital even perform catheterization procedures if there is no surgical backup?

If not, then what about all the people in the area who might die without quick access to the catheterization laboratory? Finally, is a jury of laypeople capable of sorting out these issues fairly? These are but a few questions that the above scenario raises.

Welcome to the world of medical malpractice. This chapter will attempt to review the most common types of medical malpractice claims arising out of percutaneous coronary procedures. It will further suggest strategies to help minimize the risk of such claims. The data for this chapter was readily obtained from a national search, using Westlaw, of trial court jury verdicts and appellate decisions involving percutaneous procedures.

2. General Principles of Medical Malpractice Law

It is not the intent of this chapter to discuss in great detail the law of medical malpractice. However, in order to put the chapter into context, some understanding of malpractice law is necessary.

2.1. Medical Negligence

In simplest terms, a malpractice claim asserts that a doctor or other healthcare provider was negligent, or careless, in the treatment of a patient and that such negligence caused injury. What is negligence in a medical case? It could be an orthopedic surgeon drilling a screw into the popliteal space and lacerating an artery; an obstetrician not responding quickly to troubling fetal monitoring strips; a family doctor failing to recognize that anemia could mean colon cancer in a man over 50 with no previous history; an emergency room doctor diagnosing new onset angina and sending the patient home with orders to follow up with a primary care doctor; or an interventional cardiologist not listening to an assistant's warnings during a procedure.

2.1.1. Standard of Care

The term *standard of care* is used to define the physician's conduct. The doctor must comply with the standard of care. A deviation from the standard of care that causes injury is negligence and subjects the doctor to liability for injury caused by the deviation.

The standard of care is often amorphous. In many cases, there is no set standard for any particular situation. One can glean the standard of care from the physician's education and training as well as knowledge and advances in medicine, as evidenced by the literature. Sometimes, authoritative organizations have published guidelines that can be strong evidence of the standard of care.

To prove a malpractice claim, one must normally retain the services of an expert witness. The expert must review the medical record and other factual information then render an opinion on the standard of care. Each side of the case has its own experts, with the full opportunity to cross-examine the other side's experts. The only time expert witnesses are not required is in the rare case when the malpractice is so self-evident that a jury needs no assistance to discern it, such as when the wrong leg has been amputated. Even then, an expert might be helpful to establish whether the responsibility to identify the correct leg to operate was with the doctor or the hospital nursing staff.

Malpractice claims are tried to lay juries in most every state. Normally, during the jury selection process, the lawyers strike from the jury panel those with significant backgrounds in medicine. The end result is that juries deciding these claims represent a clean slate, with little to no preconceived notions.

The medical record is of the utmost importance in any malpractice claim. In reality, it is a legal document that memorializes the actions of the healthcare providers. In a malpractice suit, every aspect of the record is analyzed, digested, and summarized. Lawyers often examine the record to determine if any doctor has altered it after the fact. Important parts of the record will be enlarged for trial. The medical record is the foundation of any malpractice case.

2.2. Informed Consent and Battery

An important, but somewhat rare, subset of medical malpractice claims are claims for battery. The legal theory of battery is an unpermitted touching. In the law, one may not touch another person in a significant way without permission.

In the medical setting, the patient must give informed consent before a doctor is allowed to invade the patient's body. If a doctor fails to provide informed consent, the patient has a claim for battery.

While this sounds theoretical, it comes to life in the case of a surgical procedure with complications. Normally, in a malpractice case, known complications are not malpractice if the doctor otherwise complied with the standard of care. However, if the patient did not give informed consent, the patient can sue for battery, alleging the patient would not have had the surgery if the doctor had fully informed the patient of the risks.

2.3. The Doctor–Patient Relationship

In any malpractice case, the patient must establish the existence of a doctor–patient relationship. Absent that relationship, the doctor has no legal duty to the patient and cannot be liable for malpractice. This point seems obvious, but there are many types of relationships in medicine, and not all of them are direct.

For example, if an on-call cardiologist receives a telephone call from an emergency room doctor, who provides facts about a patient to the cardiologist and the cardiologist then gives advice to the emergency room doctor about the patient, does the cardiologist have a doctor–patient relationship with the patient? What if the cardiologist is walking down the hall of the hospital and encounters an emergency room nurse, who expresses discomfort that the emergency room doctor is about to discharge a patient with chest pain? If the nurse shows the cardiologist the ECG and the cardiologist concurs with the discharge based on the ECG, has the cardiologist formed a relationship with the patient?

More and more, cases from around the country answer these questions affirmatively. The theory is that once the physician renders advice, the physician knows, or should know, that the advice will affect patient care. Thus, a sufficient relationship exists for the patient to sue if the advice turns out to be wrong.

In *Diggs v Arizona Cardiologists* [198 Ariz. 198, 8 P.3d 386 (App. 2000)], an emergency room doctor "bumped into" a cardiologist who was in the emergency department and "briefly discussed" a patient the emergency physician was treating at the time. The ER physician presented the cardiologist with the clinical history, the results of the physical examination, and with the ECG results.

Based upon the information the ER doctor presented, the cardiologist agreed that the patient could be discharged, concluding the patient had a case of pericarditis that could be treated with indomethacin. The cardiologist agreed the patient should follow up with her family practice physician immediately.

The patient died 3 hours later of cardiopulmonary arrest. A subsequent read of the ECG interpreted it as showing a myocardial infarction.

The trial court ruled, as a matter of law, that the cardiologist could not be liable. It found the discussion between the two doctors was "informal," that there was no relationship between the cardiologist and patient and thus that the cardiologist had no duty to the patient. The Arizona Court of Appeals, however, rejected this reasoning and ruled that a sufficient relationship existed to impose a duty of care upon the cardiologist.

The court explained that the cardiologist was in a "unique position" to prevent harm to the patient. The emergency physician relied upon the opinions of the cardiologist. The advice the cardiologist gave implied to the emergency physician that it was safe to discharge the patient. The cardiologist testified that had this patient been his own, he would have done cardiac enzyme tests to rule out myocardial infarction (MI). The court noted the cardiologist did not give this advice to the ER doctor and consequently increased the risk of harm to the patient by advising that it was appropriate to discharge the patient. The court concluded that by giving advice affecting patient care, the cardiologist became a treating doctor. He thus had a duty of reasonable care, just as if he had seen and examined the patient.

3. Case Studies Involving Percutaneous Procedures

This section is divided into groups according to the alleged misconduct of the physician, beginning with having never seen the patient and ending with delayed performance of a procedure.

3.1. The Doctor–Patient Relationship in Percutaneous Procedures

3.1.1. Percutaneous Procedures Where the Physician Never Sees or Examines the Patient

The case of *Bovara v St. Francis Hospital* [298 Ill App. 3d 1025, 700 N.E. 2d 143 (1998)] exemplifies that doctors involved in percutaneous coronary procedures need not see or treat (or even bill) the patient to have a relationship. Albert Bovara met with Dr. Pascale at St. Francis Hospital. Mr. Bovara brought with him an angiogram that had been performed at another hospital. Dr. Pascale had no training in reading angiograms and did not perform angioplasty. Dr. Pascale testified that it was interventional cardiologists who made the decision on whether angiogram was indicated.

Dr. Pascale provided the angiogram to a staff member, who passed it on to two interventional cardiologists, Drs. Edgett and Bliley, who reviewed the study. Drs. Edgett and Bliley reviewed no other records of Mr. Bovara, and they never examined the patient. They also did not bill for their services.

Dr. Pascale received a message back that angioplasty was indicated, though Dr. Pascale could not recall if he spoke directly with one of the reviewing doctors. Dr. Pascale then informed Mr. Bovara that "his people" thought Mr. Bovara was a good candidate for the procedure.

At the time of the procedure, neither Dr. Bliley nor Dr. Edgett was available. A fourth doctor, Dr. Allocco, performed the procedure. Before doing so, he reviewed the angiogram and determined that Mr. Bovara was a good candidate for the procedure. Mr. Bovara went into full cardiac arrest during the procedure and died.

Mr. Bovara's survivors sued, alleging that Mr. Bovara was not truly a candidate for angioplasty. The family attached to the lawsuit affidavits of expert physicians stating that his lesion was not the type on which angioplasty should have been performed. The plaintiffs included in this suit Drs. Bliley and Edgett, alleging they failed to recognize the risks Mr. Bovara faced in this procedure.

After suit was filed, the trial court granted summary judgment to Drs. Bliley and Edgett, on the basis that they had no doctor–patient relationship with the patient. The Illinois Court of Appeals disagreed with the trial court and reversed the decision. The court first ruled that though the doctor–patient relationship is a consensual one, such a relationship exists where a physician contacts another physician on behalf of the patient. Such a contact occurred in this case.

The appellate court stated:

The facts of *Reynolds* are distinguishable. While the consulting physician in *Reynolds* just suggested a test and was not responsible for any portion of the patient's diagnosis or treatment, [defendants] reviewed test results and interpreted them.

The *Bovara* court also noted that after reviewing the angiogram, defendants followed up by meeting with Dr. Pascale. At that meeting, they discussed Bovara's history, after which the decision was made to recommend angioplasty. In addition, Dr. Pascale recorded on the decedent's hospital chart that "catheterization reviewed by [defendants]." The *Bovara* court determined from said evidence that a genuine issue of material fact existed as to whether a physician–patient relationship was formed between defendants and the decedent and whether they owed a duty of care to the decedent and breached that duty.

More importantly, Drs. Bliley and Edgett rendered opinions that "they knew or should have known" would be passed on to the patient. Though the doctors claimed their opinion was "informal," the court said that did not mean there was no doctor–patient relationship. The indications for the angioplasty were at the heart of the case, and the court concluded that the doctors' opinion contributed to the procedure going forward.

3.1.2. The Need for Some Contact

In *Gathings v Muscadin* [318 Ill App. 3d 1091, 743 N.E. 2d 659 (2001)], the patient's treating doctor attempted to contact Dr. Muscadin to come to the hospital to consult on the case. However, Dr. Muscadin never received the call and was out of town. He could not have come to the hospital even had he received the call.

In this situation, the court ruled that there was no doctor–patient relationship. One can say, then, that if a doctor does not get a call and is out of town, there is no doctor–patient relationship. However, anytime one receives a call and renders advice, a relationship exists, even when the advice is informal and there is no billing.

3.2. Informed Consent Cases

3.2.1. Failure to Obtain a Signed Form

In *Wilkerson v Mid-America Cardiology* [908 S.W. 2d 691 (Mo. App. 1995)], nobody obtained a specific informed consent for the procedure in question. The patient, Mr. Wilkerson, refused to sign an informed consent for an angioplasty until someone explained the procedure to him. The court's opinion stated that an "orderly" who provided the form to the patient stated that someone would eventually do so.

Mr. Wilkerson had earlier undergone a diagnostic angiogram. There was no question the cardiologist had discussed that procedure with Mr. Wilkerson and had obtained and documented the informed consent for that procedure. The angiogram revealed significant blockages in the coronary arteries.

Mr. Wilkerson and family contended, however, that no one discussed the risks and benefits of the angioplasty procedure. They alleged that the cardiologist who had performed the angiogram (a noninterventional cardiologist) came to the hospital room twice before the procedure but never provided informed consent because the cardiologist had to attend to other patients. The doctor's progress notes reflect no discussion of informed consent regarding the angioplasty.

Thus, by the time Mr. Wilkerson arrived in the catheterization laboratory, no one had provided informed consent regarding the angioplasty. In this case, a coronary bypass surgery would have been a viable alternative for the patient. No one informed Mr. Wilkerson of this fact. Shortly after arriving in the catheterization laboratory, Mr. Wilkerson was provided Valium, and the procedure went forward.

During the procedure, the interventional cardiologist, whom the patient had never met before, inadvertently dissected the left main artery. This caused decreased cardiac output and cardiac arrest. Emergency surgery was then performed. While the patient survived, he suffered brain injury resulting from the cardiac arrest.

The trial court granted a "directed verdict" (meaning the court granted judgment to the defense without submitting the case to the jury for decision) based on the fact that the plaintiff never proved what he would have done had someone provided informed consent. In other words, the plaintiff never asserted that he would have refused the procedure if someone had informed him of the risks.

The Missouri Court of Appeals reversed this decision. It ruled that the plaintiff did not have to prove what he would have done. Rather, the court ruled that the question was what a "reasonable person" would have done. Under the facts of the case, the court decided that a reasonable person could have decided to forego angioplasty in favor of coronary bypass. Thus, the court reversed and sent the case back to the trial court for a new trial.

3.2.2. Failure to Use Specific Language

The case of *Harris v Tatum* [216 Ga. App. 607, 455 S.E. 2d 124 (1995)] again highlights the importance of obtaining *specific* informed consent. The plaintiff underwent a diagnostic angiogram performed by Dr. Harris. Later that same day, Dr. Harris performed a balloon angioplasty. During the course of that procedure, plaque from the treatment site dislodged, then traveled to the legs, forming clots in the left leg and right foot. Ultimately, the patient's right foot was amputated.

The patient sued, alleging he had not given informed consent for the angioplasty. He had provided a written consent for the angiogram, which alluded to the fact that other procedures might need to be performed:

I understand that during the course of the procedure described above [the angiogram] it may be necessary or appropriate to perform additional procedures which are unforeseen or not known to be needed at the time this consent is given. I consent to and authorize the persons described herein to make the decisions concerning such procedures. I also consent to and authorize the performance of such additional procedures as they deem necessary and appropriate.

A jury trial resulted in a $500,000 verdict for the plaintiff. The physician appealed, but the Georgia Court of Appeals affirmed the judgment. The court reasoned that the informed consent was vague and ambiguous whether any additional procedures had to be both necessary *and* appropriate or necessary *or* appropriate. The court further ruled that there was a question of fact for the jury to decide whether the angioplasty was necessary. Thus, the decision of the jury stood.

3.2.3. Known Risks

In *Yurick v Cleveland Clinic* [2001 WL 1042061 (2001)] the patient died of an intracerebral bleed as the result of anticoagulation medicine given in conjunction with an angioplasty. The plaintiff alleged negligence in the provision and monitoring of the medicine, but the defense contended that the bleed was a rare, but known risk. The jury found for the defendant.

If a patient is informed of the risks of the procedure and the related medications, there is no liability if such a complication occurs, without evidence of malpractice. Unfortunately, as this case demonstrates, it may be necessary for healthcare providers to proceed to trial to establish this point.

3.2.4. Failure to Offer a Risky Option

Perhaps a corollary of informed consent is the concept that a physician must discuss all available options with a patient. However, what if the physician does not think the patient is a good candidate for the procedure? Will the law require the doctor to discuss the option anyway?

This issue was raised in *Rocco v Anonymous Defendants* [10 Zarin MLA 1:19, 2001 WL 1855076 (Unknown State Court) (Verdict date May 2001)]. There, the patient, in his 40s, suffered blockage in three arteries as well as diabetes. He underwent a bypass operation in which both his right and left mammary arteries were used as donor vessels. The patient admitted that use of such vessels was appropriate. However, he contended that postoperatively he suffered intractable chest pain and that he could not get relief.

The plaintiff contended that he was not advised of the risk of permanent chest pain, nor was he advised of the option to undergo angioplasty instead of bypass. The defendants disputed the notion that the plaintiff was not advised of the risk of chest pain. Further, defendants asserted that the plaintiff was not a candidate for angioplasty because he had multivessel disease and because of his diabetes. Thus, they argued, they had no obligation to advise the patient of the option of having this procedure.

The jury in this case ruled in favor of the defendant doctors. The fact is that angioplasty was not a valid option.

3.3. Alleged Poor Technique

3.3.1. Stent Sizing

A Florida case entitled *Kohel v Anonymous Defendant* [11 Fla. J.V.R.A. 3:C2, 2000 WL 33713252 (Unknown State Court) (Verdict date October 9, 2000)] concerned the proper sizing of a stent during an angioplasty procedure. The patient suffered a cardiac arrest during the angioplasty procedure from a ruptured coronary artery. After the arrest, the patient was rushed into emergency open heart surgery. She lingered for several weeks in the hospital but died from encephalopathy.

The plaintiff's expert cardiologist testified that that the defendant doctor used a stent that was oversized and that also exceeded maximum balloon inflation, resulting in a rupture of the artery. The plaintiff's expert emphasized that the artery ruptured at the very point where the balloon was overinflated.

The defendant contended that a rupture of the coronary artery is a well-known complication of angioplasty and stenting procedures and that the patient's injury occurred in the absence of negligence. The defense maintained that the stent used in the procedure was properly sized and that the balloon inflation was proper. The defense expert testified that there may have been a calcified lesion that caused the tear of the vessel.

In support of his case, the plaintiff relied upon the manufacturer's manual. The defendant countered that subsequent medical literature and clinical practice superseded the manual. The defense argued that this was an early stent that required oversizing and overinflation. The defense submitted a great deal of medical literature, which was not refuted, establishing that if the stent was not oversized and overinflated, the patient was at significant risk for acute vessel closure and myocardial infarction.

Nevertheless, the jury found in favor of plaintiff, awarding $1,216,000. This case exemplifies that in many malpractice actions, there is a legitimate dispute over important issues. Often, credible experts on both sides clash over the exact mechanism of injury. It is then up to a lay jury to determine the facts.

3.3.2. Balloon Rupture/Stent Release into Bloodstream

Another large verdict occurred in *Estate of Washington v Chait* [2001 WL 823202] arising out of an angioplasty in 1994. During this procedure, the balloon ruptured, and the stent was released into the bloodstream. The stent had to be removed in a subsequent surgery by another surgeon.

The plaintiff alleged that the patient's heart problems could not be properly addressed after the first procedure and that he died as a result. The defendant asserted that the patient's death was unrelated to the surgical complications but to ongoing coronary artery disease. The jury found in favor of plaintiff and awarded $1,000,000.

3.3.3. Broken Guidewire

In *Purdon v Locke* [807 So.2d 373 (Miss. 2001)], the patient, Mr. Locke, underwent an angioplasty. During the course of the procedure, a piece of the guidewire broke off inside an artery.

The physician, Dr. Purdon, changed his version of the facts on several occasions. Initially, he stated that the wire broke. Later, he contended that he cut the wire. He reversed himself again, claiming that the wire broke due to a malfunction of the mechanism. Mr. Locke was immediately transferred to surgery, where a surgeon removed the wire fragment and performed a bypass.

Further, despite denials from Dr. Purdon, operating room witnesses and surgical notes indicate that Dr. Purdon went into the operating room and took the fractured wire after it was removed. The wire was never recovered.

There was no indication in this case that the bypass surgery was unsuccessful. Nevertheless, Mr. Locke sued contending he was sore and uncomfortable, that he suffered emotional instability after surgery, that his marital relationship was damaged, and that his "attitude and personality" had suffered. The jury returned a verdict for the plaintiff in the amount of $650,000.

Dr. Purdon appealed to the Mississippi Supreme Court on a number of grounds. The court rejected his arguments entirely. Dr. Purdon's strongest argument may have been that the damages were excessive. Appellate courts, however, give great deference to jury damage awards. So long as the verdict is not grossly excessive and manifestly the result of passion and prejudice, the appellate court will not reduce the verdict.

One can surmise that in this case, Dr. Purdon's conduct had something to do with the verdict. His changing stories and his activities in the operating room undoubtedly motivated the jury to assist the plaintiff in any way possible.

3.3.4. The Kissing Balloon Technique

In *Estate of Allen v Anonymous HMO* [JVR No. 186507, 1996 WL 695851 (Cal.Superior)], the patient, a 39-year-old man, had two significantly stenosed coronary arteries. He underwent angioplasty using the kissing balloon technique. During the procedure, he suffered dissections of both arteries and subsequently died the next day.

The family alleged that the cardiologist should have stopped the procedure once he realized the arteries were dissected, that the kissing balloon technique was inappropriate for the case, and that immediate bypass surgery was indicated once the dissections occurred.

The defendant doctor countered that it was appropriate to continue with the angioplasty despite the dissection and that bypass was not indicated. Moreover, the doctor argued that the patient's coronary health was already poor due to obesity and diabetes. This case settled for $850,000.

3.4. Timing Cases

3.4.1. Delay in Performing the Procedure

This was the allegation in a Michigan trial involving an anonymous 42-year-old male (2000 WL 33313836) resulting in a $3.5 million settlement on August 29, 2000. In this case, the patient presented to the defendant hospital after experiencing a heart attack. The emergency department stabilized the patient and admitted him to the hospital. The patient then experienced 1 day free of chest pain, but then his pain resumed. A cardiologist examined the patient and determined that the pain was not cardiac related. However, over the next 3 to 4 hours, the patient's condition worsened, and it was determined that the patient needed an angioplasty. Three additional hours passed, and the patient died after experiencing a cardiac arrhythmia.

3.4.2. Failure to Recognize Signs and Symptoms Resulting in Delay

The case of *Campbell v Prieto* [12 Fla. J.V.R.A. 5:C5, 2001 WL 1910941 (Unknown state court) (Verdict date January 18, 2001)] involved a family doctor who allegedly did not recognize the signs and symptoms of myocardial infarction soon enough for a percutaneous procedure to work. The patient had been seeing the defendant doctor for 3 years prior to his death. He saw the defendant on a regular basis for diabetes, high blood pressure, and high cholesterol.

In February 1997, the patient reported to his doctor complaints of left arm numbness and tingling. The defendant doctor diagnosed arthritis and prescribed anti-inflammatory medication. The patient returned a week later, reporting that his symptoms were worsening and he additionally suffered pain below his sternum and was unable to sleep at night. The defendant thought maybe the anti-inflammatory medicine was causing an upset stomach.

The next day, the patient returned and reported pain in both arms. The doctor performed an ECG on the patient for the first time in 2 years. There was no question the ECG was abnormal. In response, the physician scheduled the patient for an appointment with a cardiologist that afternoon. The cardiologist immediately hospitalized the patient.

Shortly thereafter, the cardiologist performed an angioplasty, which was apparently successful. However, the patient suffered a myocardial infarction in the recovery room and died.

The jury returned a verdict against the family doctor for $505,000. The doctor had tried to blame the cardiologist for not doing a good angioplasty. The jury, however, rejected that argument.

3.5. Infections

Of course, infections are a complication of any surgical procedure and any informed consent paperwork will include this risk. Nevertheless, patients have often sued healthcare providers, alleging malpractice caused a postsurgical infection.

The plaintiff in *Mazurowski v Garrett* [JVR No. 102702, 1990 WL 483965 (Pa.Com.Pl.) Trial date April 1990] had an artificial hip. She underwent an angioplasty.

Shortly thereafter, she began showing signs of an infection at the surgical site. The infection eventually spread to her artificial hip.

The cardiologist who performed the angioplasty was on vacation, but one of his associates ordered a blood culture which came back 4 days later, showing an infection. The physician then ordered antibiotic treatment. The plaintiff had to have her infected artificial hip replaced. The new hip dislocated. As a result, the plaintiff suffered a shortening of her left leg by one-half inch.

The patient's experts contended that the attending doctor fell below the standard of care by failing to prescribe an interim antibiotic pending blood culture results. Had such antibiotics been prescribed earlier, the experts contended that the second hip replacement would have been unnecessary. Though the defense experts disputed these propositions, the defense ultimately settled this case for $300,000.

A $500,000 settlement occurred in *Legg v Atkisson* [JVR No. 138327, 1994 WL 676908 (Unknown State Ct.)] based upon a fulminant infection following an angiography and angioplasty. The patient alleged that there was a delay in diagnosis of the infection. As a result, she suffered permanent vascular damage, permanent femoral nerve impairment, scarring and deformity of the groin and thigh, and permanent limitation of motion.

3.6. Delay in Giving Adrenaline

In one case, the patient's family successfully sued the physician for failing to timely give adrenaline following an allergic reaction to dye [*Estate of Rothstein-Siesser v Lincoln*, JVR No. 188342, 1996 WL 746886 (Md.Cir.Ct.) (Trial date June 1996)]. The plaintiff asserted that waiting 40 minutes to administer adrenaline was excessive and resulted in the patient's death. A jury awarded the plaintiff $275,000.

3.7. Femoral Nerve Damage

Damage to the femoral nerve is undoubtedly a known complication of percutaneous procedures. In *Maynard v George Washington University Hospital*, however, the patient successfully sued and received a major award of $5,000,000 [JVR No. 56588, 1990 WL 458729 (D.C. Super.) (Trial date January 1990)]. There, the plaintiff was a previously disabled individual. She alleged her right femoral nerve was punctured by a needle or sheath and then left in place for a 24-hour period. As a result she contended she lost the ability to walk, except with a walker.

The defendant hospital contended there was never any contact with the nerve and that the patient's problems were due to preexisting conditions. Following the jury award, the parties settled the case for an undisclosed amount. Not all injuries result in awards or settlements, however.

In *Prince v Shawl*, the patient was not so successful [JVR No. 172385, 1995 WL 816459 (Md.Cir.Ct.) (Trial date June 1995)]. The patient was a woman in her 60s who underwent angioplasty. The patient contended that the cardiologist failed to perform the appropriate procedure to remove the catheter, resulting in nerve damage. The cardiologist argued that he used proper technique, that nerve injury was not forseeable, and that any nerve problems the patient had were due to her diabetes. The jury agreed with the defendant doctor and rendered a defense verdict.

3.8. Complications of Anticoagulation

Estate of Peterson v Daniel Freeman Hospital [JVR No. 76532, 1995 WL 816459 (Md.Cir.Ct.) (Trial date June 1995)] concerned a complicated course following angioplasty. The patient suffered a minor heart attack during the procedure, requiring further catheterization. Postprocedure management included anticoagulation for 3 days with heparin. The patient developed a piercing headache. No doctor visited the patient during the evening hours. Hospital staff discovered the patient comatose in the wee hours of the morning. The patient died of a brain bleed.

The family argued that the heparin was excessive and that the doctors failed to react properly to the severe headache. The defendants argued that the case was complicated and that heparin treatment was required. The jury returned a verdict in favor of the defendants. [See also *Yurick v The Cleveland Clinic*, 2001 WL 1043061 (2001)] discussed previously.

3.9. Sexual Abuse Allegations

Claims of sexual abuse are potentially dangerous in any context, but often more so in medicine.

The case of *Piedmont Hospital, Inc. v Palladino* [276 Ga. 612, 580 S.E.2d 215 (2003)] demonstrates that such claims are possible in percutaneous coronary procedures. In this case, Mr. Palladino underwent an angioplasty. A hospital employee was responsible for providing postsurgical treatment to the patient. The employee was authorized to enter the hospital room, check the patient's groin area for any bleeding or complications, clean the area, and, if necessary, to move the patient's testicles in order to perform these tasks.

Mr. Palladino alleged that following his surgery, he awoke to discover the employee rubbing Mr. Palladino's penis with both hands and that the employee's mouth was positioned near Mr. Palladino's penis.

The legal issue in this case was whether the hospital could be liable for the alleged actions of the employee.

The Georgia Supreme Court decided that the hospital should not be liable. Although the employment relationship gave the employee access to the hospital room and the opportunity to commit the tortious acts, the wrongful conduct was well outside the scope of employment.

Despite the ruling of this court, whether an employer is liable for the intentional wrongdoing of the employee is often a question for the jury to decide.

3.10. Radiation Exposure

In a jury trial that took place in May 2000, the issue was whether the defendant doctors had exposed the patient to excessive radiation during angioplasty procedures [*Nicklow v. Anonymous Defendants*, 10 Zarin MLA 3:16, 2000 WL 33739879 (Verdict date May 19, 2000)].

The patient underwent a first angioplasty in October 1996. The cardiologist used X-ray fluoroscopy to visualize the catheter. The procedure lasted 5.5 hours, and the patient was exposed to 172 minutes of fluroscopy. Within 4 weeks of the first procedure, the patient developed a burn on his back which he testified developed into a rash by January 1997.

In February 1997, the patient underwent a second angioplasty. This procedure lasted 3.5 hours, with 68 minutes of fluroscopy exposure. The rash that the plaintiff had earlier suffered developed into an open wound, a radiation burn. The patient had to undergo reconstructive surgery. His doctors testified that he suffered cell damage and was at higher risk for cancer.

The plaintiff contended that the Food and Drug Administration had earlier warned doctors of the dangers of radiation burns in long angioplasty procedures. They alleged that the doctors should have taken precautions against radiation. The plaintiff's experts opined that the plaintiff had received radiation equivalent to 50,000 chest X-rays. The plaintiff also admitted into evidence a study of angioplasties in the 1980s where the maximum fluoroscopy time was 90 minutes.

The defendants countered that the procedures were indeed long and complicated but that they were performed properly. They contended that the patient needed the fluoroscopy for the angioplasties to be done safely. The alternative was bypass surgery, which was more risky. The defense also contended that the patient was already at high risk for cancer due to his smoking two to three packs of cigarettes for more than 50 years.

The jury rendered a verdict for the plaintiff in the amount of $1,000,000. The jury found the first cardiologist 90% negligent and the hospital 10%. The jury exonerated the second cardiologist. In this case, it could well be that the Food and Drug Administration warnings and prior angioplasty studies convinced the jury that this patient received more than the appropriate level of radiation.

4. Strategies to Minimize Malpractice Claims

There is no magic to avoiding malpractice claims. Sometimes, despite the best practices, one will face a claim. At the outset, one must understand that it is difficult for a lawyer to provide anything but the most practical advice regarding this issue. Even lawyers who specialize in malpractice law have only the most superficial knowledge of medicine. It is impossible for a lawyer to tell a doctor how to practice medicine.

Thus, the following advice deals mainly with matters surrounding what the evidence will be in a medical malpractice case.

4.1. Complete, Accurate, and Detailed Medical Records

The best defense in a medical malpractice case is often a complete, detailed, and accurate medical record. The existence of such a record will permit the physician to explain, with credibility, the care that was rendered and the rationale the doctor utilized.

In contrast, a poor medical record with information gaps can severely hamper the defense of a medical malpractice claim. Moreover, credible evidence that the doctor altered the medical record after the fact will destroy the defense, even in an otherwise defensible case.

It seems some doctors pride themselves on cryptic and difficult-to-read notes. Such notes are often harmful in a medical malpractice case. They create ambiguity. Ambiguity means there is room to argue what happened. That is fodder for a malpractice case.

4.2. Complete, Detailed, and Timely Informed Consent

As we have seen, a fair number of cases turned on the informed consent issue. One must obtain a complete, timely, and detailed informed consent. All possible procedures should be listed with specificity. All risks, however, rare, must be stated. The patient must read and sign the informed consent in front of a doctor or nurse before the administration of any mind-altering medication.

Furthermore, if the procedure is not emergent and is preceded by office visits, it is a good idea for the doctor to obtain written informed consent in the office chart before hospitalization. This practice will serve as a backup to any informed consent obtained in the hospital setting.

4.3. The Informal Consult

We have seen that doctors can be held liable even if they never see a patient when they give informal advice to another physician about the second doctor's patient. How can one avoid liability in such a scenario?

At least with cardiologists, the answer may be to avoid giving advice on incomplete information. If a doctor bumps into a cardiologist in the hospital and expresses concern about an ECG, the cardiologist should not advise definitive action without obtaining detailed clinical information.

4.4. Timely Action Based upon Diagnostic Information

Timeliness was the issue in several of the cases discussed above. This appears to be an obvious point, but physicians must act with required speed when the condition requires it. Scheduling difficulties and the shuffling of patients between doctors can often result in undue delay and harm to the patient.

4.5. Adherence to or Knowledge of Current Recommendations

This author has seen numerous cases where doctors have not kept up with recent changes and recommendations by authoritative medical organizations. While there may be good clinical reasons to not follow such recommendations on occasion, their presence must always be weighed in making clinical decisions. Physicians should be well aware of current recommendations, and if they choose not to follow them, they should explain to patients, as best as possible, why this is. Such discussions should be well documented in the record.

The cases described above, where government and devicemaker recommendations were at the core of the case, might have been avoided had the doctors explained to the patients, before the procedures, what the recommendations were, and why the doctor chose to deviate.

If discussing such matters with the patient is not possible, then the doctor should at least document the chart as to why the doctor is deviating from known recommendations. Put simply, a contemporaneous statement of rationale by the doctor carries much more weight than an argument put forth by a lawyer in a subsequent malpractice case.

13
Cardiac Arrest and Resuscitation During Percutaneous Coronary Interventions

Karl B. Kern and Hoang M. Thai

The ultimate percutaneous coronary interventional complication is death. Acute hemodynamic collapse and resultant cardiac arrest is a dramatic pathway, though not always an irreversible pathway, to this dreaded complication.

A 68-year-old male was transported by ambulance to the emergency department with complaints of severe chest pain and shortness of breath. Symptoms began about 4 hours earlier after coming home from work as a night watchman. In the emergency department, a 12-lead electrocardiogram (ECG) revealed ST-segment elevation in leads V2–V4 with inferior ST-segment depression. On physical examination his heart rate was 102 beats per minute (bpm) and blood pressure was 98/60 mm Hg. In addition, a S3 gallop and soft systolic murmur radiating to the left axilla were heard and elevated neck veins with diffuse pulmonary rales were noted.

In the cardiac catheterization laboratory, the patient's chest pain worsened despite the earlier administration of morphine. An intra-aortic balloon pump was placed in the descending aorta via the left femoral artery and coronary angiography revealed a normal right coronary, a total occlusion of the left anterior descending coronary artery (LAD), and a circumflex vessel with a 30% lesion in the proximal segment. After the final angiogram of the left coronary system, the patient developed ventricular fibrillation. One asynchronous shock delivered at 300 J converted the patient back into sinus tachycardia.

A L4 Sherpa guide was then used to provide access to the LAD. After giving the patient 7000 U of unfractionated heparin to achieve an activated clotting time (ACT) of 325 seconds, a High Torque Floppy guidewire was used to cross the proximally occluded LAD. A compliant 3.0-mm. balloon was then used to reopen the LAD using several short inflations. Thrombolysis in myocardial infarction (TIMI) grade 2 flow was re-established and flow improved after intracoronary nitroglycerin and verapamil. A coronary stent was deployed relatively easily and TIMI grade 3 flow was soon restored. Despite this,

the patient's chest pain persisted as did the evidence of cardiogenic shock.

A 12-lead ECG done in the catheterization laboratory revealed only slight improvement in the ST-elevations and 5 minutes following the withdrawal of the guide catheter, the patient suddenly went into ventricular fibrillation again. Two asynchronous shocks at 300 and 360 J were needed to convert the rhythm back into sinus tachycardia. The patient was then intubated, but within 3 minutes following induction a pulse was no longer detected, despite a rhythm of sinus tachycardia on the cardiac monitor. During Advanced Cardiac Life Support for electrical mechanical dissociation, an emergent cardiac echocardiogram revealed a circumferential pericardial effusion. Pericardiocentesis was performed with an initial volume of 120 mL of a bloody effusion withdrawn via the needle and 80 mL was later drained via a pigtail catheter. The patient's hemodynamic status improved and the patient subsequently was stabilized and sent to the intensive care unit. Follow-up echocardiography did not reveal reaccumulation of pericardial fluid and the pigtail drain was pulled 48 hours later. The patient was extubated 72 hours later and was discharged to home 10 days after his initial presentation.

The immediate consequence of cardiac arrest is the cessation of systemic blood flow with resultant unconsciousness and concurrent total body ischemia. In the interventional suite, death can be avoided in many instances of cardiac arrest if circulatory support is provided, followed by the timely accomplishment of definitive treatment. Immediate action is the key to preventing or minimizing any long-term sequelae, particularly to the central nervous system and the myocardium. Irreversible central nervous system (CNS) damage can occur within 7 to 10 minutes from the onset of untreated normothermic, normovolemic cardiac arrest.[1] Such CNS damage need not result if timely supportive and definitive therapy is applied. Reports of patients surviving cardiac arrest with long-term neurologically intact function are well documented.[2–4] The keys for successful long-term neuro-logically intact resuscitation are early recognition, early defibrillation of ventricular fibrillation, early institution of forceful chest compressions with minimal interruptions, and correction of the underlying cause of cardiac arrest. Each of these steps should be imminently more feasible for cardiac arrests occurring in the interventional cardiac laboratory than for those occurring in other locations within the hospital or in the community.

1. Death Associated with Percutaneous Coronary Intervention

The incidence of death associated with percutaneous coronary intervention (PCI) has been widely reported from numerous series and registries to be 0.4%–1.4%.[5–10] This in-hospital death rate is quite consistent among a number of reports and has not changed dramatically over time. Hannan and colleagues reported on perhaps the largest database to date (62,670 percutaneous interventions in New York State between 1991 and 1994) and found an in-hospital mortality rate of 0.9%.[7] Investigators from northern New England reporting on a series of nearly 35,000 interventions performed over a 7-year period (1990–1997) found no change in the in-hospital death rate over time, in spite of a significant improvement in overall clinical outcomes [driven mainly by the decreasing rate of emergency coronary artery bypass graft (CABG)].[10] They noted a death rate of 1.2% in 1990–1993; 1.1% in 1994–6/1995; and 1.1% in 7/1995–1997. King and colleagues compared in-hospital death rates from a National Heart, Lung, and Blood Institute (NHLBI) 1985–1986 registry with that from a second NHLBI 1990–1994 registry in which 45% received intervention with newer devices [directional coronary atherectomy (DCA), transluminal extraction atherectomy (TEC), rotational atherectomy, lasers, and stents

TABLE 13-2. Clinical characteristics associated with in-hospital death with elective percutaneous coronary intervention.

Older age
Female gender
Diabetes
Prior myocardial infarction
Multivessel coronary disease
Left main disease
Poor left ventricular function
Single remaining coronary
Large area of myocardium in jeopardy
Renal dysfunction

(approximately 4% of the total)].[8] No significant difference in in-hospital mortality was found between these two eras (0.7% vs. 0.9%). Table 13-1 summarizes these data.

Such registries have also helped establish who is at greatest risk for in-hospital death, and what complications during acute coronary intervention most often lead to in-hospital mortality (Table 13-2). Those at greatest risk for in-hospital death include the elderly, females, diabetics, those with a prior myocardial infarction (MI), multivessel coronary artery disease (CAD), left main CAD, poor left ventricular function, a large area of myocardium at jeopardy, and preexisting renal dysfunction.[11] Death as a result of PCI is usually associated with an acute coronary occlusion producing profound ischemia and resultant left ventricular failure.[11] Malenka and coworkers of the Northern New England Cardiovascular Study Group found that of 121 patients dying during their acute hospitalizations for PCI, 54% could be directly attributed to a procedural complication.[12] Most deaths occurred after leaving the catheterization laboratory (83%) and were associated with low-output failure. Of those who died in the catheterization suite, 19 of 20 died of hemodynamic collapse. Only one patient died from a refractory arrhythmia.[12]

2. Cardiac Arrest Associated with Percutaneous Coronary Intervention

The incidence of cardiac arrest with or without subsequent death during PCI is much more difficult to ascertain. In an isolated report, Webb and colleagues examined the incidence, correlates, and outcome of cardiac arrest from a PCI database of 4366 patients during 1996–1999.[13] They identified 57 cardiac arrests on the day of the procedure for an overall incidence of 1.3%. Cardiac arrest was defined as cardiovascular collapse requiring cardiopulmonary resuscitation with or without defibrillation. Over half (53%) of the cardiac arrests occurred after leaving the cardiac catheterization suite.

TABLE 13-1. Incidence of death with percutaneous coronary intervention.

Authors	Years	n	In-hospital death
Hannan et al.[5]	1991	5,827	0.6%
Kimmel et al.[6]	1992	10,622	0.4%
	1993	10,030	0.5%
Hannan et al.[7]	1991–1994	62,670	0.9%
King et al.[8]	1985–1986	2,311	1.0%
	1990	1,985	1.8%
O'Connor et al.[9]	1994–1996	15,331	1.1%
McGrath et al.[10]	1990–1993	13,014	1.2%
	1994–1995	7,248	1.1%
	1995–1997	14,490	1.1%
Overall		1,279/137,701	0.9%

TABLE 13-3. Major percutaneous coronary intervention complications associated with cardiac arrest.[13]

Significant side-branch occlusion
No-reflow
Stent thrombosis
Perforation with cardiac tamponade

Among those experiencing cardiac arrest during PCI, a wide variety of initial arrhythmias were found. The majority were tachyarrhythmias, including ventricular fibrillation (36%) and ventricular tachycardia (28%), but a substantial number had bradycardia (24%) or asystole (2%) as their initial cardiac arrest arrhythmia. The majority of cardiac arrests occurred after the initial balloon inflation (60%), with a few after the initial injection of radiographic contrast (12%) and a few others after the deployment of a stent (12%). Intraprocedural complications most often associated with subsequent cardiac arrest were significant side-branch occlusion, no-reflow, stent thrombosis, and perforation with cardiac tamponade (Table 13-3). No particular culprit vessel predominated, with the right coronary artery involved in 46%, the LAD in 44%, and the circumflex in 25% (total percentages exceed 100% due to multivessel disease). Clinical predictors of cardiac arrest were emergent PCI, PCI for acute myocardial infarction, and PCI for cardiogenic shock. Indeed, of the recorded cardiac arrests, 72% were associated with patients presenting with an acute myocardial infarction and 60% with patients presenting with cardiogenic shock. Cardiac arrest was uncommon in stable, elective patients undergoing coronary intervention (only 1 of the 57 cases of cardiac arrest). Cardiac arrest associated with PCI was certainly not benign, with a 24-hour mortality rate of 63%. Predictors of death after cardiac arrest were no-reflow ($P < 0.001$), age ($P < 0.006$), intraprocedural cardiac arrest ($P < 0.05$), side-branch occlusion ($P < 0.05$), and shock ($P < 0.05$). Others have noted that tamponade from PCI resulting in cardiac collapse or arrest is likewise associated with a mortality rate of 40%.[14]

3. Prevention of Cardiac Arrest During Percutaneous Coronary Intervention

Prevention of cardiac arrest is obviously preferable to the chaotic scene surrounding emergent cardiopulmonary resuscitation efforts being performed in the PCI suite. General principles of the preinterventional thought process of weighing benefits against risks cannot be overemphasized in this regard. Understanding the typical precedent events leading to acute cardiac collapse and cardiac arrest with PCI allows one to consider appropriate preparations to avoid such scenarios. Obviously, one cannot change the patients' clinical presentation, that is, acute MI with cardiogenic shock, but knowing that such is more likely to result in cardiac arrest can lead to certain preparations that could make a crucial difference if it does occur. Readily available defibrillators, pacing equipment, and circulatory support systems such as intra-aortic balloon counterpulsation or percutaneous cardiopulmonary bypass, should be considered before cardiac arrest occurs.

4. Treatment of Cardiac Arrest During Percutaneous Coronary Intervention

Cardiac arrest during PCI can and should be treated according to the underlying cause and etiology. Though initial evaluation cannot always provide the definitive approach, several different scenarios can quickly be distinguished, allowing more specific treatments to be done.

4.1. Acute Hemodynamic Collapse

Sudden loss of circulatory support with subsequent hypotension can result from profound vasodilatation (vasovagal), anaphylaxis, medication overdose, acute arrhythmias (both fast and slow), overwhelming myocardial ischemia from abrupt closure of a coronary or no-reflow phenomenon, cardiac tamponade, or extensive, ongoing bleeding. Treating the underlying cause is paramount and when done in a timely fashion can prevent a spiraling downward course leading to cardiac arrest. An organized approach to sudden hypotension during PCI can be invaluable in such stressful moments (Table 13-4).

TABLE 13-4. Approach to the hypotensive patient during percutaneous coronary intervention.

1. Ensure that the guide catheter is removed from the coronary ostium and that the system is airtight (the Y connector is tightened down)
2. Administer fluids*
3. Raise legs
4. Reverse any potentially offending medications
5. Administer a vasoconstrictive medication
   a. Phenylephrine 100 mcg bolus or >10 mcg/min infusion (max. 200 mcg/min)
   OR
   b. Epinephrine 1–10 mcg/min infusion (max. 200 mcg/min) or for suspected anaphylaxis 0.1 mg of the 1:10,000 solution)
   OR
   c. Dopamine 5–20 mcg/kg/min infusion
6. Support the rate
   a. Cardiovert for fast tachyarrhythmias
   b. Pacing for significant bradycardia if unresponsive to atropine (1 mg)
7. Search for specific cause and treat accordingly

* Volume can be administered both intravenously and intra-arterially (hand-delivered boluses through the arterial sheath) simultaneously.

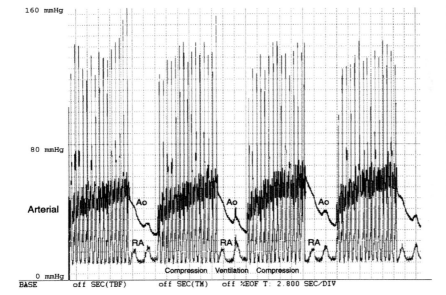

FIGURE 13-4. Aortic and right atrial pressures during standard (15:2) CPR. Coronary perfusion pressure during CPR is defined as the pressure gradient between the aortic diastolic (decompression) pressures (darkened line is the AoD) and right atrial diastolic pressure (the lowest pressure illustrated). Note with each ventilatory interruption of chest compressions the aortic diastolic pressure falls and must be rebuilt to achieve its maximal level during the next cycle of chest compressions. Maximal coronary perfusion pressure is present only a third of each complete 15:2 cycle. (Reprinted from Kern et al.[30] Copyright 1998, with permission of Elevier.)

chest compressions are interrupted coronary perfusion pressure falls and then must be rebuilt, usually requiring 5 to 10 compressions/decompressions to achieve the previous level.[30–31] Figure 13-4 illustrates that even with ideal ventilation (taking only 4s to deliver the two breaths), the resultant chest compression interruption results in maximal coronary perfusion pressure only one-third of the time during the resuscitation effort.

The use of vasoconstrictive medications (i.e., epinephrine as 1mg IV bolus every 3–5min) during cardiopulmonary resuscitation can dramatically increase the coronary perfusion pressure.[32] Epinephrine causes peripheral vasoconstriction of the small arterioles, thereby raising central aortic pressure, particularly during the diastolic or relaxation phase of rhythmic chest compressions/decompressions. Figure 13-5 shows this increase of coronary perfusion pressure during CPR following the intravenous administration of 1mg of epinephrine. High-dose epinephrine during cardiopulmonary resuscitation is no longer recommended for routine use.[32] Epinephrine administered during CPR can result in significant hypertension and potential myocardial ischemia if the resuscitation is successful. Nonetheless, during cardiac arrest the first and foremost goal must be resuscitation, and improving coronary perfusion pressure can be crucial to successful resuscitation.

Vasopressin (40U IV bolus) has been recommended as a potential alternative to epinephrine during ventricular fibrillation cardiac arrest.[32] Because vasopressin is not an adrenergic agonist but works through specific vasopressin receptors that are neither inotropic nor chronotrophic, the postresuscitation period may be less difficult in the

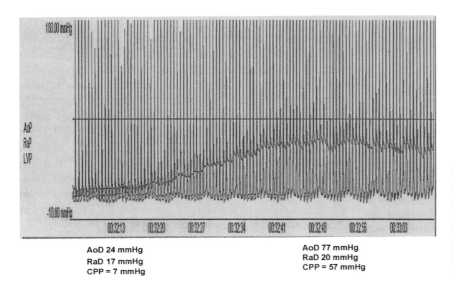

FIGURE 13-5. Epinephrine and coronary perfusion pressure during CPR. Epinephrine administration (at 00:32:13) results in a marked increase in aortic diastolic pressure, with little effect on right atrial diastolic pressure during CPR. The result is an increase in coronary perfusion pressure during the resuscitation.

PCI patient, but specific data are still lacking. Due to vasopressin's longer half-life, a single bolus is recommended. Due to the lack of data for multiple doses of vasopressin during cardiac arrest, if additional vasoconstrictive support is needed after the initial administration of vasopressin, epinephrine should then be used.

Additional drug therapy should be considered if, after several minutes of chest compressions, repeated attempts at defibrillation fail. Two prospective, randomized, double-blind clinical trials have now shown that amiodarone administered during ongoing chest compressions for refractory ventricular fibrillation cardiac arrest can improve defibrillation success and short-term survival.[33,34] Both trials administered amiodarone as a 300 to 350 mg bolus IV (over 20–30 s) during the performance of chest compressions for refractory ventricular fibrillation cardiac arrest. The mean relative improvement in short-term survival for these two studies was over 50%. Use of aminodarone during CPR is unfortunately not easy secondary to several limitations. Current formulations come only as 150-mg vials requiring two vials (glass) to be broken and the solutions mixed into one syringe. The available formulation is not water soluble, and comes combined with Tween-80, a diluent to keep the drug in solution. This additive can foam if agitated, hence care must be given in preparing the syringe and in its administration. Intravenous boluses of amiodarone can result in hypotension and bradycardia. Experimental work has shown that concurrent administration with epinephrine is feasible and prevents any adverse effect on CPR-generated coronary perfusion pressure.[35] Attention postresuscitation must be given to treat any persistent symptomatic bradycardia or hypotension.

A unique form of CPR, cough CPR, was first described in treating VF cardiac arrest (VFCA) in the angiographic suite.[36] Rhythmic coughing every 1 to 3 seconds upon the recognition of ventricular fibrillation and prior to unconsciousness produced systolic aortic pressures of 140 ± 4 mmHg and preserved consciousness for up to 40 seconds in some patients. This technique can be successfully used to maintain cerebral perfusion during VF until the defibrillation equipment is readied and applied. Our experience suggests that instructing the patient to stop coughing once the defibrillator is charged and paddles are ready for application results in rapid loss of consciousness and thereby avoids delivering a shock to an awake patient, while still providing excellent CNS support until the very moment of defibrillation. We have noted the avoidance of any grand mal seizure activity prior to defibrillation with this approach in several patients suffering VF during PCI. A second advantage of this approach is the avoidance of any trauma to recently placed intracoronary stents. Though not common, case reports of stent compression occurring with chest compressions during CPR have been published.[37,38] Proximal LAD stents appear to be the most vulnerable to mechanical compression from standard anterior–posterior chest compressions during cardiopulmonary resuscitation.[37,38]

4.5. Fixing the Cause of Cardiac Arrest

Throughout the ongoing efforts at treating the cardiac arrest, paramount is consideration and treatment of the underlying cause. Though often difficult to do both perform quality cardiopulmonary resuscitation and complete a PCI, the very opportunity and ability to do so makes cardiac arrest in the PCI suite unique. Such procedures are more likely to be successful in the PCI suite than in any other location in or out of the hospital. If a catastrophic left main dissection and occlusion occurred it must be successfully crossed and reopened if long-term resuscitation success is to be accomplished. Similarly, if abrupt occlusion of another vessel, or profound no-reflow to the remaining viable myocardium led to the ventricular fibrillation cardiac arrest, they must be reversed while ongoing resuscitation efforts continue. Injection of a calcium channel antagonist into a culprit vessel with no-reflow or recannulating and tacking up an occlusive dissection may be challenging during chest compressions, but it can and has been done successfully. Remember: the less that chest compressions are interrupted the better the myocardial perfusion, but if the vessel is occluded or the microcirculation essentially nonfunctional, these must be successfully treated or all the CPR-generated coronary perfusion pressure will not result in any meaningful myocardial perfusion.

4.6. Intra-Aortic Balloon Counterpulsation During Cardiac Arrest

The role of counterpulsation during actual cardiac arrest is limited, particularly because there is no consistent pressure wave or electrocardiographic signal to coordinate the auxiliary pumping. Experimental reports have highlighted the usefulness of ascending or high descending aortic occlusion during chest compressions to enhance blood flow to the CNS and the myocardium during CPR.[39,40] Hence, if an aortic balloon is in place, inflation with maintenance of constant inflation in the thoracic aorta could be of some value. Postresuscitation may be an ideal time to consider the use of intra-aortic counterpulsation for support of stunned ventricular function (see Postresuscitation Care).

4.7. Percutaneous Cardiopulmonary Bypass During Refractory Cardiac Arrest

Because cardiac arrest during PCI is generally associated with a remediable underlying cause in a location where invasive options are readily available, the use of ultimate circulatory support, percutaneous cardiopulmonary bypass (PCPB), for refractory cardiac arrest has been espoused. Several small series of using PCPB in such cases have been reported.[41-44] Shawl reported on 3 patients with abrupt closure post–coronary angioplasty who failed to respond to standard ACLS therapy.[41] Percutaneous cardiopulmonary bypass was begun emergently after 10 to 25 minutes of unsuccessful cardiopulmonary resuscitation effort. A mean aortic pressure of 92 mmHg and an average of 4.8 L/min flow was achieved. All three survived after undergoing revascularization following stabilization with PCPB. Overlie reported 10 patients with cardiac arrest in the PCI suite after failed PTCA.[42] Five of 10 survived long-term. Mooney reported the use of emergent CPB support in 5 patients in whom cardiac arrest resulted as a complication of PCI.[43] All were successfully stabilized, subsequently underwent successful revascularization, and survived. Redle and colleagues reported on 8 additional patients treated with PCPB after developing refractory hemodynamic collapse with PTCA.[44] Five of eight survived to hospital discharge. A summation of this experience shows both the feasibility of such therapy, and also a long-term survival rate of 69% (18/26). Early institution after failed initial CPR is vital. All successfully treated long-term survivors were successfully revascularized postresuscitation, again emphasizing the importance of a reversible and remediable cause of the underlying cardiovascular collapse and cardiac arrest.

4.8. Technique for Using Percutaneous Cardiopulmonary Bypass in the Percutaneous Coronary Intervention Suite for Refactory Cardiac Arrest

Some knowledge of the insertion and removal techniques warrants attention.[45] The usual site has been the left femoral artery and vein. The venous cannula is large, hence progressive dilatation with 8F, 12F, and 14F is recommended as is the use of a stiff 0.038-inch J guidewire to guide the sheath and dilator into the right atrium. Tension on the guidewire can facilitate passage to the right atrium. Pressure should be externally applied to the abdomen at the time of removal of the inner dilator to create positive venous pressure and avoid incoming air. The sheath is then clamped with the attached line clamp. The arterial sheath is inserted in a similar fashion including progressive dilatations. Air is purged through a side port and the sheath clamped. Heparin should be given (300 U/kg) with an ACT goal of more than 400 seconds.

During the operation of the PCPB system, 4 to 5 L/min flow with a nonpulsatile mean arterial pressure of 70 to 100 mmHg should be obtainable. Significant vasodilata-

tion can result from the nonpulsatile flow and volume replacement, or vasoconstricting medications may be required. No left ventricular venting occurs with this system (as opposed to standard CPB in the operating room), hence left ventricular distension can occur and must be considered if long runs of PCPB are anticipated.

Potential complications include air embolism, vascular trauma, bleeding, and anemia (large blood volume can be lost with the priming of the system). It cannot be overemphasized that PCPB is a temporizing therapy to stabilize until definitive revascularization therapy can be accomplished. Mortality approaches 100% when no definitive revascularization can be accomplished.

5. Non–Ventricular Fibrillation Cardiac Arrest

5.1. Brady–Asystole or Pulseless Electrical Activity

The most important initial therapy for brady–asystole or pulseless electrical activity (PEA) cardiac arrest is to provide myocardial perfusion through the generation of optimal coronary perfusion pressure. The same principles apply as to VF cardiac arrest. Uninterrupted or minimally interrupted chest compressions are crucial in this regard. Epinephrine or vasopressin should be considered early and the need for additional doses determined by following the aortic pressure generated with cardiopulmonary resuscitation. Because no other timely therapy (such as defibrillation) is helpful, sustained perfusion is the only real option, and cough CPR is not a viable option for these patients.

Identifying the underlying etiology of brady–asystolic or PEA arrest is critical. Some treatable causes can occur with PCI. It is important to consider tamponade early in the differential diagnosis. Tamponade is an uncommon complication associated with perforations during PCI, but has been reported to be increased with the use of newer atheroablative therapies.[46] A review of the William Beaumont Hospital PCI database found 31 cases of tamponade after 25,697 PCI procedures for an incidence of just over 0.1%.[47] A little over half were diagnosed in the PCI suite, while 45% were diagnosed after leaving the laboratory, approximately 4 to 5 hours later. All the acute cases were documented to have occurred after coronary perforation. The majority had substantially large pericardial effusions by echocardiography, and 19 of 30 were successfully treated with pericardiocentesis alone. However, the other 40% required surgical intervention. Tamponade from perforation during PCI was associated with a significant mortality (60% for those recognized in the PCI suite) and morbidity. In spite of pericardiocentesis, volume therapy, reversal of anticoagulant therapy, and inotropic support when needed, the mortality of this complication can be high. Other series suggest a more benign course, but such have typically not confined their cases to post-PCI complications.[48] In the PCI suite where cardiac arrest has occurred, the prudent course seems to perform cardiopulmonary resuscitation aggressively until ready for emergent pericardiocentesis, at which time chest compression must stop and the pericardiocentesis be performed. Once safe, that is, once the needle is removed from the thorax, then chest compressions may be critical again to assist the return of myocardial mechanical function.

Another possible cause of non–ventricular fibrillation in the PCI suite is profound volume loss (Table 13-4). Occult bleeding especially in the well-anticoagulated patient receiving multiple antiplatelet therapies can be another potentially reversible cause of non-VF cardiac arrest in the PCI suite. Always consider the possibility of retroperitoneal or other bleeding.

6. Postresuscitation Care

Restoration of a self-sustained pulse and blood pressure is a very welcome event following cardiac arrest during PCI coronary intervention. But after a sigh of relief, remember the job is not yet done. Resuscitation does not necessarily translate into long-term survival for the majority of those successfully resuscitated. A series of reports for out-of-hospital cardiac arrest suggests that over 66% of all initially resuscitated victims of sudden cardiac death succumb postresuscitation during their hospital stay.[49–51] No data exists on the postresuscitation period for those surviving cardiac arrest in the PCI suite, but general principles learned from out-of-hospital cardiac arrest probably pertain to this population as well. Central nervous system damage and postresuscitation myocardial failure account for about two-thirds of all postresuscitation deaths. After years of failure, two recent randomized clinical trials suggest that mild hypothermia after resuscitation can improve neurological outcome.[52,53] Similarly, there is now good experimental and clinical data to suggest that global myocardial stunning occurs after cardiac arrest[54–56] and can be treated, once recognized or anticipated, with dobutamine support[57] or perhaps intra-aortic balloon counterpulsation.[58] Timely consideration of both these therapies for the successfully resuscitated victims of cardiac arrest during PCI may further improve long-term outcomes.

7. Summary

Cardiac arrest in the PCI suite is an uncommon but very dramatic event. Such occurrences are almost always precipitated by a complication of the intervention itself, usually in a very high-risk clinical setting. Nevertheless, a timely, methodical approach to both immediate application of cardiopulmonary resuscitation techniques while searching for and treating the underlying cause can save lives. The very location and circumstances surrounding cardiac arrest in the PCI suite provide important advantages for successful resuscitation, especially the ability to monitor aortic pressure during chest compressions (the indirect gauge of coronary perfusion pressure). Hemodynamic feedback during the performance of chest compressions is invaluable for optimizing the resuscitation and successful outcome. Opportunities for correcting the underlying cause of cardiac arrest and for aggressive institution of total circulatory support (PCPB) exist in the PCI suite, while they are rarely feasible for cardiac arrest victims elsewhere.

References

1. Bass E. Cardiopulmonary arrest: pathophysiology and neurologic complications. Ann Intern Med. 1985;103:920–927.
2. Earnest MP, Yarnell PR, Merrill SL, et al. Long-term survival and neurologic status after resuscitation from out-of-hospital cardiac arrest. Neurology. 1980;30:1298–1302.
3. Longstreth WT, Inui TS, Cobb LA, et al. Neurologic recovery after out-of-hospital cardiac arrest. Ann Intern Med. 1983;98:588–592.
4. Bedell SE, Delbanco TL, Cook EF, et al. Survival after cardiopulmonary resuscitation in the hospital. N Engl J Med. 1983;309:569–576.
5. Hannan EL, Arani DT, Johnson LW, et al. Percutaneous transluminal coronary angioplasty in New York State. Risk factors and outcome. JAMA. 1992;268:3092–3097.
6. Kimmel SE, Berlin JA, Strom BL, et al. Development and validation of a simplified predictive index for major complications in contemporary percutaneous transluminal coronary angioplasty practice. J Am Coll Cardiol. 1995;26:931–938.
7. Hannan EL, Racz M, Ryan TJ, et al. Coronary angioplasty volume-outcome relationships for hospitals and cardiologists. JAMA. 1997;277:892–898.
8. King SB, Yeh W, Holumkov R, et al. Balloon angioplasty versus new device intervention: clinical outcomes. J Am Coll Cardiol. 1998;31:558–566.
9. O'Connor GT, Malenka DJ, Quinton H, et al. Multivariate prediction of in-hospital mortality after percutaneous coronary interventions in 1994–1996. J Am Coll Cardiol. 1999;34:681–691.
10. McGrath PD, Malenka DJ, Wennberg DE, et al. Changing outcomes in percutaneous coronary interventions. J Am Coll Cardiol. 1999;34:674–680.
11. Smith SC Jr, Dove JT, Jacobs AK, et al. ACC/AHA guidelines for percutaneous coronary intervention: a report of the American College of Cardiology/American Heart Association Task Force on Practice Guidelines (Committee to revise the 1993 Guidelines for Percutaneous Transluminal Coronary Angioplasty). J Am Coll Cardiol. 2001;37:2239i–lxvi.

12. Malenka DJ, O'Rourke D, Millar MA, et al. Cause of in-hospital death in 12,232 consecutive patients undergoing percutaneous transluminal coronary angioplasty. Am Heart J. 1999;137:632–638.

13. Webb JG, Solankhi NK, Chugh SK, et al. Incidence, correlates, and outcomes of cardiac arrest associated with percutaneous coronary intervention. Am J Cardiol. 2002;90:1252–1254.

14. Fejka M, Kahn JK. Diagnosis, management, and clinical outcome of cardiac tamponade complicationg percutaneous coronary intervention. Cardiovasc Rev Rep. 2003;24:416–420.

15. Weisfeldt ML, Becker LB. Resuscitation after cardiac arrest: a 3-phase time-sensitive model. JAMA. 2002;288:3035–3038.

16. American Heart Association in collaboration with the International Liaison Committee on Resuscitation. Guidelines 2000 for Cardiopulmonary Resuscitation and Emergency Cardiovascular Care: International Consensus on Science, Part 6 Advanced Cardiovascular Life Support. Circulation. 2000;102(suppl 1):I-90–I-94.

17. Ewy GA, Taren D. Relative impedance of gels to defibrillator discharge. Med Instrum. 1979;13;295–296.

18. Pagan-Carlo LA, Spencer KT, Robertson CE, et al. Transthoracic defibrillation: importance of avoiding electrode placement directly on the female breast. J Am Coll Cardiol. 1996;27:449–452.

19. Schneider T, Martens PR, Paschen H, et al. Multicenter, randomized, controlled trial of 150-J biphasic shocks compared with 200- to 300-J monophasic shocks in the resuscitation of out-of-hospital cardiac arrest victims. Circulation. 2000;102:1780–1787.

20. Assar D, Chamberlain D, Colquhoun M, et al. Randomized controlled trials of staged teaching for basic life support: skill acquisition at the bronze level. Resuscitation. 2000;45:7–15.

21. Heidenreich JW, Higdon TA, Sanders AB, et al. Chest compression performance is better with chest compression-only than standard CPR. Circulation. 2002;106(suppl II):II663–II664.

22. Kern KB. Limiting interruptions of chest compressions during cardiopulmonary resuscitation. Resuscitation. 2003;58:273–274.

23. Ralston SH, Voorhees WD, Babbs CF. Intrapulmonary epinephrine during prolonged cardiopulmonary resuscitation: improved regional blood flow and resuscitation in dogs. Ann Emerg Med. 1984;13:79–86.

24. Michael JR, Guerci AD, Koehler RC, et al. Mechanism by which epinephrine augments cerebral and myocardial perfusion during cardiopulmonary resuscitation in dogs. Circulation. 1984;69:822–835.

25. Halperin HR, Tsitlik JE, Gueric AD, et al. Determinants of blood flow to vital organs during cardiopulmonary resuscitation in dogs. Circulation. 1986;73:539–550.

26. Kern KB, Lancaster LD, Goldman S, et al. The effect of coronary artery lesions on the relationship between coronary perfusion pressure and myocardial flow during cardiopulmonary resuscitation. Am Heart J. 1990;120:324–333.

27. Kern KB, Ewy GA, Voorhees WD, et al. Myocardial perfusion pressure: a predictor of 24-hour survival during prolonged cardiac arrest in dogs. Resuscitation. 1988;16:241–250.

28. Kern KB, Hilwig RW, Ewy GA. Retrograde coronary blood flow during cardiopulmonary resuscitation in swine: intracoronary Doppler evaluation. Am Heart J. 1994;128:490–499.

29. Pierpont GL, Kruse JA, Nelson DH. Intra-arterial monitoring during cardiopulmonary resuscitation. Catheter Cardiovasc Diagn. 1985;11:513–520.

30. Kern KB, Hilwig RW, Berg RA, et al. Efficacy of chest compression-only BLS CPR in the presence of an occluded airway. Resuscitation. 1998;39:179–188.

31. Berg RA, Sanders AB, Kern KB, et al. Adverse hemodynamic effects of interrupting chest compressions for rescue breathing during CPR for ventricular fibrillation cardiac arrest. Circulation. 2001;104:2465–2470.

32. American Heart Association in collaboration with the International Liaison Committee on Resuscitation. Guidelines 2000 for Cardiopulmonary Resuscitation and Emergency Cardiovascular Care: International Consensus on Science, Part 6 Advanced Cardiovascular Life Support. Circulation. 2000;102(suppl 1):I-129–I-135.

33. Kudenchuk PJ, Cobb LA, Copass MK, et al. Amiodarone for resuscitation after out-of-hospital cardiac arrest due to ventricular fibrillation. N Engl J Med. 1999;341:871–878.

34. Dorian P, Cass D, Schwartz B, et al. Amiodarone as compared to lidocaine for shock-resistant ventricular fibrillation. N Engl J Med. 2002;346:884–890.

35. Paiva EF, Perondi MBM, Kern KB, et al. Effect of intravenous amiodarone on CPR hemodynamics—an experimental study in a canine model of resistant VF. Resuscitation. 2003;58:203–208.

36. Criley JM, Blaufuss AH, Kissel GL. Cough-induced cardiac compression. Self-administered form of cardiopulmonary resuscitation. JAMA. 1976;236:1246–1250.

37. Vogtmann T, Volmar J, Kronsbein H, et al. Deformation of a coronary stent as a sequel of resuscitation. Z Kardiol. 1999;88:296–299.

38. Windecker S, Maier W, Eberli FR, et al. Mechanical compression of coronary stents: potential hazard for patients undergoing cardiopulmonary resuscitation. Catheter Cardiovasc Interv. 2000;51:464–467.

39. Paradis NA, Rose MI, Garwrl MS. Selective aortic perfusion and oxygenation: an effective adjunct to external chest compression-based cardiopulmonary resuscitation. J Am Coll Cardiol. 1994;23:497–504.

40. Tang W, Weil MH, Noc M, et al. Augmented efficacy of external CPR by intermittent occlusion of the ascending aorta. Circulation. 1993;88:1916–1921.

41. Shawl FA, Domanski MJ, Wish MH, et al. Emergency cardiopulmonary bypass support in patients with cardiac arrest in the catheterization laboratory. Catheter Cardiovasc Diagn. 1990;19:8–12.

42. Overlie PA. Emergency use of portable cardiopulmonary bypass. Catheter Cardiovasc Diagn. 1990;20:27–31.

43. Mooney MR, Arom KV, Joyce LD, et al. Emergency cardiopulmonary bypass support in patients with cardiac arrest. J Thorac Cardiovasc Surg. 1991;101:450–454.

44. Redle J, King B, Lemoe G, et al. Utility of rapid percutaneous cardiopulmonary bypass for refractory hemody-

namic collapse in the cardiac catheterization laboratory. Am J Cardiol. 1994;73:899–900.

45. Tommaso CL. Use of percutaneously inserted cardiopulmonary bypass in the cardiac catheterization laboratory. Catheter Cardiovasc Diagn. 1990;20:32–38.

46. Ellis SG, Ajluni SC, Arnold AZ, et al. Increased coronary perforation in the new device era: incidence, classification, management, and outcome. Circulation. 1994;90: 2725–2730.

47. Fejka M, Dixon SR, Safian RD, et al. Diagnosis, management, and clinical outcome of cardiac tamponade complicating percutaneous coronary intervention. Am J Cardiol. 2002;90:1183–1186.

48. Von Sohsten R, Kopistansky C, Cohen M, et al. Cardiac tamponade in the "new device" era: evaluation of 6,999 consecutive percutaneous coronary interventions. Am Heart J. 2000;140:279–283.

49. Schoenenberger RA, von Planta M, von Planta I. Survival after failed out-of-hospital resuscitation. Arch Intern Med. 1994;154:2433–2437.

50. Brain Resuscitation Clinical Trial I Study Group. A randomized clinical study of thiopental loading in comatose survivors of cardiac arrest. N Engl J Med. 1986;314: 397–403.

51. Brain Resuscitation Clinical Trial II Study Group. A randomized clinical study of a calcium-entry blocker (lidoflazine) in the treatment of comatose survivors of cardiac arrest. N Engl J Med. 1991;324:1125–1131.

52. The Hypothermia after Cardiac Arrest Study Group. Mild therapeutic hypothermia to improve the neurologic outcome after cardiac arrest. N Engl J Med. 2002;346: 549–556.

53. Bernard SA, Gray TW, Buist MD, et al. Treatment of comatose survivors of out-of-hospital cardiac arrest with induced hypothermia. N Engl J Med. 2002;346:557–563.

54. Kern KB, Hilwig RW, Rhee KH, et al. Myocardial dysfunction following resuscitation from cardiac arrest: an example of global myocardial stunning. J Am Coll Cardiol. 1996;28:232–240.

55. Tang W, Weil MH, Sun S, et al. Progressive myocardial dysfunction after cardiac resuscitation. Crit Care Med. 1993;21:1046–1050.

56. Gazmuri RJ, Weil MH, Bisera J, et al. Myocardial dysfunction after successful resuscitation from cardiac arrest. Crit Care Med. 1996;24:992–1000.

57. Kern KB, Hilwig RW, Berg RA, et al. Post resuscitation left ventricular systolic and diastolic dysfunction: treatment with dobutamine. Circulation. 1997;95:2610–2613.

58. Tennyson H, Kern KB, Berg RA, et al. Treatment options for post resuscitation myocardial failure: intraaortic counterpulsation versus dobutamine. Resuscitation. 2002;54: 69–75.

14
Adverse Event Reporting: Physicians, Manufacturers, and the Food and Drug Administration

Eva B. Manus

1. A Serious Injury Report

Stent deployment was attempted on a stenosis in the left circumflex artery. However, the stent would not cross the lesion. During withdrawal of the device from the left coronary system, the stent separated from the delivery system at the bifurcation of the circumflex and the left main artery. Attempts to remove the stent were unsuccessful and the patient was sent for emergent cardiac surgery.[1] The sales representative for the device was notified of the event and the details of the procedure were forwarded to the manufacturer. The Food and Drug Administration (FDA) subsequently received a report that a serious patient injury occurred during the use of the device (Figure 14-1). The stent delivery system was not returned to the manufacturer for investigation.

Unforeseen and unfavorable events will inevitably occur during some interventional procedures. Some of the potential complications that arise may or may not be related to a device failure or malfunction. This chapter presents some typical problems that may be encountered with the most common interventional devices, focusing on what role the various levels of healthcare providers, manufacturers, and the FDA play in this process.

In the United States, the FDA regulates and monitors the safety and efficacy of medical devices. Manufacturers are required by law to monitor the performance of their products and report incidents to the FDA in which a serious injury or death occurred during their use, or which may have posed a health or safety risk to the patient.[2] Significant fines have been imposed on medical device companies for failure to report adverse events within strict deadlines mandated by the FDA. Corporations are at risk of having certain products removed from the market or even being shut down temporarily or permanently. Consequently, remaining in compliance with FDA regulations is a priority for all medical device manufacturers.

2. MedWatch

The Center for Devices and Radiological Health (CDRH) division of the FDA developed and implemented MedWatch, the FDA Safety Information and Adverse Event Reporting Program.

MedWatch is the system that is used by device manufacturers and user facility risk management personnel to report device-related adverse events for early detection and correction of product problems. Access to the MedWatch reporting system is also available to healthcare professionals and consumers directly through the FDA or their website (http://www.fda.gov) along with definitions and detailed instructions for correctly interpreting and completing the form (Figure 14-2).

A collective database of reportable adverse events and malfunctions has been established, also accessible through the FDA website (http://www.fda.gov/cdrh/maude.html) that is available for review as a matter of public record. The Manufacturer and User Facility Device Experience Database (MAUDE) from manufacturer's reports goes back as far as August 1996. An online search can be performed for deaths, injuries, and malfunctions related to specific products from all medical device companies. Once again, many physicians, as well as consumers, do not know that this database is readily available and user friendly. It is a valuable tool for tracking device failures and the situations that caused them (Figure 14-3).

3. Device Expectations

The manufacture and marketing of devices for coronary interventions is a complex process. By the time the finished product reaches the customer, it has developed from various plastics and metals into a highly sophisticated tool, neatly packaged in an attractive, often color-

Adverse Event Report

MEDTRONIC AVE, INC. MEDTRONIC AVE S7 OTW OTW CORONARY STENT SYSTEM

back to search results

Issue Unknown (for use when the patient's condition is not known)

Manufacturer Response

Eval, results: "other-lack of info": unknown details of how the stent dislodged and lesion morphology. "failure to follow instructions": for removal of undeployed stent. "inherent risk of procedure": dislodgement listed in ifu. Eval, conclusion: "other-lack of inherent": unknown details of how the stent dislodged and lesion morphology. The returned goods investigation revealed the stent delivery catheter was separate from the stent. The stent was damaged and was returned attached to a snare device. All stent welds and segments were accounted for. The delivery balloon had adequate evidence to indicate the stent had been correctly mounted.

Problem Description

A 3. 5mm diameter by 24mm length s7 stent delivery system was inserted for treatment of a proximal lesion in the right coronary artery. The incident occurred in 2002. Despite repeated attempts to obtain further info from the user facility, no info is available. It is reported that the instructions for use may have not been followed for removal of an undeployed stent. There is no additional info from the user facility regarding this event.

Search Alerts/Recalls

new search | submit an adverse event report

Brand Name	MEDTRONIC AVE S7 OTW
Type of Device	OTW CORONARY STENT SYSTEM
Baseline Brand Name	MEDTRONIC AVE S7 WITH DISCRETE TECHNOLOGY OVER-THE-WIRE CORONARY STENT SYSTEM
Baseline Generic Name	OTW CORONARY STENT SYSTEM
Baseline Catalogue Number	S73524W
Baseline Device Family	NA
Baseline Device PMA Number	P970035
Baseline Shelf Life Information	Yes
Is Baseline 510(K) Number Provided?	No
Baseline Preamendment?	No
Transitional?	No
510(K) Exempt?	No

Shelf Life(Months)	12
Date First Marketed	04/05/2001
Manufacturer (Section F)	MEDTRONIC AVE, INC. 3576 Unocal Pl. Santa Rosa CA 95403
Manufacturer (Section D)	MEDTRONIC AVE, INC. 3576 Unocal Pl. Santa Rosa CA 95403
Manufacturer Contact	Nick Parker, Manager 3576 Unocal Place Santa Rosa , CA 95403 (707) 591 -7094
Device Event Key	419090
MDR Report Key	430101
Event Key	406899
Report Number	2953200-2002-00052
Device Sequence Number	1
Product Code	MAF
Report Source	Manufacturer
Source Type	Health Professional,Company Representative
Event Type	Injury
Type of Report	Initial
Report Date	10/29/2002
1 Device Was Involved in the Event	
1 Patient Was Involved in the Event	
Date FDA Received	11/27/2002
Is This An Adverse Event Report?	Yes
Is This A Product Problem Report?	Yes
Device Operator	Health Professional
Device EXPIRATION Date	08/28/2003
Device Catalogue Number	S73524W
Device LOT Number	1H18E02
Was Device Available For Evaluation?	Device Not Returned To Manufacturer
Date Returned to Manufacturer	10/22/2002
Is The Reporter A Health Professional?	Yes
Was the Report Sent to FDA?	No
Date Manufacturer Received	10/29/2002
Was Device Evaluated	

FIGURE 14-1. This is a typical adverse event report that can be found on the Manufacturer and User Facility Device Experience Search (MAUDE) website. See text for description.

ful box with an intriguing name displayed on the label. It has been factory sealed on the outside, a second pouch is sealed on the inside, and the product is contained in another secure dispenser. Removing the device itself, after peeling through several layers, is almost like uncovering a prize.

There is an impression and unconscious expectation, perhaps, that the device is somehow perfectly constructed and will not, or should not, fail. The reality is that inter-ventional devices are composed of many intricate components and are hand-assembled by humans. During preparation and then delivery in a patient, they are subject to anatomical challenges and stresses, as well as highly variable user manipulations. The manufacturer ensures, through appropriate product testing and numerous quality control processes, that safe and effective devices are released for distribution for their FDA-approved proper use.

U.S. Department of Health and Human Services

Form Approved: OMB No. 0910-0291, Expires: 03/31/05
See OMB statement on reverse.

MEDWATCH

The FDA Safety Information and
Adverse Event Reporting Program

For VOLUNTARY reporting of
adverse events and product problems

Page _____ of _____

FDA USE ONLY

Triage unit
sequence #

A. PATIENT INFORMATION

1. Patient Identifier	2. Age at Time of Event:	3. Sex	4. Weight
In confidence	or _____ Date of Birth:	☐ Female ☐ Male	_____ lbs or _____ kgs

B. ADVERSE EVENT OR PRODUCT PROBLEM

1. ☐ Adverse Event   and/or   ☐ Product Problem (e.g., defects/malfunctions)

2. Outcomes Attributed to Adverse Event (Check all that apply)
☐ Death: _____ (mo/day/yr)
☐ Life-threatening
☐ Hospitalization - initial or prolonged
☐ Disability
☐ Congenital Anomaly
☐ Required Intervention to Prevent Permanent Impairment/Damage
☐ Other: _____

3. Date of Event (mo/day/year)

4. Date of This Report (mo/day/year)

5. Describe Event or Problem

6. Relevant Tests/Laboratory Data, Including Dates

7. Other Relevant History, Including Preexisting Medical Conditions (e.g., allergies, race, pregnancy, smoking and alcohol use, hepatic/renal dysfunction, etc.)

PLEASE TYPE OR USE BLACK INK

C. SUSPECT MEDICATION(S)

1. Name (Give labeled strength & mfr/labeler, if known)
#1
#2

2. Dose, Frequency & Route Used
#1
#2

3. Therapy Dates (If unknown, give duration) from/to (or best estimate)
#1
#2

4. Diagnosis for Use (Indication)
#1
#2

5. Event Abated After Use Stopped or Dose Reduced?
#1 ☐ Yes ☐ No ☐ Doesn't Apply
#2 ☐ Yes ☐ No ☐ Doesn't Apply

6. Lot # (if known)
#1
#2

7. Exp. Date (if known)
#1
#2

8. Event Reappeared After Reintroduction?
#1 ☐ Yes ☐ No ☐ Doesn't Apply
#2 ☐ Yes ☐ No ☐ Doesn't Apply

9. NDC# (For product problems only)
_____ - _____

10. Concomitant Medical Products and Therapy Dates (Exclude treatment of event)

D. SUSPECT MEDICAL DEVICE

1. Brand Name

2. Type of Device

3. Manufacturer Name, City and State

4. Model #	Lot #	5. Operator of Device
Catalog #	Expiration Date (mo/day/yr)	☐ Health Professional ☐ Lay User/Patient
Serial #	Other #	☐ Other: _____

6. If Implanted, Give Date (mo/day/yr)

7. If Explanted, Give Date (mo/day/yr)

8. Is this a Single-use Device that was Reprocessed and Reused on a Patient?
☐ Yes ☐ No

9. If Yes to Item No. 8, Enter Name and Address of Reprocessor

10. Device Available for Evaluation? (Do not send to FDA)
☐ Yes ☐ No ☐ Returned to Manufacturer on: _____ (mo/day/yr)

11. Concomitant Medical Products and Therapy Dates (Exclude treatment of event)

E. REPORTER (See confidentiality section on back)

1. Name and Address   Phone #

2. Health Professional? ☐ Yes ☐ No

3. Occupation

4. Also Reported to:
☐ Manufacturer
☐ User Facility
☐ Distributor/Importer

5. If you do NOT want your identity disclosed to the manufacturer, place an "X" in this box: ☐

FDA

Mail to: **MEDWATCH**
5600 Fishers Lane
Rockville, MD 20852-9787
-or-
FAX to:
1-800-FDA-0178

FORM FDA 3500 (12/03)   Submission of a report does not constitute an admission that medical personnel or the product caused or contributed to the event.

FIGURE 14-2. This is the MedWatch form used when reporting device or other safety issues to the FDA. It is available at http://www.fda.gov/medwatch/how.htm.

ADVICE ABOUT VOLUNTARY REPORTING

Report adverse experiences with:

- Medications *(drugs or biologics)*
- Medical devices *(including in-vitro diagnostics)*
- Special nutritional products *(dietary supplements, medical foods, infant formulas)*
- Cosmetics
- Medication errors

Report product problems - quality, performance or safety concerns such as:

- Suspected counterfeit product
- Suspected contamination
- Questionable stability
- Defective components
- Poor packaging or labeling
- Therapeutic failures

Report SERIOUS adverse events. An event is serious when the patient outcome is:

- Death
- Life-threatening *(real risk of dying)*
- Hospitalization *(initial or prolonged)*
- Disability *(significant, persistent or permanent)*
- Congenital anomaly
- Required intervention to prevent permanent impairment or damage

Report even if:

- You're not certain the product caused the event
- You don't have all the details

How to report:

- Just fill in the sections that apply to your report
- Use section C for all products except medical devices
- Attach additional blank pages if needed
- Use a separate form for each patient
- Report either to FDA or the manufacturer *(or both)*

Confidentiality: The patient's identity is held in strict confidence by FDA and protected to the fullest extent of the law. FDA will not disclose the reporter's identity in response to a request from the public, pursuant to the Freedom of Information Act. The reporter's identity, including the identity of a self-reporter, may be shared with the manufacturer unless requested otherwise.

If your report involves a serious adverse event with a device and it occurred in a facility outside a doctor's office, that facility may be legally required to report to FDA and/or the manufacturer. Please notify the person in that facility who would handle such reporting.

Important numbers:

- 1-800-FDA-0178 -- To FAX report
- 1-800-FDA-1088 -- To report by phone or for more information
- 1-800-822-7967 -- For a VAERS form for vaccines

To Report via the Internet:

http://www.fda.gov/medwatch/report.htm

Fold Here-   -Fold Here-

The public reporting burden for this collection of information has been estimated to average 30 minutes per response, including the time for reviewing instructions, searching existing data sources, gathering and maintaining the data needed, and completing and reviewing the collection of information. Send comments regarding this burden estimate or any other aspect of this collection of information, including suggestions for reducing this burden to:

Department of Health and Human Services
Food and Drug Administration
MedWatch; HFD-410
5600 Fishers Lane
Rockville, MD 20857

Please DO NOT
RETURN this form
to this address.

OMB statement:
"An agency may not conduct or sponsor, and a person is not required to respond to, a collection of information unless it displays a currently valid OMB control number."

U.S. DEPARTMENT OF HEALTH AND HUMAN SERVICES
Food and Drug Administration

FORM FDA 3500 (12/03) (Back)   Please Use Address Provided Below -- Fold in Thirds, Tape and Mail

DEPARTMENT OF
HEALTH & HUMAN SERVICES

Public Health Service
Food and Drug Administration
Rockville, MD 20857

Official Business
Penalty for Private Use $300

BUSINESS REPLY MAIL
FIRST CLASS MAIL   PERMIT NO. 946   ROCKVILLE MD

POSTAGE WILL BE PAID BY FOOD AND DRUG ADMINISTRATION

MedWatch
The FDA Safety Information and Adverse Event Reporting Program
Food and Drug Administration
5600 Fishers Lane
Rockville, MD 20852-9787

NO POSTAGE
NECESSARY
IF MAILED
IN THE
UNITED STATES
OR APO/FPO

Figure 14-2. *Continued.*

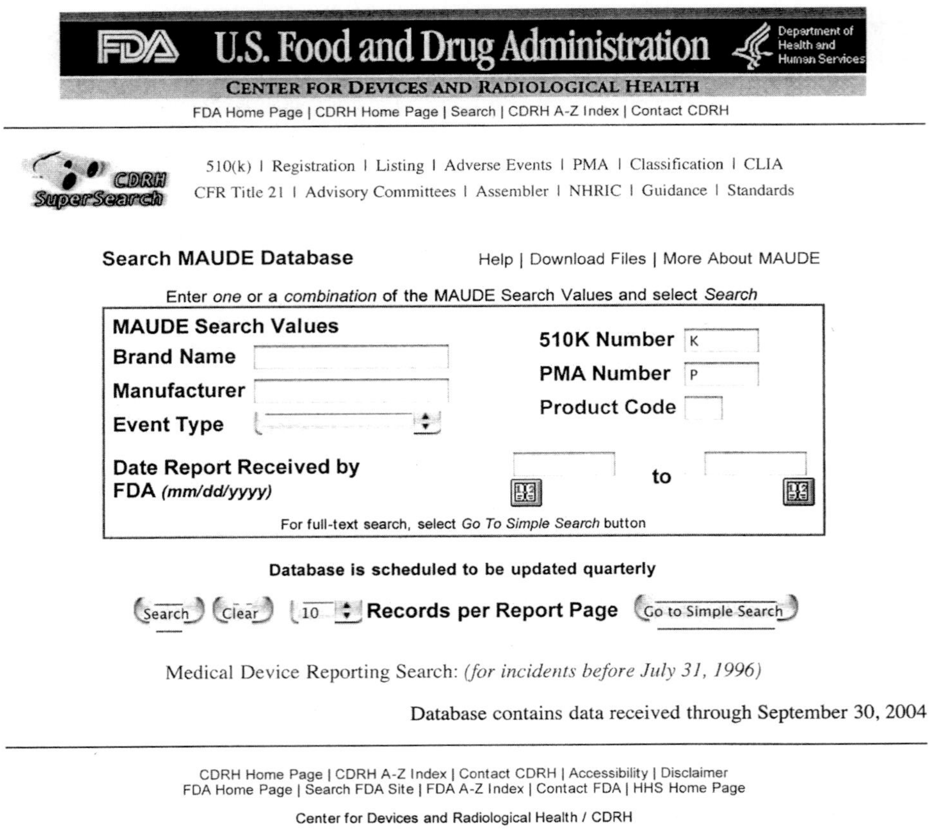

FIGURE 14-3. The web page for the MAUDE search engine is available at http://www.accessdata.fda.gov/scripts /cdrh/cfdocs/cfMAUDE/search.cfm?s earchoptions = 1.

4. Instructions for Use

Physicians learn how to use interventional devices in a number of ways: by formal training programs, proctoring, or company representative in-service programs. The instructions for use (IFU), which is provided in the packaging of every device, is an important tool in the proper use of the product. The IFU is regulated by the FDA and, like the device itself, needs to be submitted and approved before market release. Even slight changes or modifications to the document must be approved by the FDA after release of the product.

The IFU spells out the approved and recommended applications, patient indications and contraindications, warnings regarding handling and use, adverse effects, proper device preparation prior to use, and directions for use. It is the document that is referenced by the manufacturer and the FDA when evaluating reportable events for indications of user error. The FDA defines user error simply as an error made by any person using a device. A user error may contribute to or be the direct cause of a reportable event. It can be either a failure to perform a step or process specified in the IFU, or a use of the device in a manner or application that is contraindicated in the IFU. The recognition of user errors by the FDA relevant to adverse events is not to assign blame. A user error may

alert the FDA of possible inadequacies in the directions for use and the need for improved device labeling in the warnings or instructions in order to prevent future injuries.[3]

Although it may seem time-consuming, the IFU should be reviewed before use of a device. **Whether or not it is read, the physician is accountable for the information contained in it.** In the event there is a device failure as a result of a user error that may have led to a serious injury or death, the actions of the physician with regard to proper device usage should be able to hold up to legal scrutiny. Attention to the details of the IFU can avert many reported complications. With this in mind, the IFU has been created for the protection of both the patient and the physician.

It cannot be overemphasized that all individuals handling any device from the time of its unpacking through its use in the patient should familiarize themselves with the information contained within the IFU. Damage to the device may be overlooked or ignored under frequently stressful or high-pressure situations, such as in low lighting, or during complex and/or emergency procedures. It may be perceived that the product issue is minor or inconsequential; however, failure to follow the IFU directions can result in a cascade of negative events.

FIGURE 14-3. *Continued.*

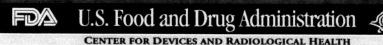

FDA Home Page | CDRH Home Page | Search | CDRH A-Z Index | Contact CDRH

510(k) | Registration | Listing | Adverse Events | PMA | Classification | CLIA
CFR Title 21 | Advisory Committees | Assembler | NHRIC | Guidance | Standards

1   2   3   >

59 records meeting your search criteria returned - **Manufacturer:** *"GUIDANT"* **BrandName:** *"PIXEL"* **EventType:** *"Malfunction"* **ReportDateFrom:** *"01/01/2000"*
ReportDateTo: *"09/30/2004"*

New Search   Help | Download Files | More About MAUDE

Manufacturer	Brand Name	Date Report Received
GUIDANT VASCULAR INT	MULTI-LINK RX PIXEL	03/10/2004
GUIDANT VASCULAR INT	MULTI-LINK RX PIXEL	02/26/2004
GUIDANT VASCULAR INT	MULTI-LINK OTW PIXEL	09/26/2003
GUIDANT VASCULAR INT	MULTI-LINK OTW PIXEL	05/07/2003
GUIDANT VASCULAR INT	MULTI-LINK RX PIXEL	04/22/2003
GUIDANT VASCULAR INT	MULTI-LINK RX PIXEL	04/17/2003
GUIDANT VASCULAR INT	MULTI-LINK RX PIXEL	04/16/2003
GUIDANT VASCULAR INT	MULTI-LINK RX PIXEL	04/03/2003
GUIDANT VASCULAR INT	MULTI-LINK RX PIXEL	03/06/2003
GUIDANT VASCULAR INT	MULTI-LINK RX PIXEL	02/26/2003
GUIDANT VASCULAR INT	MULTI-LINK RX PIXEL	01/30/2003
GUIDANT VASCULAR INT	MULTI-LINK RX PIXEL	01/22/2003
GUIDANT VASCULAR INT	MULTI-LINK OTW PIXEL	01/17/2003
GUIDANT VASCULAR INT	MULTI-LINK RX PIXEL	01/17/2003
GUIDANT VASCULAR INT	MULTI-LINK RX PIXEL	01/16/2003
GUIDANT VASCULAR INT	MULTI-LINK OTW PIXEL	01/15/2003
GUIDANT VASCULAR INT	MULTI-LINK RX PIXEL	01/15/2003
GUIDANT VASCULAR INT	MULTI-LINK OTW PIXEL	01/14/2003
GUIDANT VASCULAR INT	MULTI-LINK OTW PIXEL	12/19/2002
GUIDANT VASCULAR INT	MULTI-LINK RX PIXEL	10/30/2002
GUIDANT VASCULAR INT	MULTI-LINK RX PIXEL	10/25/2002
GUIDANT VASCULAR INT	MULTI-LINK RX PIXEL	10/11/2002
GUIDANT VASCULAR INT	MULTI-LINK RX PIXEL	10/09/2002
GUIDANT VASCULAR INT	MULTI-LINK OTW PIXEL	10/03/2002
GUIDANT VASCULAR INT	MULTI-LINK RX PIXEL	09/09/2002

1   2   3   >

5. Common User Errors

While coronary interventional devices vary slightly from one another in specifications or applications, most of the IFUs pertaining to the devices have similar warnings and precautions regarding their correct use. The most common IFU violations, or user errors, specifically associated with the use of interventional devices are identified in Table 14-1. Any of the listed device misuses can potentially result in unexpected procedure complications or patient injury, and even a seemingly small discrepancy can lead to a bigger issue.

5.1. Examples of Common User Errors

5.1.1. Use of Device after Damage Has Been Observed

In one particular instance, not difficult to imagine, it was reported that the shaft of a catheter became slightly kinked during preparation for use. Nonetheless, the device was placed in the patient, positioned in the lesion, and the stent was deployed without difficulty. However, during removal from the patient, the shaft of the catheter separated into two pieces at the location of the initial kink, which

TABLE 14-1. Top 10 user errors with interventional devices.

Advancement or removal of a device against resistance
Application of excessive force
Inflation above rated burst pressure (RBP)
Incorrect removal of devices
Incorrect device preparation
Use of the device after damage has been observed
No predilatation (when required)
Treatment of proximal lesions before distal ones (stents)
Off-label use
Contraindicated patient

resulted in the use of a snare device to remove the distal portion.[1]

From a manufacturer's perspective, catheter shaft kinks have long been known to risk total separations with further handling. The physician is not expected to understand the behavior or characteristics of product materials; however, most IFUs warn against using damaged devices. From a regulatory standpoint, the aforementioned event would require a report to the FDA because additional medical intervention was used to prevent permanent impairment. The report would reflect that a user error caused or contributed to the adverse event.

Device discrepancies identified during the preparation process may not be conveyed to the physician by the individual who performed that function. While a kink is usually visible to the user prior to the device's introduction in the patient, a leak in the system caused by a hole in the balloon or inflation lumen may not be noticed. This issue may be identified during device preparation while negative pressure is applied to the catheter. A hasty performance of this step could lead to the failure of the balloon to inflate once it was positioned inside the patient. While this issue might not result in patient injury, it certainly will lead to the additional steps of device removal and exchange, a luxury in a complex or urgent procedure. This could also subject the patient to inadvertent injection of air into the coronary artery, potentially leading to further complications and interventions.

The physician may not be aware that negative pressure was applied incorrectly, or not performed at all. However, inadequate device preparation, or prepping the catheter inside the patient, can lead to serious injury. This particular IFU violation has been associated with balloon ruptures, inflation irregularities, deflation difficulties, device component separations, and air embolism.

5.1.2. Incorrect Device Preparation

An actual reported event involved a balloon catheter that was not prepped outside the patient and was subsequently positioned in a lesion. During the inflation, the balloon could not be seen under fluoroscopy because it was filled with air. Believing the balloon had not inflated, it was then pressurized above the rated burst pressure, resulting in a balloon rupture and consequent vessel dissection, which required the implantation of an unplanned stent.[1] A serious injury MedWatch report was filed in this case that indicated that device misuse caused or contributed to the adverse event.

5.1.3. Application of Excessive Force

This kind of device misuse can be understood from a report of two guidewires that were used to access a lesion in a patent ductus arteriosus (PDA) via a saphenous vein graft. A stent was successfully deployed and the stent delivery system was removed. During attempts to remove the guidewires from the artery, resistance was encountered and force was used to pull the guidewires out of the vessel, resulting in tip separations of both guidewires in the artery. Attempts to recover the tips with a retrieval device were unsuccessful and they were left in the patient. The use of excessive force is a common user error associated with device separations. It may be difficult for the physician to gauge exactly how much force is too much. Examination of the device by the manufacturer can confirm stress overload with the use of advanced photography methods, which utilize high-powered magnification techniques to study the damaged segments.

The IFU will provide directions, suggestions, and recommendations regarding applications in the patient and proper use to prevent device malfunctions, but it will not provide direction or assistance when a device failure has occurred and the physician is trying to control and correct complications. It makes sense to be proactive and take steps to avoid complications before they occur by becoming familiar with the IFU and ensuring that all personnel involved in the procedure are properly educated on the handling of the device.

6. Medical Device Reporting

Prior to 1990, a widespread underreporting of serious injuries, deaths, and certain device malfunctions led to the initiation of the Safe Medical Device Act (SMDA) of 1990.[2] Although manufacturers had already been required to submit reports of adverse events since 1984, the user facility where an incident occurred was not required to report those events to the manufacturer. Under this regulation, hospitals, distributors, and outpatient treatment facilities are now required to do so within 10 working days. Although the FDA can enforce the filing regulation, no appointed regulatory representative physically monitors or performs routine audits of interventional procedures; therefore, the organization depends on the voluntary cooperation of the healthcare providers in order to accomplish the regulatory objectives.[3]

The FDA does, however, conduct lengthy and intense audits of the manufacturers' regulatory and quality assurance teams to verify compliance with filing regulations. Manufacturers must file a report to the FDA within 30 calendar days after receiving information that reasonably suggests there has been a device-related death or serious injury, or a device malfunction that may lead to a death or serious injury. Accounts of these events are commonly brought to the attention of the manufacturer by a company representative or hospital staff member, at which time the 30-day reporting timeframe begins.

The FDA expects the company to make a reasonable attempt to obtain the necessary information within that period in order to submit a report that provides accurate details of the event. The physician and individuals involved during the case can expect to be approached with follow-up questions from the company representative or the manufacturer. It is frequently difficult to recall specifics regarding the chronology of events during complicated procedures, so timely retrieval of any information is vital in the investigation of the event and the filing process.

7. Health Insurance Portability and Accountability Act Privacy Rules and MedWatch

Any person can submit a MedWatch report, not just a device manufacturer or a healthcare facility. If the physician becomes aware that the patient has experienced a postprocedure adverse effect that may qualify as a device-related serious injury according to the FDA guidelines, a MedWatch report can be initiated (Figure 14-2).

Health insurance portability and accountability act (HIPAA) privacy rules allow for the communication of adverse events both to the manufacturer and to the FDA, and does not discourage the reporting of those events. Any MedWatch report filed by the device company or directly to the FDA may be the key that prompts a change or modification in the use or design of the product leading to improved patient safety.

8. The Reporting Process

8.1. The Complaint

The reporting process starts with a complaint. All medical device manufacturers are responsible for documenting complaints against the product and evaluating them for reportability. Technically, a complaint is any written, elec-

tronic, or oral communication that alleges deficiencies related to the identity, quality, durability, reliability, safety, effectiveness, or performance of a device after it is released for distribution. For example, if a device failed to meet quality or performance expectations, including labeling or packaging errors, it should be reported to the manufacturer.

The physician plays a key role in providing the important details of the complaint to the appropriate device company. Those details are often filtered through technical staff by the time they reach the manufacturer and it may be difficult to recall the specifics about a particular event as time goes by. Therefore, a timely and accurate description of the actual procedure details, product performance, and patient's status is critical in determining whether a MedWatch report is necessary. The physician will typically have the clearest understanding of what was actually happening during the procedure, how the device was behaving, and why certain decisions were made in regard to treatment. Often, a few moments spent sharing key information as soon as possible with the sales representative will go a long way in affecting necessary device changes or tracking devices that may have manufacturing issues.

8.2. Processing the Complaint

When problems arise with particular interventional tools, procedures are in place locally by the physician, the hospital (user facility), and the staff to define what error or missteps took place. Similarly, the FDA and good business practices mandate methods to identify and then improve on faulty equipment, be it in design, assembly, or materials.

When a complaint is received by the manufacturer, it is evaluated for reportability by quality assurance or regulatory staff. Investigation of the event involves clarification of the case details and product performance issues, as well as patient injury and treatment, if any. Angiographic images of the procedure may be requested to aid in the clinical comprehension of the case. If the used device is available for examination, it will be visually inspected, applicable measurements will be taken, and functional tests will be performed, if possible. In addition to enhanced photographic images, chemical analysis of materials may also be used at times. Laboratory bench testing of returned products can be an invaluable source of information, giving truer insight to the root cause of a device failure, at times, than what was reported. After the product investigation is complete and clinical correlation is applied, a root cause may be able to be determined and follow-up to the physician can be provided.

For example, in one particular experience by Dr. Butman, a coronary cutting balloon could not pass over a guidewire at the entry point into the coronary artery.

A standard balloon also could not pass over the wire, leading to the removal of both wire and balloon; however, the case was completed with a new wire and alternate devices with a satisfactory result. The wire was examined outside the patient and then sent to the manufacturer for a more detailed examination to rule out a manufacturing defect.

The response was a detailed analysis with close-up photography, which revealed that the original wire was not to blame, but that the twisting and torquing required to traverse the complex anatomy had led to some bunching or offsetting of the coils at the guiding catheter intubation point of the coronary artery (Figure 14-4). The reduced clearance of these very low profile tools does not allow for any widening of the wire due to bunching or collection of blood or contrast on the wire. In this case, the detailed inspection provided new insight into the true limits of our tools and reaffirmed the directions for use, which do not support torquing or twisting of the wires in one direction without correction.

This is a good illustration of the complaint handling process from the beginning to the end. If there had been a reportable device malfunction or serious injury, a MedWatch report would have been filed by the manufacturer. The success of this process could be attributed to diligence in returning the device in question back to the manufacturer, along with a clear description of the event. A thorough and complete examination of the

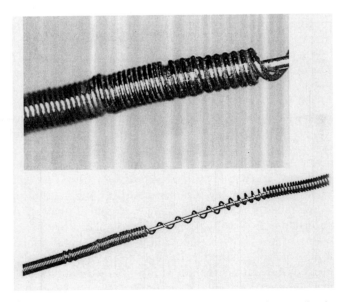

FIGURE 14-4. This is a photomicrograph of a damaged wire removed during a coronary interventional procedure. Due to excessive torque and twisting, the coils lost their low profile and made advancement over the wire device difficult. See text for description of the event.

device is dependant upon the return of the product in as close to the condition it was in when it was removed from the patient as possible. If the product issue was observed before use in the patient, the same would be true, as well. Although it may be tempting for the physician or staff to examine the device in question with closer scrutiny in the catheterization laboratory, the actions could prevent appropriate follow-up bench testing on the product for that issue of concern. The product should be returned to the manufacturer carefully and promptly, and if a device has separated, all segments should be returned, if possible.

MedWatch reports are often filed based on investigational findings. It is not uncommon for the manufacturer to receive a complaint detailing an event that did not appear to be reportable based on the information that was initially provided, but the investigation of the returned device identified a malfunction that could have caused a serious injury. In some hospitals, the risk management department may retain a device, either temporarily or indefinitely, that was involved in a case that resulted in a serious injury or death. The manufacturer will try to recover the device, if at all possible, in order to evaluate its relationship to the adverse event.

8.3. Determining Reportability

Once the complaint has been received by the manufacturer, the details that were provided are examined for indications that an adverse event occurred. A MedWatch report will be filed if the information reasonably suggests that the device may have caused or contributed to a death or serious injury. Additionally, if a device malfunction occurred which would be likely to cause or contribute to a death or a serious injury, the event would be reported.

The FDA allows, in some cases, for medical opinion to be considered when determining the reportability of the complaint. Specifically, manufacturers are not required to report events when information is available that would cause a person qualified to make a medical judgment (e.g., a physician, nurse, risk manager, or biomedical engineer) to conclude that the device did not cause or contribute to the adverse event.[2] For example, if a serious injury or death occurs during an interventional procedure, the event should be reported to the manufacturer of the device(s) involved. If the physician can conclude that the device was not responsible for the patient's deterioration and did not cause the event, a report may not be required by the FDA. In the absence of specific details for a reported complaint where the potential for serious injury is questionable or unknown, the manufacturer may rely on the opinion of clinical and medical experts to determine the reportability of the event.

TABLE 14-2. FDA-defined serious adverse events.

Serious adverse event	Definition	Example
Death	Suspected as a direct outcome of the adverse event	
Life threatening	Patient was at substantial risk of dying at the time of the adverse event	Cardiac arrest, resuscitation
Hospitalization (initial or prolonged)	Patient admitted to hospital or prolonged hospital stay resulted	
Disability	Adverse event resulted in a significant, persistent, permanent change, impairment, damage or disruption in the patient's body function/structure, physical activities, or quality of life	Infarctions, permanent neurological events, device fragment remains in patient
Requires intervention to prevent permanent impairment or damage	Use of the device resulted in a condition that required medical or surgical intervention to preclude permanent damage or impairment	Use of additional stents, balloon dilatations, snare/retrieval devices, cardiac surgery, surgical cutdowns, certain medical treatment

9. The Adverse Events: Death, Serious Injury, and Malfunction of a Device

Adverse events can be broken down into three main categories: death, serious injury, and malfunction of a device. The five specific types of serious adverse events associated with coronary interventional procedures, along with their definitions assigned by the FDA, are described in Table 14-2.

9.1. Serious Injury

The determination that an adverse event resulted in a serious injury is made based on the patient outcome.[3] A serious injury is generally defined by the FDA as one that is life threatening, even if temporary in nature; results in a permanent impairment of a body function or damage to a body structure; or necessitates medical or surgical intervention to preclude permanent impairment of a body function or permanent damage to a body structure.

9.2. Malfunction

Not all product malfunctions or failures identified with an interventional device are reportable to the FDA, even if they inconvenience or irritate the physician, or cause unexpected delays in or modifications to the procedure. A device malfunction is reportable if it is likely to cause or contribute to a death or serious injury should the malfunction recur.[2] More specifically, a malfunction of an interventional device should be reported if the chance of a death or serious injury occurring as a result of a recurrence of the malfunction is not remote; the consequences of the malfunction affect the device in a catastrophic manner that may lead to a death or serious injury; or it causes the device to fail to perform its essential function and compromises the device's therapeutic or diagnostic effectiveness, which could cause or contribute to a death or serious injury.

Table 14-3 illustrates a few device malfunctions that have been reported in the MAUDE database. These device issues are observed across the board with all manufacturers of interventional products. Keep in mind that these issues have been reported, even though there was no injury associated with them during a particular event. In contrast to a serious injury, a reportable device malfunction does not result in a patient injury either because of fortunate circumstances or due to the quick thinking of a skilled interventionalist; they may even happen outside of the anatomy. The likelihood of a future injury is determined by evaluating injury trends related to the particular device in question. This is done by the manufacturer and is based on product performance data, the results of clinical risk and health hazard assessments, and consultations with clinical experts.

From a physician's perspective, any device issue has the potential to cause or contribute to an injury. However, the potential for injury from a regulatory standpoint differs in that an injury has to have occurred due to the device issue in order for the potential or likelihood for injury to exist. To put it simply, once an injury occurs, the FDA then presumes the device malfunction will recur and is likely to result in an injury. Conversely, if there has been no injury, the issue is not likely to result in one. Using this definition as a guideline, the malfunctions listed in Table 14-3 have resulted in a serious injury at some time, which means the device failure is likely to

TABLE 14-3. Examples of Reportable Device Malfunctions.

Stents	Balloons	Guidewires
Shaft separation	Shaft separation	Core separation
Stent dislodgement	Deflation difficulty	Tip separation
Deflation difficulty	Mislabeled device	
Postdeployment resistance: SDS removal from stent difficulty		
Mislabeled device		

result in an injury again and events involving those product issues should be reported.

Device manufacturers may choose to report an event or device failure from a conservative standpoint, even if a serious injury did not, or has never, resulted from the issue. Finally, if 2 years should pass without a particular reportable malfunction resulting in another injury, the manufacturer is no longer required to file a report to the FDA for that malfunction.

Table 14-3 also indicates that mislabeling is a device malfunction. Packaging or device mislabeling is an issue that has been known to contribute to possible serious injury, specifically, when the packaged stent or balloon was larger than indicated on the labeling. Manufacturers are sensitive to product mislabeling and corrective action may need to be taken immediately to ensure that affected lot numbers are identified and removed from circulation or prevented from being shipped, if appropriate. Confirming the size of the device relative to its packaging is a good step to take as part of the unpacking process and a thorough device prep.

It should be noted that the FDA does not expect healthcare providers to be experts in regulatory law. If the physician has successfully completed the case without patient injury in spite of device complications, the necessity of reporting the event to the company might be forgotten amid the sighs of relief or busywork that follows a challenging procedure. However, user facilities are still required by the FDA to file reports of serious injuries or deaths within the required 10-day deadline.

10. Injury Without Device Malfunction

In some cases, the device behaves and performs perfectly well without any product issues; however, an injury still results. Every patient is unique and even with the most experienced physician, the use of any device within a coronary artery might result in an adverse event. If a serious injury occurs in the absence of a product malfunction, a MedWatch report is required if the event reasonably suggests that the device caused or contributed to the injury. Vessel dissections, perforations, and thrombosis are examples of this. Usually, the injury also results in additional intervention, which also makes the event reportable.

11. Global Reporting Requirements

Global marketing of cardiac products necessitates the filing of several reports by the manufacturer for one adverse event in some cases. Outside the United States, regulatory agencies similar to the FDA, collectively known as competent authorities (CA), govern the distribution and sale of products in the medical device marketplace within specific geographies. Although the primary goal of public safety is the same, CA guidelines for device reporting are unique and often differ from those outlined by the FDA.

European countries usually receive approval to market interventional devices before the United States. The device manufacturer is responsible for reporting all adverse events associated with the use of their product and filing reports with the CA in the country where the event occurred, if required, even if the product is not approved for use in the United States. Japan monitors the activity of all products that are approved for use in that country, and may require a report of an adverse event that did not even occur in Japan. Conversely, many countries that market interventional devices do not have a governing regulatory body and adverse events are reported only to the FDA.

12. Clinical Trial Event Reporting

Frequently, clinical trials are still being conducted in the United States while the device is being sold and used in broader applications elsewhere. Devices that are used in clinical trials in the United States are exempt from reportability; however, the FDA does require that all adverse events associated with clinical products be tracked and documented appropriately according to regulations governing clinical trials.

13. Conclusions

The successful execution of interventional procedures involves the coordination of multiple processes and the expertise and attention of all individuals who come in contact with the devices. The products used for coronary interventions in the United States can be used confidently with the knowledge that those devices are being closely monitored and regulated at multiple levels from a safety standpoint; however, even a device that meets 100% of the manufacturing specifications can behave unpredictably when it is subject to forces that exceed its design limitations.

Dealing with unexpected complications related to device issues is a challenge that all interventionalists face. Ultimately, responsible usage of interventional devices will reduce the likelihood of patient injury, and conscientious regulatory reporting will ensure that appropriate corrective actions can be taken to design better and safer products.

References

1. Manufacturer and User Facility Device Experience (MAUDE) Database. Food and Drug Administration website. Available at: http://www.accessdata.fda.gov/scripts/cdrh/cfdocs/cfMAUDE/search.cfm. Accessed February 6, 2004.

2. Medical Device Reporting for Manufacturers. Rockville, MD: Department of Health and Human Services, Public Health Service and Food and Drug Administration, Center for Devices and Radiological Health; March 1997.

3. Food and Drug Administration. Code of Federal Regulation. Vol. 60, No. 237. Washington, DC: US Government Printing Office; December 1995.

Index